I0069975

The Patient Self-Determination Act

Meeting the Challenges in Patient Care

CLINICAL MEDICAL ETHICS

Editors

H. TRISTRAM ENGELHARDT, JR., The Center for Ethics, Medicine and Public Issues, Baylor College of Medicine, Houston, Texas

KEVIN WILDES, S.J. Department of Philosophy, Georgetown University, Washington, D.C.

Editorial Advisory Board

GEORGE J. AGICH, School of Medicine, Southern Illinois University, Springfield, Illinois

DAN W. BROCK, Department of Philosphy, Brown University, Providence, Rhode Island

BARUCH A. BRODY, Center for Ethics, Medicine and Public Issues, Baylor College of Medicine, Houston, Texas

ALLEN E. BUCHANAN, School of Medicine, University of Wisconsin at Madison, Madison, Wisconsin

ANTONIO M. GOTTO, JR., Department of Medicine, Baylor College of Medicine, Houston, Texas

ANGELA R. HOLDER, School of Medicine, Yale University, New Haven, Connecticut

JAY KATZ, Yale Law School, Yale University, New Haven, Connecticut

LORETTA M. KOPELMAN, Department of Medical Humanities, School of Medicine, East Carolina University, Greenville, North Carolina

EDMUND D. PELLEGRINO, Director, Center for Clinical Bioethics, Georgetown University, Washington, D.C.

STEPHEN WEAR, Department of Philosophy, State University of New York at Buffalo, Buffalo, New York

Previous Books in the Series

The Patient Self-Determination Act

Meeting the Challenges in Patient Care

Lawrence P. Ulrich, Ph.D.
The University of Dayton

GEORGETOWN UNIVERSITY PRESS / WASHINGTON, D.C.

Georgetown University Press, Washington, D.C. 20007
©1999 by Georgetown University Press, all rights reserved
Printed in the United States of America
10 9 8 7 6 5 4 3 2 1 1999

Library of Congress Cataloging-in-Publication Data

Ulrich, Lawrence P.
   The Patient Self-Determination Act : meeting the challenges in
patient care / Lawrence P. Ulrich.
      p. cm. — (Clinical medical ethics)
   Includes bibliographical references and index.
   ISBN 0-87840-747-2 (cloth). — ISBN 0-87840-748-0 (paper)
   1. Right to die—United States. 2. Patients—Legal status, laws,
etc.—United States. I. Title. II. Series: Clinical medical
ethics (Washington, D.C.)
   [DNLM: 1. Treatment Refusal—legislation & jurisprudence—United
States. 2. Patient Advocacy—legislation & jurisprudence—United
States. 3. Advance Directives—legislation & jurisprudence—United
States. 4. Bioethics—United States. W 32.5 AA1 U19p 1999]
R726.U39 1999
174'.24—dc21
DNLM/DLC
for Library of Congress   99-19307
                                                                   CIP

To my dear wife, Renate,
who continually gives
a renewing spirit to my life and work,
this book is gratefully dedicated.

Contents

Acknowledgments

No effort of this sort is undertaken without the support of many friends and colleagues. The merits of this venture are owed in a large part to them. Its shortcomings, alas, are mine alone. I would like to give my thanks to the following who have been particularly instrumental in whatever achievement this book enjoys: To the anonymous reviewers whose critical comments in the early manuscripts of this book challenged me and contributed in numerous ways to the final product; to Kevin Wildes, S.J., Ph.D. who has managed the earlier manuscripts through the maze of reviewers; to Klem Bartosik of Holy Cross Care Services who prompted my extensive analysis of the Patient Self-Determination Act with an invitation to do my first workshop on the law and its impact on caregivers; to David Kinsey who, on that fateful Easter Sunday in 1991, held my workshop documents in his hand and said "this is pure gold"—from that moment he and I happily embarked on the joint project of developing an extensive handbook for implementing the Patient Self-Determination Act by caregivers in healthcare facilities; to all those physicians and other healthcare providers and bioethicists who have encouraged my work over the last 25 years; to the many hospitals and healthcare organizations that have given me the opportunity to exercise and develop my abilities in clinical ethics; to the physicians of the Columbus Physicians Ethics Circle, particularly its co-founder with me, Vincent Barresi, M.D., who continue to stimulate and challenge me and who show me the redeemed promise of the virtues of medical practice; to David Goldberg, D.O. whose guidance persists and who gives me hope in the future of medicine; to Hagop Nersoyan, Ph.D., a treasured colleague, whose appraisals of ancestral versions of this manuscript have moved me forward; to Raymond Herbenick, Ph.D., a most trusted and beloved colleague and friend, whose untimely death as this volume was nearing completion set in relief the enthusiastic support he gave me at every stage of the project; to H. Tristram Engelhardt, Jr., M.D., Ph.D. who saw the promise of this volume and who offered encouragement when discouragement began to rule the day; to Sr. Carmencita, C.S.C who always showed unflinching confidence in my work; and to Scott Loman, without whose extensive assistance in researching many areas of this book, it could never have seen the light of day. Friends and colleagues alike, thank you.

The Patient
Self-Determination Act

Meeting the Challenges in Patient Care

Introduction

At first glance this book may seem to be an attempt to make the simple into something quite complex. But upon reflection it should become apparent that the Patient Self-Determination Act is much more than a few bureaucratic requirements on a piece of paper that can be discharged by signing or exchanging other pieces of paper. What is at stake in the Patient Self-Determination Act is nothing short of the well-being of patients who frequently find themselves on the fringes of their control in healthcare institutions and programs that all too often prize efficiency and convenience above all else. The Patient Self-Determination Act emphasizes the active role of patients as they determine the direction of their healthcare, sometimes making decisions that will result in their deaths. Furthermore, this law provides a structure for integrating many of the issues with which healthcare has wrestled for the past two generations.

This book is intended for the audience of healthcare professionals who might find it useful to have a comprehensive context for implementing the Patient Self-Determination Act. Without an understanding of the context of this relatively new law, it would be easy for its implementation to be either ignored or relegated to a mere bureaucratic exercise. This book is written with the hope that neither negative outcome will occur. Rather, its ambition is to demonstrate the extraordinary impact of this rather simple piece of legislation on many facets of healthcare as it unfolds in the clinical setting. If this insight is generated, both the law and this book will be successful in refocusing attention on the patient's authority and responsibility in making healthcare decisions. For the law empowers patients in their present and future clinical decisions. This book shows the way in which healthcare professionals can contribute to that empowerment by understanding their patients better, engaging in conversations with them about the issues raised by the Patient Self-Determination Act, and helping them face the complex issues in contemporary healthcare practices.

The focus of attention will be on the provisions of the law that can actually empower patients. Thus, it concentrates on only limited features of self-determination—the right to refuse treatment and the role of advance directives in healthcare decision making. It does not attempt to map out the broad sweep of self-determination that would include a patient's right to make absolute and binding decisions about the direction of her healthcare. The distinction between "negative" self-determination (the right to *refuse* treatment) and "positive" self-determination (the right to *demand* treatment) is important not just for implementing the Patient Self-Determination Act, but also for addressing the issue of making judgments about futile care, which has become a central issue in healthcare ethics, law, and medical practice.[1] The right to refuse treatments has a long history of approval in both ethics and the law. The right to demand treatment has a much shorter history and still remains a very controversial matter. While this text does discuss comprehensive self-determination on occasion, it does so only within the context of provisions of the Patient Self-Determination Act. It does not attempt to justify every aspect of self-determination, although it will attempt to put the right to demand treatment in the context of the Patient Self-Determination Act in a brief discussion of futility.

Two major challenges to the possibility of promoting patient self-determination are underscored by two very significant features of healthcare that have come to light in the last decade. The first is the growing presence of managed care on the healthcare scene. Managed care, in itself, does not make it impossible for patients to exercise their decisional authority because it does not directly dictate to patients what they may or may not choose in determining the direction of their healthcare. However, managed care does effectively and indirectly restrict healthcare choices by refusing to pay for therapeutic interventions that lie outside what the organization considers to be part of the managed care contract. Thus, patients can exercise a wide range of self-determination provided they can pay for the interventions they select. But they often cannot exercise the same self-determination if they must operate within the confines of their managed care contracts and receive reimbursement for the interventions.

Another feature of the challenge that managed care presents to patients, which may be less noticeable to patients, lies in the conflict of interest that managed care sometimes creates for physicians.[2] Physicians practicing under a managed care contract often find themselves confronted with divided loyalties. Their fiduciary relationship requires them to provide the best care for the patient, including all information that will help the patient become a better decision maker. On the other hand, their managed care contract often requires them to limit the kind of care given to the patient as well as the information about alternative approaches.[3]

Both negative and positive forms of self-determination are jeopardized in the context of managed care if the patient (1) cannot be provided with the full range of care, (2) cannot obtain sufficient information to select care, and (3) cannot have access to care because of arbitrary financial restrictions. If the Patient Self-Determination Act is to fulfill its role of promoting self-determination in refusals of and consents to treatments, the challenges of managed care will have to be met aggressively.

The book begins with a statement of the provisions of the Patient Self-Determination Act and, what may be equally important, an attempt to formulate the spirit of the law. The latter effort is important in order to help move beyond the mere functional considerations specified in the law to understanding the goals that the law seems to be attempting to achieve. Without knowing the goals, the process for implementing the law may very possibly miss the mark.

Since no law is formulated in a vacuum, considerations leading up to the formulation of the law can shed light on its importance in our society. There is no way in a text like this to give a comprehensive treatment of the legal backdrop for the law. The four cases selected for examination, *Quinlan, Bartling, Brophy,* and *Cruzan,* were chosen because the issues with which they wrestled have a direct bearing on the specifications of the Patient Self-Determination Act. It might even be argued that, if the law had been in effect at the time these four patients were in their respective healthcare institutions, the progress of their care might have taken a decidedly different turn, and a greater sensitivity to their rights and dignity might have resulted in better care for them.

The book next turns to the social and technological issues that permeate the delivery of healthcare today. The insatiable expectations for consuming healthcare that is currently available and utilizing forms of healthcare that may have questionable benefits become major issues to address when attempting to implement the Patient Self-Determination Act. The problem of expectations arises especially around the issue of refusing treatments. The definition of the physician-patient relationship is undergoing significant reexamination in healthcare, particularly within the movement to managed care. Inadequate attention to the dynamics of this relationship could be a major contributing factor to the way the law is implemented and the manner in which the delivery of healthcare will be reoriented in the future. The problem of living in a society that views technology as the panacea for all human woes must be addressed if we are to place the delivery of healthcare in proper perspective.

Finally, no social context could be complete without developing some understanding of the current and ongoing debate of reforming healthcare. The Patient Self-Determination Act could become a major contributor to the necessary reforms insofar as it might stimulate wiser consumption of healthcare. However, the self-determination it encourages generally focuses upon refusals of treatment within a broad range of options. Reforms in healthcare may actually limit the self-determination of patients by restricting their choices. In spite of the serious problems that self-determination raises in healthcare reform, there is virtually no discussion in the public arena about the law or its role in reforming healthcare.

Though the reality of our finitude is brought to our attention on a continuing basis in many areas of our lives, its awareness is often left at the doors of healthcare facilities. This will change only when healthcare professionals face the issue squarely and realize that the Patient Self-Determination Act can help patients confront the reality of their finitude and the limitations that are an inexorable part of medical interventions. An indispensable dimension of the human context is the meaning of personal dignity. Everyone in healthcare talks about it, and all the ethics codes require its protection. But few, if any, take the trouble to give a detailed analysis of personal dignity or the matter of developing virtues, which is an integral part of it. Because of this neglect it becomes easy to violate patient dignity even though its preservation lies at the heart of the Patient Self-Determination Act.

An attempt is made to outline the way institutions can address the spirit of the Patient Self-Determination Act, through the development of conversations with patients, as well as its letter. The importance of being faithful to the spirit of the law is particularly pivotal for those institutions that have special mission and social commitments. It is also important if institutions are to manage the liability issues that this new law may have introduced into the clinical setting.

The suggestion made throughout this text in relation to both institutions and healthcare professionals is that well-designed conversations with patients or surrogates will help in a significant way to implement the Patient Self-Determination Act. And yet, it is in precisely this area that the second major challenge of the last decade to patient self-determination is situated. For the SUPPORT study published in 1995 indicates that attempts at detailed conversations with patients and surrogates by nurses in the study had little or no effect on DNR orders, pain reduction, or the implementation of advance directives.[4] Though the challenges to communication presented by the SUPPORT study are profound, they may simply indicate that more extensive and effective means of communication must be explored and developed if the Patient Self-Determination Act is to be implemented in productive ways. Some of these ways, and possible responses to the SUPPORT study, will be suggested throughout this text, particularly in chapters 5, 7, and 8.

Perhaps the core of this book is to be found in chapter 6, which attempts to lay out the ethical foundations of the Patient Self-Determination Act. In this section the ethical issues are raised directly and integrated in the context of the Patient Self-Determination Act. A complete analysis of the ethical foundations of the Patient Self-Determination Act requires an examination of the way the principles of bioethics, including virtue ethics, fit into the law and support its role in healthcare. Informed consent and decisional capacity are ongoing issues in the clinical setting that are a significant component of the law. The right to refuse treatment is singled out for special attention because the Patient Self-Determination Act seems to have this as its pivotal point. In contrast, the inclination to demand treatment is a matter of great concern in the current healthcare climate, particularly if those demands are for what some would characterize as futile care. These two related issues are given special consideration.

Much of the attention given to the Patient Self-Determination Act has focused on the dramatic issue of advance directives. Though they are an important feature of the law, they are only a part of it. An attempt is made to describe the nature and purpose of advance directives and outline the social factors that have produced them. The general problems, advantages, and disadvantages of advance directives and the way they can most effectively be written are given considerable attention. Finally, some strategies for assisting patients and potential patients in writing advance directives are explored.

The various roles of healthcare professionals vis-à-vis the implementation of the Patient Self-Determination Act in healthcare are explored. No one role has exclusive province in its implementation. Rather, the various healthcare professionals can complement one another in helping patients realize the goals of the law.

The book concludes with a seldom discussed issue in health-care—namely, the importance of being a responsible patient and the way this responsibility can be exercised in the healthcare setting. Unfortunately, healthcare often looks upon patients who wish to exercise personal responsibility in decision making as inconveniences and nuisances. The Patient Self-Determination Act, on the other hand, recognizes the authority and power of patients and presents a new vehicle for exercising them. If the Patient Self-Determination Act does nothing else, it should encourage patients to become more active participants in the decisions that set the direction of their healthcare both in refusing and in consenting to treatments.

As can be seen from this brief introduction, the scope covered by the Patient Self-Determination Act is broad although its provisions are few. It has the potential for genuinely altering the way healthcare is practiced in this country. But the law will not fulfill its purpose if healthcare professionals and institutions fail to enter into its spirit and instead treat it only as a bureaucratic inconvenience unworthy of their time. Perhaps the best way to avoid neglect of the law is for healthcare professionals to approach it from the perspective of its impact on their own lives rather than on the lives of their patients. Healthcare professionals might ask themselves questions such as the following: (1) How do *I* view the role of technology in *my* healthcare? (2) How have *I* come to grips with *my* finitude? (3) Under what conditions might *I* wish to refuse treatment? (4) When faced with a critical illness, what might *I* consider futile care? (5) How do advance directives fit into *my* healthcare plans? (6) How do *I* want to have my dignity respected when *I* become a patient? (7) How can *I* best exercise *my* responsibility as a patient? Once they ask these questions of themselves, they may better understand the significance of the Patient Self-Determination Act for those whom they serve. Such a reflective posture may place them in a better position to help others who are more vulnerable address the personal and ethical issues of the law.

NOTES

1. See the recent volume, Medical futility, edited by Zucker MB and Zucker HD and published by Cambridge University Press, 1997. This excellent volume contains sixteen essays that address the ethical, medical, legal, and social policy issues surrounding the determination of futile treatments.

2. Rodwin MA. Medicine, money, and morals: Physicians' conflicts of interest. New York: Oxford University Press, 1993, pages 8–18 and 223–234.

3. The latter problem (i.e., giving full information to the patient) has been addressed in the new Patients' Bill of Rights for medicare recipients established by executive order. See USA Today 1998; February 20.

4. Connors AF et al. (The SUPPORT Principal Investigators). A controlled trial to improve care for seriously ill hospitalized patients: The study to understand prognoses and preferences for outcomes and risks of treatments (SUPPORT). JAMA 1995; 274:1591–1598.

1

The Requirements of the
Patient Self-Determination Act

The Explicit Demands of the Law

The requirements of the Patient Self-Determination Act are deceptively simple, but they carry profound implications for the way healthcare is practiced. The law mandates that, in healthcare institutions that receive Medicare or Medicaid funding, patients must be informed in writing upon admission of (1) their right to accept or refuse treatment, (2) their rights under existing state laws regarding advance directives, and (3) any policies the institution has regarding the withholding or withdrawing of life-sustaining treatments.[1] The institutions are also required to engage in ongoing educational activities for both their employees and the general public regarding the right to accept or refuse treatment and the opportunity for drafting or signing advance directives.

The law was passed by Congress on November 5, 1990, and went into effect on December 1, 1991. It is based on the principles of informed consent. The law lays the foundation for the exercise of the patient's decision-making authority, which will affect the course of treatment for all patients whether or not they possess decisional capacity. The law extends to all healthcare institutions, including hospitals, extended care facilities, hospices, HMOs, and home healthcare agencies, and thus covers virtually all individuals seeking health-care. The only exceptions might be those few institutions where services are paid for directly by patients independently of government funding.

The law does not give any new rights to patients except the right to be informed of the stipulated matters at the time of admission to certain healthcare facilities. It generally reaffirms rights that patients already possess, such as the right to refuse treatment.[2] Unfortunately, patients have not always been aware of these rights, and for this reason they have all too often become victims of the decisions of others. The right of patients to receive adequate information about matters that will help them exercise their self-determination in health-care practices is underscored by the new duty imposed upon health-care facilities to provide specific information to them.

The Spirit of the Law

All legislation must be understood in terms of both its explicit stipu-lations and its spirit. The spirit of a law constitutes its "soul." Com-pliance with the spirit (one might go so far as to say the intent) of a law demonstrates the effectiveness of the law in a comprehensive way and the commitment of the institutions that it binds. The intent of legislators often becomes a matter for serious consideration when challenges to a law or its implementation are addressed by the courts. The many debates over constitutional issues and the intent of the drafters of the Constitution bear witness to this phenomenon. The fact is that the intent behind a law is frequently opaque because it is undocumented. It achieves partial clarity only when the courts inter-pret the law. However, one can draw inferences about the intent of the Patient Self-Determination Act by recognizing that it was initiated by Senator John Danforth of Missouri at the time the situation of Nancy Cruzan was working its way through the courts in Missouri. It would seem that Senator Danforth and those who cosponsored the bill with him wanted to ensure that a situation like Cruzan's would not happen again. Thus, the intent of the legislation seems to be the recognition and strengthening of the decisional authority of patients and their surrogates when making healthcare decisions of any sort whether they be in critical or noncritical situations.

In the Patient Self-Determination Act conformity to the letter of the law is quite simple. It can be accomplished, and often is, by simply giving patients the required notifications on paper with minimal oral presentations at the time of admission to the facility or program. When this approach is taken, the same problems arise that have plagued the informed consent process for decades.

The informed consent process has all too frequently consisted of a description on paper of the medical intervention to be undertaken, a few words of additional explanation, the inquiry "Do you have any questions?" and a signature at the end of the printed form.[3] This procedure offers no assurance that the patient truly understands what will occur in the clinical encounter or what complications could arise from the interventions being considered. At times patients have used the inadequacy of the informed consent process as a legal argument in malpractice litigation.[4] All patients have to do is make a reasonable case that they did not truly understand the issues involved even though they signed the consent form. Thus, perfunctory informed consent procedures do not accomplish the purpose for which informed consent was intended—namely, to give content to the consent that is given, thereby enhancing the authority of the decision maker.[5]

If the spirit of the Patient Self-Determination Act is to be accomplished, more than perfunctory notification will be required, and a more in-depth understanding of the advantages of the law will be necessary. To put it simply, the Patient Self-Determination Act can enable patients to become better decision makers in healthcare by accomplishing the following goals. (1) It provides clear ethical and legal recognition of the authority of patients and surrogates in the healthcare setting by affirming the control they have in making many decisions about their lives and what transpires in them. (2) By identifying the decisional authority of patients and surrogates in the healthcare setting, it provides the opportunity to reflect upon what is important to them in selecting healthcare interventions. (3) It can reinforce the opportunity to choose alternatives that will allow them to achieve their goals even after the onset of decisional incapacity. (4) Finally, it extends the ideals of political liberty into the daily decisions individuals make about one of the most central and problematic areas of their lives—namely, the direction of their healthcare. Each of the notifications and requirements contributes to these purposes.

The right of patients to consent to or refuse treatments is the basis of everything to be found in this law. This is an application of the basic liberty that we all enjoy in a democratic society. It is a common misunderstanding that the initiation of medical treatments is automatic with the onset of a pathology. Conceptually speaking, there is nothing in the concept of pathology that requires treatment. For this reason the initiation of treatment requires consent. The right to consent to treatment has a long history in the law.[6] Though the right to refuse treatment is implied in the right to consent, taking the form of withholding consent,[7] it has been extensively articulated in the law only during the last twenty years.[8] In spite of the clear identification of this right in both ethics and the law, patients often think that they must accept treatments when they are offered. In a sense the offering of treatment often "defaults" to its initiation with very little actual *reflective decision making* on the part of the patient involved. The Patient Self-Determination Act is intended to amplify autonomous decision making by helping patients clearly understand that they can take control of their healthcare even to the point of refusing any or all treatments.

The Patient Self-Determination Act attempts to take advantage of the current climate of state initiatives authorizing the utilization of advance directives in healthcare decision making. This extension of decision-making authority beyond the onset of decisional incapacity recognizes that patients have an interest in the healthcare decisions that affect them even if they are no longer able to participate in them in an active and direct way. Advance directives can enlarge the range of alternatives open to patients as they are considering the direction of their healthcare. This interest of patients in what happens to them after the onset of decisional incapacity had already been established by the courts prior to the passage of the law.[9]

Many patients have ideas about what direction they would like their healthcare to take if they are no longer able to make the decisions for themselves at the time the interventions are being considered. They express themselves on these matters in a variety of ways—some, such as Karen Quinlan and Nancy Cruzan,[10] informally and others, like Brother Fox, more formally.[11] But without special information, these patients are often ignorant of the protection that states have offered them in these circumstances and the methods they can employ to maximize this protection. A great many individuals seem to be unaware that avenues are open that allow them to articulate their treatment wishes in anticipation of decisional incapacity.

The Patient Self-Determination Act seeks to empower patients by ensuring that they receive the proper information so that they can consider the role of advance directives in their healthcare plans and make the appropriate decisions about them in view of their values and goals. *Notification* of the current state laws is only a first step in this extremely significant process, but it opens the door to other ways of qualitatively increasing the authority patients can exercise over their treatment decisions after the onset of decisional incapacity. Among the other issues related to advance directives is the encouragement of self-reflection by patients on the values and goals that guide their lives and may ultimately guide the process of their dying, as well as specific treatment approaches they may want to specify or decline.

If patients are to be empowered to forgo treatments, it is essential that they understand any restrictions that healthcare institutions may have regarding this practice. The law's requirement that facilities provide information to patients related to their policies regarding the withholding or withdrawing of life-sustaining treatments is clearly directed to making patients better decision makers. If patients find that a particular facility has certain restrictions on treatment alternatives flowing either from its mission or from other considerations, they can exercise greater control over where they will receive care. Knowledge prior to or at the time of admission may alert patients and their families to seek out a different facility if the one they have initially chosen is too restrictive of patient or family choices. This is particularly important if there will be a long-term commitment between the patient and the institution.

The final requirement of the law goes well beyond notifications given to individual patients. It places an educational obligation on healthcare institutions. The institutions are required to have ongoing educational programs to explain to their employees and members of the community their rights regarding consent to and refusal of treatments and the advance directive conditions in their state. The purpose of the educational requirement is to provide potential patients (i.e., all persons) the opportunity to learn about the stipulations of the Patient Self-Determination Act by underscoring some of their most fundamental treatment alternatives. A purely educational situation allows them to explore methods for making healthcare decisions in a climate that is less pressurized than the time of admission to a healthcare facility.

In summary, the Patient Self-Determination Act is designed to make patients better informed about many of their rights regarding treatment decisions. It underscores the role and importance of patient participation in healthcare decisions by clearly identifying the parameters of their decision-making authority. Perhaps its most important feature is the emphasis it places on the responsibility of patients for the direction their healthcare takes. In the current climate of healthcare much has been made of the obligations of healthcare professionals and the rights of patients. Little discussion has been centered on the responsibility of patients. The result of the Patient Self-Determination Act can be a focused interest on patients' taking responsibility for the course of their healthcare decisions. The hope is that enlightened and prudent patients, guided by sound assistance in reflecting on their conditions, alternatives, and possibilities will make realistic decisions within the context of their personal values. These decisions will then take the form of approaches to treatment that will truly benefit them and allow them to achieve their goals.

NOTES

1. Patient Self-Determination Act of 1990, sections 4206 and 4751 of Omnibus Reconciliation Act of 1990, Pub L No. 101-508 (November 5, 1990).

SEC. 4206. MEDICARE PROVIDER AGREEMENTS ASSURING THE IMPLEMENTATION OF A PATIENT'S RIGHTS TO PARTICIPATE IN AND DIRECT HEALTH CARE DECISIONS AFFECTING THE PATIENT. [The Patient Self-Determination Act applies] in the case of hospitals, nursing facilities, home health agencies, and hospice programs, . . . and a provider of services or prepaid or eligible organization [to] maintain written policies and procedures with respect to all adult individuals receiving medical care by or through the provider or organization—[The designated institutions are required]

(A) to provide written information to each such individual concerning—

(i) an individual's rights under State law (whether statutory or as recognized by the courts of the State) to make decisions concerning such medical care, including the right to accept or refuse medical or surgical treatment and the right to formulate advance directives . . . and

(ii) [to provide] the written policies of the provider or organization respecting the implementation of such rights;

(B) to document in the individual's medical record whether or not the individual has executed an advance directive;

(C) not to condition the provision of care or otherwise discriminate against an individual based on whether or not the individual has executed an advance directive (this shall not be construed as requiring the provision of care which conflicts with an advance directive);

(D) to ensure compliance with requirements of State law (whether statutory or as recognized by the courts of the State) respecting advance directives at facilities of the provider or organization (this shall not be construed as prohibiting the application of a State law which allows for an objection on the basis of conscience for any health care provider or an agent of such provider which as a matter of conscience cannot implement an advance directive); and

(E) to provide (individually or with others) for education for staff and the community on issues concerning advance directives. . . . The written information . . . shall be provided to an adult individual—

(A) in the case of a hospital, at the time of the individual's admission as an inpatient,

(B) in the case of a skilled nursing facility, at the time of the individual's admission as a resident,

(C) in the case of a home health agency, in advance of the individual coming under the care of the agency,

(D) in the case of a hospice program, at the time of initial receipt of hospice care by the individuals from the program, and

(E) in the case of an eligible organization . . . or an organization provided under [Medicare or Medicaid] at the time of enrollment of the individual with the organization.

. . . [T]he term "advance directive" means a written instruction, such as a living will or durable power of attorney for health care, recognized under State law (whether statutory or as recognized by the courts of the State) and relating to the provision of such care when the individual is incapacitated.

2. The right to refuse treatment will be more fully explored in chapter 6. Its constitutionality was first established in In re Quinlan. 70 N.J. 10, 355 A.2d 647 (1976), on the basis of the right to privacy and has been reiterated by many state courts on the same basis. On the federal level the right to refuse treatment was upheld in Cruzan v. Director, Missouri Department of Health. 110 S. Ct. 2841 (1990), on the basis of the liberty interest of the Fourteenth Amendment. Subsequent to the Patient Self-Determination Act, the right to refuse treatment has been emphatically upheld once again in Vacco v. Quill. 117 S. Ct. 2293 (1997), on the same basis as it was in *Cruzan*.

3. Lidz CW et al. Two models of implementing informed consent. Arch Intern Med 1988; 148:1385–1389.

4. Berman v. Allen. 80 N.J. 421, 404 A.2d 8 (1979).

5. Canterbury v. Spence. 464 F.2d 772 (D.C.C.A. 1972).

6. Schloendorff v. Society of New York Hospital. 211 N.Y. 125, 105 N.E. 92 (1914). See also Katz J. Informed consent in the therapeutic relationship: Legal and ethical aspects. In Reich WT (ed). Encyclopedia of bioethics. New York: Free Press, 1978, pages 770–778.

7. Meisel J, Kuczewski M. Legal and ethical myths about informed consent. Arch Intern Med 1996; 156:2521–2526.

8. This examination began with *Quinlan* (In re Quinlan. 70 N.J. 10, 355 A.2d 647 (1976)) and culminated in *Cruzan* (Cruzan v. Director, Missouri Department of Health. 110 S. Ct. 2841 (1990)).

9. In re Dinnerstein. 6 Mass. App. Ct. 466, 380 N.E.2d 134 (App. Ct. 1978).

10. In re Quinlan. 70 N.J. 10, 355 A.2d 647 (1976), and Cruzan v. Director, Missouri Department of Health. 110 S. Ct. 2841 (1990).

11. In re Eichner (In re Storar). 420 N.E.2d 64 (N.Y. 1981).

2

The Legal Background of the Patient Self-Determination Act

Ethics and the Law

The relationship between ethics and the law has not always been as complex at it is today in highly developed industrial and technological societies. In the early forms of human societies the relationship was fairly linear. Communities reflected on the behavior of their members and made decisions about those behaviors that would promote the good of the community and those that were detrimental to its welfare. Having made the decisions over a period of time, they passed the "mandates" on through informal ethical codes and narratives, such as hero stories, which attempted to set norms for ideal behaviors. Eventually the desired behaviors became so important to the community that legal codes were developed that outlined precisely what was to be done in certain situations and imposed penalties for behaviors that deviated from the norms established in the law.[1] Courts were established to interpret the law and its application to different circumstances.

Even a cursory study of the development of legal codes as they achieve greater degrees of sophistication reveals several striking phenomena. Laws governing behavior flow from beliefs that the members of a community hold about themselves and the ethical decisions that follow from those beliefs.[2] However, laws do not always reflect the beliefs of the entire community but often reflect the convictions of only a certain portion of the community. This portion can be a large segment, or it can be a minority, clustered around politically powerful special interests, such as landowners, military leaders, etc. When the politically powerful create and interpret laws based upon their self-interest, ordinary citizens often suffer.[3] Thus, the many dimensions of human experience and the protection of those experiences are often ignored. In such situations individuals must continually struggle for recognition of their interests and legal protection.

As the community progresses through its lived experience with the law and as its ethical reflections on certain behaviors become more finely honed, revisions in the law take place. These revisions are frequently pragmatically based. Either the law doesn't work at all, or it does not accomplish what those drafting the law had intended. Sometimes it happens that the reflective experience of the population indicates that the law is unnecessary. At other times the lived experience reveals that the issues addressed by the law are so important that the law must be refined and enlarged to cover greater complexities.

All too frequently the development of laws bypasses the extensive reflective life of the community and seeks to incorporate a particular ideology into the legal system.[4] When this occurs, alterations in the law become extraordinarily difficult because the ordinary avenues for change—namely, the community's lived experience—are ignored or discounted. When this occurs, factions develop that engage in political struggles either to initiate change in the law or to preserve the law for its ideological content. One of the first victims of these inflammatory struggles is often the ethical and reflective life of the community. Productive legislative change cannot occur until this life is restored.

The narrative of human life in any social structure beyond the most primitive reveals a very complex interaction of experience, reflection, ethical beliefs, ideological commitments, and law.[5] There is a continual feedback loop, or spiral, involving these elements. Refined and well-developed ethical beliefs will frequently lead the way. But this is not inevitably the case. Sometimes the law, through its interpreters, challenges the community to think more carefully about its ethical beliefs and enter into a period of more intensive reflection on its experience. Ideology may contribute to this process by setting forth a norm that is considered essential, but it fails to serve the process if it advances a norm that disregards human experience or is considered impervious to challenge or negotiation.

It is helpful to be aware of the above complex dynamics so that the correct foundation for social change can be identified. Ethical beliefs should not be mistaken for legal protections. Legal requirements should not necessarily be considered the embodiment of the most refined ethical position. Experience can never be discounted as an important ingredient for ethical and legal development in society. When the foundation for change has been correctly identified, then a truer course for the necessary changes can be charted.

The law cannot be relied upon to provide comprehensive guidance for human actions because it cannot address every possible situation in human life. The law paints in broad strokes rather than in infinitesimal detail. Interpretive applications of the law can and do occur to translate it into everyday human experience. But because human life is so complex, the law, even with extensive interpretation, cannot take everything into account. Human beings must rely on the process of systematic and disciplined ethical reflection to give greater guidance to the details of human experience. This ethical examination provides content, nuances, and reasoning for the law.

Though ethical reflection can often provide much supportive impetus and texture for the development and understanding of the law, legal stipulations frequently provide significant challenges to those who would engage in careful ethical reflection on the human condition. These challenges result from either attempting to promote the welfare of citizens through broad legislation or interpreting applications of the law in particular cases. In these situations the law raises issues that prompt much more extensive ethical reflection than would have occurred without the law. The *Roe v. Wade* decision of 1973 provides an interesting example.[6] By referring to the fetus as not being a person "in the whole sense," the decision generated much more extensive and sophisticated reflection on the meaning of "personhood" and its ethical ramifications than was present in the ethical literature prior to 1973.[7]

In the arena of healthcare there is frequently an alliance, albeit sometimes uneasy, of ethics and the law. Problems remain until the relevant issues are explicitly addressed in both domains. The following four cases will demonstrate the struggles encountered in attempting to bring ethics and the law into harmony on some very restricted healthcare matters.

In each case there seems to be a conflict between the law and ethics. The law takes as its fundamental commitments toward individuals the preservation of life, the prevention of suicide, the protection of third parties, and respect for the integrity of caregivers.[8] Healthcare ethics, on the other hand, takes as its fundamental commitment the promotion of the dignity and best interest of patients. The two orientations are not in essential conflict. However, because of a lack of articulation about some situations in the law and the practice patterns of caregivers, there have arisen ambiguities about the conceptual boundaries of each commitment. Sometimes the preservation of life seems to be in conflict with pursuing what some might consider the best interests of the patient. Sometimes the promotion of patient dignity will require a clarification or reinterpretation of what counts as suicide. Sometimes the relative weights of the interests of patients and those of third parties must be reconsidered and delicately balanced. Sometimes caregivers must enlarge their notion of professional integrity in order to meet the legitimate needs of dying or critically ill patients.

Each of the following four cases illustrates some significant dimension of the ambiguity involving the legal and medical approaches to the patient involved and those in similar situations. In some cases there was no legislation or judicial opinion to give any guidance at all. Each case presents some facet of care that needed to be addressed so that caregivers would feel secure in their medical approaches to the patient involved, and the judicial decision resolved some of the ambiguity between the legal and ethical approaches to the care of these patients. In rendering these decisions, the courts addressed some of the issues that would ultimately be incorporated in the Patient Self-Determination Act. Thus, these four cases over the past two and one-half decades can be seen as an important legal backdrop for the Patient Self-Determination Act of 1990. Nor are these the only cases to explore the issues relevant to the act. They provide only a sample of the judicial decisions contributing to the issues addressed in that legislation.

The following analyses are not an attempt to address all the issues raised in the four cases. Rather, they are an attempt to examine only the self-determination issues that provided the climate generating the Patient Self-Determination Act.

The Case of Karen Ann Quinlan

Court procedures surrounding the unhappy circumstances of Karen Ann Quinlan in New Jersey provided the first dramatic legal arena for examining the issues of patient self-determination and the termination of life-sustaining or life-extending technologies.[9] This case made public the struggles that many physicians, institutions, and families had faced with the development of more and more sophisticated technologies that were able to prolong the process of dying for patients who would have died more quickly from their syndromes if the technologies had not been employed. Because the ethical and legal issues surrounding the employment and limitation of these technologies had not been resolved to the satisfaction of the members of the healthcare community, relief was sought through the courts so that Karen Quinlan's best interests could be served. The family had come to terms with the limitations of technology in Quinlan's case. However, the physicians and the healthcare institution insisted on pursuing a course to preserve her life in spite of her severely compromised condition and the wishes of her parents.

Karen Ann Quinlan was twenty-one years of age in 1975 when, at a party, she stopped breathing for two fifteen-minute intervals. After she could not be roused with mouth-to-mouth resuscitation, she was taken to the hospital; there she was placed on a respirator, and a tracheotomy was subsequently performed. After three days her physician determined that she had suffered anoxia and her cortex had been severely damaged. Her EEG was not flat, and thus she was not brain dead, but it was abnormal in a way that was consistent with the anoxic state of her cortex. She soon began to exhibit all the characteristics of a chronic vegetative state, including the sleep-wake cycles consistent with this state. Consulting neurologists confirmed this condition. Attempts to wean her from the respirator were unsuccessful. She was considered totally respirator dependent and moribund. Nutrition was delivered by means of a nasogastric tube.

Karen's father, Joseph, sought the court's appointment of him as guardian of her person so that he could make the decision regarding the removal of her respirator. The superior court refused his petition,[10] but the New Jersey Supreme Court, reversing the lower court, granted it. Mr. Quinlan was supported by the traditions of the Roman Catholic Church holding that patients are not required to undergo treatments that are considered "extraordinary."[11] This term refers to treatments that will not provide a reasonable hope of benefit to the patient.[12] Since the respirator would not lead to Ms. Quinlan's recovery or even to a moderate improvement in her condition, the use of the respirator could be determined to be lacking in benefit and thus extraordinary. Mr. Quinlan claimed to be in a sound position to assert his daughter's wishes because they were grounded in their Roman Catholic religious tradition. Under the principle of autonomy it can be asserted that patients are in the best position to determine their own best interests and thus what will benefit them. It was claimed that Mr. Quinlan, acting as his daughter's surrogate and following her wishes, would be acting in her best interests.

The decision of the New Jersey Supreme Court turned on the issue of the right to privacy. The court had to decide whether the constitutional right to privacy established in *Griswold v. Connecticut*[13] and upheld in *Roe v. Wade*[14] could be extended to cases such as Ms. Quinlan's. This was the first time a court was called upon to apply the right to privacy to a situation involving the removal of life supports. The court compared a patient in this condition with a patient in a terminal condition from cancer. It asserted that there was no logical distinction between the rights of patients to make decisions in the two situations, thereby coming very close to asserting that a persistent vegetative state is a terminal condition.[15] Although the state can limit the right to privacy in the determination of medical treatments, the court indicated that the ability of the state to limit this right is directly related to the state's interest in preserving the life of the patient. In the analysis the court clearly described this relationship: "We think that the State's interest weakens and the individual's right to privacy grows as the degree of bodily invasion increases and the prognosis dims."[16] The court determined that this analysis applied to Karen Quinlan and that since she was incompetent, her father could exercise her right to privacy on her behalf.

Furthermore, the court expressed the opinion that in such cases the refusal of treatment should not be construed as suicide and the withdrawal of treatment should not be considered homicide. Rather, the court acknowledged that death in such cases occurs as the result of the natural process of the impaired condition. It also expressed the opinion that future cases of this kind need not be brought before the court for resolution. Instead, the proper place for their resolution is with the family of the patient in consultation with the physicians treating the patient and the ethics committee of the facility in which the patient is being treated.

This pioneering decision contains several of the foundation stones for the Patient Self-Determination Act. The basis of the law is established by the recognition of the right of the patient, supported by the constitutional guarantee of the right to privacy, to refuse treatment when faced with a severely life-threatening and irreversible pathophysiological condition. The patient's liberty to do so is grounded in the patient's values. The state has only a limited right to interfere with the implementation of those values. The right to self-determination overrides most state interests when healthcare options are at stake, and it is virtually absolute when the patient's prognosis is as bleak as Karen Ann Quinlan's.

The decision also supports the role of the surrogate in advancing the interests of an incompetent patient. Implied in this role is the belief that the incompetent patient does not lose her interest in what will happen to her merely because she has become incompetent.[17] The surrogate can articulate the patient's interest about the direction of her healthcare on her behalf.

An important extension of this decision and its refusal to consider the removal of treatments in conditions of this kind as homicide is the assertion of the responsibility of the patient. Since the physician is not considered to be committing homicide when patients refuse treatments in life-threatening situations, the responsibility for the end-of-life decision lies with the patient or her surrogate.[18]

Moreover, the removal of life-extending treatments in situations of this sort is considered a customary form of medical practice. The *Quinlan* court recognized that such an approach to medical practice is not only customary but even desirable: "We glean from the record here that physicians distinguish between curing the ill and comforting and easing the dying; that they refuse to treat the curable as if they were dying or ought to die, and that they have sometimes refused to treat the hopeless and dying as if they were curable."[19] In chapter 6 we will examine the principle of justice in delivering healthcare and will give a detailed analysis of this principle as it applies to the sentiment expressed by the court in this passage.

The Case of William Bartling

William Bartling was seventy years old when he entered Glendale Adventist Hospital in California in 1984[20] for treatment of depression. At the time of his admission he was known to be suffering from emphysema and arteriosclerosis. A routine physical examination revealed a tumor on his lung, and a biopsy confirmed that it was malignant. The biopsy needle caused the lung to collapse, and the emphysema prevented the lung from reinflating, causing chronic respiratory failure. Bartling was placed on a ventilator with a tracheotomy. He also had an abdominal aneurysm. Although each of these conditions could individually be lethal, Bartling was not diagnosed as terminally ill. Attempts to wean him from the ventilator were unsuccessful, and he was considered ventilator dependent. His physicians admitted that, at best, he could live for only a year if he could be weaned from the ventilator.

Initially Bartling attempted to remove the ventilator tubes but was unsuccessful. To prevent a successful attempt, he was placed in restraints so that the tubes could remain in place. Both Bartling and his wife asked the physicians to remove the ventilator, but they refused.

The Bartlings then filed a complaint against Glendale Adventist Hospital seeking damages for battery and the violation of Mr. Bartling's state and federal constitutional rights. Attached to the complaint were a living will executed by Mr. Bartling and a durable power of attorney for healthcare appointing Mrs. Bartling his attorney-in-fact. In the documents Bartling expressed a clear understanding of his healthcare condition, the distress he was in as a result of the continued ventilator support, the consequences (possible death) of the removal of the ventilator, and his unswerving desire to have the ventilator disconnected. His wife and daughter added documents releasing the hospital and his physicians from all civil liability for whatever consequences might result from following his wishes. The hospital and his physicians remained steadfast in their refusal to disconnect the ventilator both because he was not considered terminally ill and because, so they contended, the religious traditions of the hospital required that life be preserved as long as the patient had cognition, even with such a poor quality and prognosis.

The situation was complicated by Bartling's apparent vacillation. He said that he did not want to die but neither did he want to live on a ventilator. However, at times he seemed to be reconciled to his impending death. On the infrequent occasions when the tubes became accidentally disconnected he seemed to gesture to the nurses to reconnect them. Finally, there were reports by some of the physicians that Bartling had said he did not want the ventilator disconnected.

The trial court, in relying on *Quinlan,* ruled that only patients who were in a comatose, vegetative state or who were determined to be terminal could have ventilators disconnected.[21] It ruled that those who were competent—and it acknowledged that Bartling was competent—could not have their ventilators disconnected.

The appellate court overturned the trial court's decision by relying on *Cobbs v. Grant,*[22] which took the position that adults of sound mind can determine whether to submit to medical treatments as a matter of exercising control over their own bodies. Citing other legal decisions and the recognized intent of California statutes and constitutional provisions,[23] the court concluded that the right to refuse treatment extends beyond the situations of persistent coma and terminal illness to include all patients who wish to make healthcare decisions and their authorized surrogates. The court held that any medical intrusion into a patient's bodily integrity was the object of consent or refusal on the part of the patient.

In addressing the expressed interest of the hospital in preserving life as part of its Christian orientation, the court held that if the right of the patient to self-determination is to have any meaning, it must be paramount if there is an apparent conflict between the goals of the institution and the goals of the patient. As a constitutionally grounded right, self-determination must maintain freedom of choice, even if the consequences are life-threatening, regardless of the religious beliefs of an institution.[24]

With regard to the issue of suicide, the court, as in *Quinlan,* clearly stated that death resulting from the removal of a ventilator is not suicide but rather the result of the natural course of the disease.

Furthermore, the court expressed the opinion that the state's interest in preventing suicide extends only to "irrational" suicide. The refusal of treatment in cases such as Bartling's not only would not be suicide but would not be irrational.

Finally, the court judged that neither the physicians nor the hospital would be liable for Bartling's death if they followed his wishes. Since Bartling was directing the course of his care, he assumed the responsibility for its outcome.

The *Bartling* court enlarged the scope of considerations beyond those designated by *Quinlan*. It made it clear that any patient can refuse treatment whether in a terminal condition or not. But Bartling's situation underscored the importance of clear thinking when addressing the issue of terminal illness. For example, proximity in time to death may not be the best way to think about terminal illness. The severity, degeneration, and irreversibility of the disease process may be more, or at least equally, telling factors. Furthermore, the court seemed to acknowledge the importance of quality-of-life assessments in making a decision to terminate healthcare interventions. Even if Bartling would not be considered terminal, he concluded that his quality of life was so poor that it was not worth continuing, and that the continuance or introduction of any healthcare interventions would place his quality of life in further jeopardy.

The court underscored the importance of giving patients the benefit of the doubt when assessing their decisional capacity. In this it seemed to be following the suggestion of the President's Commission for the Study of Ethical Problems in Medicine and Biomedical and Behavioral Research, which, two years earlier, had set the standard of *presuming* that patients possessed decisional capacity unless it could be clearly shown that they were lacking it.[25] The court further emphasized decisional capacity by asserting the right of competent patients to refuse healthcare treatment, thereby dispelling the rather popular myth at the time that treatments could be withdrawn only for patients who were comatose with no chance of recovery and/or who were terminal. *Bartling* makes it clear that competent, nonterminal patients have the right to refuse treatments. This power extends to their refusals for any reason, including those based upon quality-of-life issues.

This decision also illustrates the role that advance directives can play in treatment refusals. Bartling developed one kind of advance directive in which he specified the reason for the decisions he was making and specified the direction he wanted the treatment to take. He gave specific directions to his attorney-in-fact so that no one could question whether she was adequately representing him in the substituted-judgment process. In taking this approach, Bartling was not only setting the course of his treatment but also giving credibility to his decisions. At the same time he was validating his decisional capacity. His approach to his treatment decisions influenced the court in determining that he did possess decisional capacity and that his approach to his treatment was rational.

The hospital's Christian commitment to preserving life was singled out by the court for special attention. Institutional concerns about the place of patients' refusals of treatment have emerged periodically in court cases about forgoing life-sustaining treatments.[26] The *Bartling* decision places patient self-determination above institutional beliefs. The Patient Self-Determination Act responds to this concern by requiring hospitals to state their policies on such matters at the time of admission. This presumably will give patients the opportunity to seek assistance in other institutions where the policies are more harmonious with their own beliefs and wishes.

But because of the secular sentiments protecting self-determination that were present in this decision, the liberty of an individual appears to be on a collision course with the religious commitments of an institution. *Bartling* would consider that the former must prevail. However, those who sponsor institutions with particular religious commitments consider their mission commitments to supersede the personal liberty of patients, particularly because of the "conscience clauses" in most advance directive legislation.[27] As will be discussed below, it would seem that *Cruzan* in 1990 laid this conflict to rest by grounding the right to refuse treatment in the constitutional liberty interest, thereby making a patient's liberty right paramount in our society. However, the specific issue of religious institutions' mission commitments and patients' liberty rights has not been addressed by the U.S. Supreme Court. Until that time the legal ambiguity described earlier prevails.

The court took an approach similar to that followed in *Quinlan* when considering two related issues in *Bartling*. It stated that no prior judicial approval was necessary to resolve conflicts between patients and caregivers or institutions. It was perfectly appropriate to resolve them at the patient's bedside among the parties involved in the patient's care, *including* the patient. It furthermore stated that physicians could not be held liable for homicide when they followed the wishes of the patient in these matters. The court's decision on both of these issues once again emphasizes the patients' responsibility in determining the direction of their care. Liability does not extend to others when they act as instruments of the patient.

The Case of Paul Brophy

In 1983 Paul Brophy, an active and athletic middle-aged firefighter in Massachusetts, suffered a ruptured aneurysm located at the apex of the basilar artery.[28] He was taken to the hospital, where surgical treatment was not successful. He had no cortical activity, however he was able to breathe on his own but was unable to chew or swallow. For this reason a nasogastric tube was inserted, which was later replaced by a gastrostomy tube as the vehicle for his receiving nutrition and hydration. He was diagnosed as being in a persistent vegetative state, which meant that he had no chance of recovery.

When Brophy's condition became firmly established, his wife and family requested that his gastrostomy tube be either clamped off or removed. They based their decision on the belief that, although Brophy had never documented his wishes in matters such as these, he had verbally stated that he would not want to continue to exist in this condition. His physicians and the hospital (New England Sinai Hospital, where he was finally transferred) refused the family's request. His physicians felt that the removal of the gastrostomy tube would be a harmful act that would directly produce death. Then began the long journey through the courts that ended in the decision of the Massachusetts Supreme Court in 1986.

Initially the probate court found that, if he had been competent, Brophy would have wanted the tube removed.[29] For it was clear from the outset, from informal statements he made, that he would not have wanted to continue to exist in his current condition. But the court refused to authorize the removal of the tube, although it did follow the recommendation of the guardian ad litem to enter a DNR order and to refrain from an aggressive treatment plan if a life-threatening infection should occur. The court found that the patient was not terminally ill and could live for several years in his persistent vegetative state.

In its review of the case the Supreme Court of Massachusetts recognized the legitimacy of Brophy's wishes as represented by the family through the exercise of substituted judgment. It authorized his guardian, Mrs. Brophy, to remove her husband to the care of a healthcare facility where his wishes would be honored. The court authorized the transfer because it respected the right of the hospital to refuse to remove or clamp the gastrostomy tube.

The supreme court supported its opinion by reiterating a number of positions that had already been articulated by other courts. It recognized the right of the patient to refuse treatment based upon the right to privacy. In doing so it quoted *Lane v. Candura,*[30] which stated that "the law protects [a person's] right to make [his] own decision to accept or reject treatment, *whether that decision is wise or unwise."* The court noted that the roots of the right to self-determination and individual autonomy lie deeply imbedded in our national history and common-law tradition.[31] Because the right to refuse treatment, out of respect for the patient's dignity, extends to both the competent and the incompetent, the decisions by the incompetent can be represented through the process of substituted judgment.

The court determined that allowing the removal of the gastrostomy tube did not undermine the state's interest in preserving life in this case. However, it did recognize the state's interest as a legitimate one in those cases where the patient could expect full recovery to a functional life. Although it avoided an assessment of Brophy's quality of life, it did indicate that the intrusiveness of the tube, along with the time that it could be in place, clearly constituted a situation where the interests of the patient in avoiding an existence contrary to his wishes outweighed the state's interest in preserving life. In this matter it followed *Quinlan* very closely.

It also followed *Quinlan* and *Bartling* on the issue of the prevention of suicide. The removal of the gastrostomy tube, it was held, would not be the "death-producing agent." Rather, when death occurs after the removal of life-sustaining treatments, the death is attributable to natural causes in the disease process. Thus, the disease is allowed to run its natural course.

When considering the standard test of whether the removal of life-sustaining treatment from such patients violates the integrity of the medical profession, the court was not so generous to Brophy. It departed substantially from *Bartling* on this point. The court determined that the removal of the tube would not violate the integrity of the institution provided the institution was not required to remove it. Thus, the tube could be removed if Mrs. Brophy could find an institution that would do it. The hospital was required to assist her in finding such a facility. The court based its judgment in this matter on the controversial nature of tube feedings at the time of the judgment (1986) and the disagreements in the medical profession about the requirement to continue tube feedings in such cases.[32] The court recognized that, in such a climate, there was good reason to allow the hospital to follow its commitments to continue tube feedings as a matter of principle.

One of the central issues raised by *Brophy* is that of advance directives. Although the courts reviewing his case acknowledged that he would not want to continue existing in his condition, they did so as a result of the informal statements he made to others. There was no documentation of his wishes in the form of a written advance directive. Without the formal documentation the courts could just as easily have discounted the statements of his family as not meeting a clear and convincing evidence standard. This is what happened in *Cruzan,* as we shall see below. The only way for a patient to rest assured that her wishes would be honored would be to place them in writing in the form of an advance directive. Had Brophy done so, the issue of the hospital's compliance would not have been resolved completely, but his position would certainly have been more compelling if it could have been demonstrated that he had formally established his self-determination and the reasons for his wishes. Faced with a formal advance directive, the hospital might have been less reluctant to follow his wishes.

On the other hand, it could be argued that *Brophy* demonstrates that a verbal advance directive can express the wishes of a patient just as surely as a written one. The major problem with a verbal advance directive is that in situations where there is a difference of opinion about the patient's wishes or her intentions, there is no document to resolve the dispute. In Brophy's case everyone agreed as to what his wishes were. Had he never spoken his mind on the matter, as happens so often with patients, it might have been even more difficult to remove his gastrostomy tube.

The court's protection of the hospital's refusal to remove the tube once again raises the issue of the hospital's right to limit the patient's self-determination as a matter of policy. We saw in *Bartling* that the hospital was not permitted to do so. One year after *Brophy,* in New Jersey's *In re Jobes,*[33] the hospital was also compelled to follow the wishes of the patient as advanced by her surrogate. Because *Brophy* does not place such an obligation on the hospital, it may therefore lay the basis for the stipulation in the Patient Self-Determination Act that a hospital must articulate its policies regarding the removal or withholding of life-sustaining treatments. According to the act, a hospital would have to tell patients or their families upon admission that it would not, as a matter of principle, remove tube feedings from patients under certain circumstances. Those needing healthcare, then, would have the option of seeking it elsewhere. *Brophy* places in sharp relief the significance of this provision of the Patient Self-Determination Act and the controversy surrounding it.

The Supreme Court of Massachusetts found justification for protecting the right of the hospital to refuse the removal of Brophy's feeding tube in the controversial nature of the intervention itself. Indeed, there were many disputes about the nature and appropriateness of tube feedings while the Brophy case was being discussed and heard between 1983 and 1986. Though all the contentions around tube feedings have not been laid to rest even at this time, there have been significant advances in the medical, ethical, and legal communities in understanding the rights of patients to refuse them. The American Medical Association[34] and the Society of Critical Care Medicine[35] among others, acknowledge that it is proper to withhold or withdraw tube feedings under many circumstances. The ethical community has gained some important perspectives on the matter.[36] Finally, the legal community has been well served by the U.S. Supreme Court's decision in *Cruzan,* which took the position that artificial nutrition and hydration are *medical* interventions. It would be much more difficult after the Patient Self-Determination Act for the court's justification respecting the hospital's rights in *Brophy* to stand. Other justifications would have to be developed to allow the same sort of decision.

Finally the role of the responsible patient once again emerges in this case. There is the recognition of the patient's right to self-determination and the acknowledgment of the patient's right to choose death by natural processes rather than waiting for technology to fail, as it surely must. The patient can take control of the direction of his healthcare and can plot its course along the vector of his values and wishes. *Brophy* is very clear that these values do not have to be agreed to by everyone. It is sufficient for them to be the patient's values even if others see them to be "unwise."

The Case of Nancy Cruzan

The most immediate catalyst for the Patient Self-Determination Act was the case of Nancy Cruzan. Although the act followed by about five months the U.S. Supreme Court's *Cruzan* decision in June of 1990,[37] it was already being considered prior to the decision. Cruzan's situation had achieved such attention as it made its way through the courts that the U.S. Congress began to respond to the issues it raised prior to and independently of the court's decision. But the Patient Self-Determination Act will always be linked to *Cruzan* because of the similar issues it addresses.

In January of 1983 Nancy Cruzan (aged 25) suffered severe injuries as a result of an automobile accident. The estimate was that her brain had been deprived of oxygen for about twenty minutes, and this anoxia left her in a persistent vegetative state. She was not ventilator dependent but was dependent on a gastrostomy tube to deliver nutrition and hydration.

In 1985 her parents petitioned the probate court to remove the tube and allow her to die a natural death. They claimed that Cruzan had indicated on several occasions that she would not want to live in this kind of condition and would not want continued nourishment by artificial means. The trial court seemed to interpret loosely Missouri's clear and convincing evidence standard for the removal of life-sustaining treatments from an incompetent and accepted the testimony of her parents and her friends as sufficient evidence of Cruzan's wishes. Accordingly, the court ordered the gastrostomy tube removed.[38]

The attorney general appealed the decision, and the case went directly to the Missouri Supreme Court, which overturned the lower court with its decision in 1988.[39] In this decision the state supreme court discounted the testimony about Cruzan's wishes. It stated that her verbal statements did not constitute clear and convincing evidence, according to the state's public policy standards, which would be necessary to discontinue the gastrostomy feedings. The court also held the gastrostomy feeding not to be medical treatment; it was not treatment of a disease but rather was sustaining a life that could continue for thirty more years. The most telling part of the decision was the position that, because Missouri had taken such a strong policy stand in its living will statute favoring life regardless of its quality, the state's interest in preserving Cruzan's life outweighed her right to privacy and her right to refuse treatment, particularly when there was any uncertainty about her wishes. In summary, the Missouri Supreme Court went against the decisions in *Quinlan, Bartling,* and *Brophy* as well as a host of others that had been decided by various states between 1975 and 1988.

The case was appealed to the U.S. Supreme Court, which agreed to hear it in 1989 as the first such "right to die" case to come before it. The decision was handed down on June 25, 1990, at the conclusion of the Court's term. The Court held that the U.S. Constitution does not forbid Missouri or any state from adopting a clear and convincing evidence standard of an incompetent patient's wishes if life-sustaining treatments are to be withdrawn. It also held that competent persons have a liberty interest guaranteed by the Fourteenth Amendment to refuse any and all medical treatments. However, this interest must be balanced against relevant state interests. An incompetent patient may not have the same right as a competent one to refuse treatment because of the lack of informed consent, but surrogates may be empowered to make such decisions for patients. The Court further ruled that the state may refuse to consider the patient's quality of life in decisions to terminate treatment. Finally, the Court ruled that the Constitution does not require that family members automatically become authorized surrogates in cases like Cruzan's. States can impose their own requirements for surrogacy.

In its decision the Supreme Court acknowledged a number of powers that patients have in the current healthcare climate. They are powers related to the participation of patients in their healthcare decisions whether they are competent or not. The right of the competent patient to refuse any and all treatments is central to its analysis of the *Cruzan* case. Though the Court did not go as far as many state courts had previously done in grounding the right to refuse treatment in the penumbral right to privacy (First, Fourth, Fifth, Ninth, and Fourteenth Amendments),[40] the Court did ground this right in the Constitution, namely, in the due process clause (Fourteenth Amendment). Thus, it is now clear that after *Cruzan,* patients can be said to have a constitutionally based right to refuse treatment regardless of the number of amendments used to support that right.

The *Cruzan* decision underscored that informed consent is central to the decisional process in healthcare. Informed consent is essential for competent patients who are immediately facing a particular healthcare decision and those who need to anticipate healthcare decisions in the future. One can infer from the Court's decision that patients even need to be informed to some extent about the option of drafting advance directives to cover future contingencies.

The Court strengthened the substituted-judgment standard as applied to healthcare decisions for incompetent patients. By placing a strong emphasis on the patient's rights in making healthcare decisions, it gave new importance to the wishes of the patient. For this reason, any attempt to make decisions for incompetent patients must reflect the decision the patient would have made if she had been able to do so. However, this standard, as articulated by the Court, may require an explicit indication of the patient's wishes. The drawing of inferences from more tangential statements made by the patient or the patient's behaviors may not be sufficient to qualify as clear and convincing evidence.

The Court's analysis could lead to the conclusion that the best-interest test will not qualify for the removal of life-sustaining treatments if the state requires a clear and convincing evidence standard. The best-interest test has often been seen as a reasonable alternative when substituted judgment cannot be utilized.[41] Serious questions arise about the use of the best-interest test in the traditional practice of medicine as a result of this decision. One interpretation might allow states to abolish the test altogether, a strategy that could prove disastrous for sound medical practice, particularly in a climate that is preoccupied with healthcare reform. This excess could lead to the practice of required treatment for incompetents unless the patients have indicated desires to the contrary, or continuing treatment for incompetents unless decisions are made in advance about their termination. In view of the low incidence of advance directives and their lack of specificity, an impossible situation will arise if the Court's attitude toward substituted judgment and best interest is taken too strictly.[42]

The Supreme Court accelerated the public and legislative interest in advance directives. These documents, which barely six years before had often been casually dismissed, were given central importance in healthcare.[43] The Court encouraged patients to express their wishes about life-sustaining treatment in advance of decisional incapacity. It indicated that barring an outweighing state interest, the expressed wishes of incompetent patients must be honored. Finally, the Court indicated that advance directives can act as clear and convincing evidence of an incompetent patient's wishes regarding life-sustaining treatments if they are specific with regard to the condition the patient might face and the treatments that might be considered. Unfortunately, this condition may set an impossibly high standard, which will have to be revisited or at least reinterpreted by the courts.[44]

One remarkable aspect of *Cruzan* is the Court's consensus identifying tube feedings and hydration as *medical* interventions.[45] We saw before in both *Bartling* and *Brophy* that the controversy about the moral and "therapeutic" status of tube feedings led to many of the complications in those petitions and decisions. *Cruzan* seems to have laid to rest the judicial issue about the medical status of tube feedings. They are of equal status with CPR, dialysis, surgeries, chemotherapy, etc.

The decision gives rise to another issue, however. If tube feedings are legally indistinguishable from other forms of medical interventions, does the clear and convincing evidence standard apply equally to all life-sustaining interventions for the incompetent? What was said above about the best-interest test may again be relevant here. One should not do CPR on every dying patient. Medical standards exempt certain classes of patients, such as the terminally ill, from CPR attempts.[46] Evidence is also mounting that CPR should not be done on most elderly patients.[47] Nor should dialysis be employed in every case of renal failure.[48] Impossible situations can arise if the *Cruzan* decision is taken too strictly—that is, if clear and convincing evidence of a patient's wishes can be required before withdrawing or forgoing life-sustaining treatments. For sometimes clinicians simply *must* act in the best interests of their patients following the appropriate medical indicators for treatment, or nontreatment, in order to avoid harm to the patient.[49] The pursuit of the patient's best interest is a primary concern to physicians regardless of a lack of expression of the patients' wishes.

The major strength of the *Cruzan* decision is the strong stand that the Court takes toward the autonomy of patients in spite of the restrictions that can be placed on healthcare conditions in states with a clear and convincing evidence standard for removing life-sustaining treatments for incompetents. But even in those states the Court has strengthened autonomy by emphasizing advance directives. The focus on patient autonomy again underscores the role of the responsible patient.

Because of its powerful stand on patient autonomy, *Cruzan* lays the constitutional cornerstone for the Patient Self-Determination Act. It also has given a much needed impetus to and respect for advance directives whether they take the form of living wills or appointments under a durable power of attorney for healthcare. By encouraging patients to use this avenue of decision making, it encourages more extensive participation in healthcare decisions through the process of informed consent, greater reflection on the part of patients, and the exercise of increased responsibility on the part of patients in the clinical situation.

If Nancy Cruzan had had an advance directive, her care could have been terminated six and one-half years before it was actually terminated in December of 1990. Unfortunately, she is like the approximately 85 percent of Americans who do not have advance directives and like many more who do not have advance directives that meet the standards of specificity regarding conditions and treatments that are strict enough to satisfy a rigid clear and convincing evidence rule.[50] With an advance directive Nancy Cruzan could have died without a court battle in most states. Without it she fell into a situation similar to those of Karen Quinlan, William Bartling, and Paul Brophy.

After the *Cruzan* decision and the implementation of the Patient Self-Determination Act, patients in the United States are in much better positions when life-sustaining treatments become an issue. The decision and the law give patients authority and strategies to have their wishes followed. It is now up to healthcare facilities and programs to implement the law. The decision also challenges physicians and other caregivers to assist patients in utilizing the law and to respect their decisions. Finally, the law invites patients to take responsibility for their healthcare in new and often unfamiliar ways.

General Implications

These four cases provide both the broad outlines and some central details for healthcare decision making.[51] Each case breaks significant ground or affirms fundamental beliefs about the way patients should be able to participate in making decisions about their healthcare and the respect that must be accorded them even though their decisions might result in an earlier death than they might otherwise experience. *Quinlan* emphasizes the right to refuse treatment and the right of surrogates to make decisions on behalf of incompetents. *Bartling* illustrates the right to refuse treatment by a competent patient in a nonterminal condition based upon quality of life considerations. It also focuses attention on the matter of advance directives and the obligation of healthcare institutions to follow the wishes of patients in refusing treatment regardless of the mission commitments of the institution. *Brophy* highlights the issue of advance directives and the concerns around tube feedings as a form of life-sustaining treatments. *Cruzan* directs attention to the constitutional right to refuse treatment, the central role of informed consent and advance directives, and the conditions for surrogate decision making. It also resolves the legal issue of tube feedings as medical treatments. Some general implications may be derived from this cluster of cases as a ready reference for understanding the legal background of the Patient Self-Determination Act.

(1) Competent patients are always empowered to refuse any and all treatments for themselves regardless of the threat to the extension of their lives, provided they do not have minors who are dependent upon them.[52] No form of treatment is exempt from this provision. Legally this principle is seen as a constitutional right based minimally on liberty rights guaranteed by the Fourteenth Amendment or maximally on the right to privacy derived from the First, Fourth, Fifth, Ninth,

and Fourteenth Amendments. Ethically this is based upon the right to make decisions and follow through on them autonomously. Ideologically it is based on the commitment to thoroughgoing self-determination that lies at the heart of the beliefs of a democratic society.[53]

(2) Competent patients do not forfeit their interests in refusing treatments merely by the onset of decisional incapacity. Patients have the right to participate in decision making while possessing decisional capacity. If they have some values they wish to pursue or goals they wish to accomplish, the onset of decisional incapacity does not preclude their right to enjoy the fruition of these desires. Healthcare professionals have a fiduciary duty to engage in such actions so as to promote the patient's interest in these matters.

(3) For patients who have not made provisions for the direction of their healthcare through a well-documented advance directive or the appointment of a surrogate, it may be difficult to have treatments terminated even though the treatments are not significantly benefiting the patient. It is not impossible in these cases to withhold or withdraw treatments, but it is much more difficult in the current healthcare climate to do so without some form of instructions from the patient. Unfortunately, many myths abound that add to the difficulty of terminating treatments.[54]

(4) Healthcare decision-making surrogates for patients who lack decisional capacity may take a variety of forms: guardian, attorney-in-fact in a durable power of attorney appointment, or next of kin either designated by statute or as part of the common-law tradition. Such surrogates have virtually the same decision-making authority as patients do in refusing treatments. In order to guarantee this authority patients should explicitly appoint surrogates in a well-documented fashion and give explicit instructions to them about the direction they wish their healthcare to take.

(5) Explicit documentation by patients about their wishes, values, and goals is not absolutely essential for the withholding or withdrawing of treatments. However, such documentation will make end-of-life decisions a great deal easier by eliminating guesswork and challenges on the part of those who are involved in the patient's care.

(6) Though decisions about end-of-life situations in advance of the onset of decisional incapacity are difficult, they take on increasing importance as more and more individuals become involved in the

patient care process and the decisions become increasingly complex. The more detail incorporated in such decisions, or the more specific the appointment of a surrogate, the better.[55] These decisions made in advance may carry the same constitutional weight and certainly the same moral authority as decisions made by a patient who is directly and consciously involved in making them. Without making decisions in advance, patients are causing themselves to be vulnerable to a large variety of other interests and agendas that may not benefit them. The prolongation of a very undesirable dying process may often be the result.

In addition, it is important to remember the following:

(1) The right to refuse treatment in no way implies the right to demand treatment.[56] Any right to demand treatment would require an entitlement that very likely would not be *carte blanche* but would carry some restrictions as the allocation of healthcare resources becomes more and more of a problem.

(2) Patients should be cautious about entering healthcare institutions or programs whose policies may be at odds with their beliefs and wishes. Though it is not clear that the policies of the institutions will override patients' wishes, it is equally unclear that the right of self-determination in healthcare will always override institutional policies that conflict with it, particularly if the patient knows in advance about the policies.

Over time the American judicial system has developed a patchwork of decisions that have addressed the conditions of end-of-life decisions in our society. In doing so it has prompted legislative initiatives that, while not always successful, have moved decidedly in the direction of patients' active participation in their healthcare decisions. This has led to a clear emphasis on the authority and responsibility of patients in the decisional process. The decisions of the courts, though not always consistent in every detail, have nonetheless emphasized the importance and role of patient self-determination in the decisional process in clinical situations.

Though there is no explicit right to die in our society, the four cases examined in this chapter affirm in no uncertain terms the right of individuals to make healthcare decisions that may result in their deaths. The restraint upon the state and upon healthcare professionals and families is clear when patients, whether they are competent or not, are making distinct decisions about the direction of their health-care, even in extreme situations. Patients who wish to take responsibility for the direction of their healthcare and preserve this right have ample vehicles available to them as a result of the courageous efforts of the Quinlans, the Bartlings, the Brophys, and the Cruzans. If patients now become victims of the institutions of healthcare or family discord, or if their lives are prolonged through extensive court battles, they generally have only themselves to blame.

NOTES

1. Redfield R. How human society operates. In Shapiro HL (ed). Man, culture, and society. New York: Oxford University Press, 1971, pages 431–433.

2. Wilson EO. The biological basis of morality. Atlantic Monthly 1998; April, pages 53–70.

3. Mill JS. On liberty. Indianapolis, IN: Bobbs-Merrill Co. Inc., 1956. Mill asserts that the liberty of majorities ("the tyranny of the majority") and minorities can be usurped and suppressed by the power of one individual or a large, but not universally representative, group. "If all mankind minus one were of one opinion, mankind would be no more justified in silencing that one person than he, if he had the power, would be justified in silencing mankind" (page 21). Such a tyranny becomes detrimental to the welfare of individuals who may have a set of interests different from those of the politically powerful.

4. Marx K, Engels F. The German ideology. New York: International Publishers, 1972, pages 64–65.

5. Arendt H. Between past and future. New York: Viking Press, 1968, pages 197–226.

6. Roe v Wade. 410 U.S. 113, 93 S. Ct. 705 (1973).

7. An example of this embellished discussion is Joseph Fletcher's Human-hood: Essays in biomedical ethics, Buffalo, NY: Prometheus Books, 1979, and the extensive reaction this single volume generated.

8. These four concerns are addressed in each of the four following cases, *Quinlan* (1976), *Bartling* (1984), *Brophy* (1986), and *Cruzan* (1990). They have also been addressed in other cases such as Bouvia v. Superior Court. 179 Cal. App. 3d 1127, 225 Cal. Rptr. 297 (April 1986). Most recently they have been addressed by the Ninth and Second Circuit Courts of Appeals in examining the issue of physician-assisted suicide. (See Compassion in Dying

v. Washington. 79 F.3d 790 (9th Cir. 1996) and Quill v. Vacco. 80 F.3d 716 (2d Cir. 1996).)

9. In re Quinlan. 70 N.J. 10, 355 A.2d 647 (1976).

10. In re Quinlan. 137 N.J. Super. 227, 348 A.2d 801 (1975).

11. United States Catholic Conference. Ethical and religious directives for Catholic health facilities. Washington, D.C., 1971. These directives were revised in 1975 and again in 1994. They are consistent in holding the position on extraordinary means of extending life. Cf. directive 57 in the 1994 revision and published in 1995.

12. Kelly G. Medico-moral problems. St. Louis, MO: Catholic Health Association, 1957, page 129.

13. Griswold v. Connecticut. 381 U.S. 479, 85 S. Ct. 1678, 14 L. Ed. 2d 510 (1965).

14. Roe v. Wade. 410 U.S. 113, 153, 93 S. Ct. 705 (1973).

15. This is at odds with a position later articulated by the American Academy of Neurology asserting that a persistent vegetative state is *not* a terminal condition. American Academy of Neurology. Position of the American Academy of Neurology on certain aspects of the persistent vegetative state patient. Neurology 1989; 39:125–126.

16. In re Quinlan. 70 N.J. 10, 355 A.2d 647 (1976), page 663.

17. The point was explicitly addressed later in In re Colyer. 660 P.2d 738 (Wash. 1983).

18. The ethical issues surrounding the responsibility of patients will be more extensively explored in chapter 9.

19. In re Quinlan. 70 N.J. 10, 355 A.2d 647 (1976), page 667.

20. Bartling v. Superior Court. 163 Cal. App. 3d 186; 209 Cal. Rptr. 220 (1984).

21. Superior Court of Los Angeles County, No.C500735, Lawrence C. Washington, Judge.

22. Cobbs v. Grant. 8 Cal. 3d 229, 242, 104 Cal. Rptr. 505, 502 P.2d 1 (1972).

23. Notably Lane v. Candura. 6 Mass. App. 377, 376 N.E.2d 1232, 93 A.L.R.3d 59 (1978), and Barber v. Superior Court. 147 Cal. App. 3d 1006, 195 Cal. Rptr. 484 (1983). See also the policies of the Natural Death Act (Health & Saf. Code, § 7185 et seq.).

24. It is this issue that gives rise to the concerns addressed in the Patient Self-Determination Act requiring healthcare facilities to inform patients of their policies regarding the withholding or withdrawing of life-sustaining treatments.

25. President's Commission for the Study of Ethical Problems in Medicine and Biomedical and Behavioral Research. Making health care decisions: The

ethical and legal implications of informed consent in the patient-practitioner relationship. Washington, D.C.: U.S. Government Printing Office, 1982, page 62.

26. In some cases, although it is not publicly acknowledged or practiced frequently, some religiously oriented institutions, rather than legally contest such matters, have transferred patients to other institutions where their wishes can be followed in order to avoid the dilemma presented by situations similar to Mr. Bartling's. When the religiously oriented institution is the only institution in the immediate geographical area, patients' wishes are sometimes honored at the religious institution even though they may run counter to the institution's commitments. Such practices can be justified on the basis of the principles of autonomy, beneficence, fidelity, and justice due to the fiduciary pledge of the institution to meet the patient's needs and wishes in particular cases, even though the principles of the institution might be compromised in rare cases. The removal of feeding tubes in terminal patients may be an example of such situations.

27. Choice in Dying. Non-compliance provision maps. New York: Choice in Dying, Inc. 1997. Thirty-one states have noncompliance provisions allowing both healthcare institutions and individual providers to refuse to honor the provisions of a living will. Similarly, thirty-five states have such provisions regarding healthcare agents. Fifteen states have such provisions permitting individual providers to refuse to honor the provisions of a living will. Eight states allow individual providers to refuse to comply with the instructions of a healthcare agent. Professional codes have applied the "conscience clause" approach to healthcare professionals as well. Council on Ethical and Judicial Affairs, AMA. Code of medical ethics: Current opinions with annotations. Chicago, IL: American Medical Association, 1996, Opinion 2.20.

28. Brophy v. New England Sinai Hospital, Inc. 398 Mass. 417, 497 N.E.2d 626 (1986).

29. The Norfolk (MA) Division of the Probate and Family Court, David H. Kopelman, J. (1985).

30. Lane v. Candura. 6 Mass. App. Ct. 377, 383, 376 N.E.2d 1232 (1978), page 1245. (Emphasis added)

31. This position continues to be an ongoing theme in judicial decisions about end-of-life decisions. Compassion in Dying v. Washington. 79 F.3d 790 (9th Cir. 1996).

32. The American Medical Association began to lay this controversy to rest with its opinion 2.18 in 1986 (now 2.20 in Council on Ethical and Judicial Affairs, AMA. Code of medical ethics: Current opinions with annotations. Chicago, IL: American Medical Association, 1996), where, in re-

sponse to the Brophy case it held that, in accordance with patients' wishes, the removal of feeding tubes in patients who were terminally ill or in a persistent vegetative state violated the integrity of neither the medical profession nor healthcare institutions.

33. In re Jobes. 108 N.J. 394 (1987). *Jobes* differs from *Brophy* in that the healthcare institution in *Jobes* was required to remove the feeding tube; Mr. Jobes did not have to find another institution to do it.

34. Council on Ethical and Judicial Affairs, AMA. Code of medical ethics: Current opinions with annotations. Chicago, IL: American Medical Association, 1996, Opinion 2.20.

35. Task Force on Ethics of the Society of Critical Care Medicine. Consensus report on the ethics of foregoing life-sustaining treatments in the critically ill. Crit Care Med 1990; 18:1435–1439.

36. Lynne J. By no extraordinary means: The choice to forgo life-sustaining food and water. Bloomington, IN: Indiana University Press, 1986. This entire volume of twenty-seven essays is devoted to exploring the use of feeding tubes.

37. Cruzan v. Director, Missouri Department of Health. 110 S. Ct. 2841 (1990).

38. Teel CE Jr., Judge. Circuit Court, Jasper County, Probate Division (1987).

39. Cruzan, By Cruzan v. Harmon. 760 S.W.2d 408 (Mo. en banc 1988).

40. This penumbra was first identified in Griswold v. Connecticut. 381 U.S. 479, 85 S. Ct. 1678, 14 L. Ed. 2d 510 (1965) and was applied in that case to the use of contraceptives. The penumbra was first applied to end-of-life decisions in In re Quinlan. 70 N.J. 10, 355 A.2d 647 (1976).

41. While "substituted judgment" attempts to replicate the wishes of the incompetent, the "best interest" standard makes no substantial reference to the wishes of the incompetent. See Jonsen AR. Clinical ethics: A practical approach to ethical decisions in clinical medicine. 4th edition. New York: McGraw-Hill, Inc., 1998, page 87. Instead, the best-interest standard assumes the position of a "reasonable" observer who weighs all the factors in the patient's situation and makes a decision (albeit based on an evaluation and balancing of the factors involved) that is deemed to promote the best interest of the patient. Thus, the best-interest standard may not reflect the wishes of the patient, if those wishes were known. Similarly, the substituted-judgment standard may not reflect the best interest of the patient unless one takes the position that the patient, through her surrogate, is in the best position to judge what is in her best interests.

42. The problems attendant to advance directives will be examined in chapter 7.

43. American College of Physicians. Ethics manual. 1st edition. Philadelphia: American College of Physicians, 1984, pages 29–30.

44. The issues of specificity and the difficulty of achieving it in an advance directive will be examined in chapter 7. In view of the challenges faced in this matter, the Court may have set an unsuitably high standard, which very few advance directives can achieve.

45. Cruzan v. Director, Missouri Department of Health. 110 S. Ct. at 2867 (1990).

46. Council on Ethical and Judicial Affairs, American Medical Association. Guidelines for the appropriate use of do-not-resuscitate orders. JAMA 1991; 265:1868–1871.

47. Murphy DJ et al. Outcomes of cardiopulmonary resuscitation in the elderly. Ann Intern Med 1989; 111:199–205. See also Taffet GE et al. In-hospital cardiopulmonary resuscitation. JAMA 1988; 260:2069–2072. See also Schneider AP. In-hospital cardiopulmonary resuscitation: a 30-year review. J Am Brd Fam Prac 1993; 6:91–101.

48. Council on Ethical and Judicial Affairs, American Medical Association. Code of medical ethics: Current opinions with annotations. Chicago: American Medical Association, 1996, Opinion 2.20.

49. Pellegrino ED, Thomasma DC. For the patient's good: The restoration of beneficence in health care. New York: Oxford University Press, 1988, pages 26–27. The principle of nonmaleficence is the fundamental principle in healthcare. Because of this principle physicians are often required to act in certain ways even though they may not know their patients wishes and, occassionally, must act contrary to the known wishes of the patient.

50. Hanson, LC et al. The use of living wills at the end of life. Arch Intern Med 1996; 156:1018–1022.

51. Other cases, which fall outside the scope of this investigation, add texture to the legal background of the Patient Self-Determination Act. As was previously noted, these four have been chosen because they raise key points that are addressed in the Patient Self-Determination Act.

52. Even if minor dependents are affected by the decision, there are situations where the patient has been permitted to refuse treatment. See, e.g., a Jehovah's Witness case in Ohio, Perkins v. Lavin. 648 N.E. 2d 839 (1994).

53. President's Commission for the Study of Ethical Problems in Medicine and Biomedical and Behavioral Research. Making health care decisions: The ethical and legal implications of informed consent in the patient-practitioner relationship. Washington, D.C.: US Government Printing Office, 1982, pages 44–48.

54. Meisel A. Legal myths about terminating life support. Arch Intern Med 1991; 151:1497–1502.

55. Schneiderman LJ. Relationship of general advance directive instructions to specific life-sustaining treatment preferences in patients with serious illness. Arch Intern Med 1992; 152:2114–2122.

56. Meisel A. The right to die. 2nd edition, vol. 2. New York: John Wiley & Sons, 1995, page 546. The right to refuse treatment is a negative right conferring on an individual the right to act without interference. The right to demand treatment would be a positive right; such a right has not been upheld by the courts to this point. See Gilgunn v. Massachusetts General Hospital, no. 92–4820 (Mass. Super. Ct. Civ. Action Suffolk Co. April 22, 1995). In re Conservatorship of Wanglie, No PX-91-283 (Minn. Dist. Ct. Hennepin Co. July 1991) although seeming, at first glance, to protect a right to demand treatment, actually only established Mr. Wanglie's right to make decisions for his incompetent wife. (Mrs. Wanglie died three days after the decision was rendered.) The decision in the Baby K. case, while ordering treatment, did so only for admission in emergency situations until the infant was stabilized; the decision was made on an extended interpretation of EMTALA and the Americans with Disabilities Act. In re Baby K. 16 F.3d 590 (4th Cir.), cert. denied sub nom. Baby K ex rel. Mr. K v. Ms. H 115 S. Ct. 91 (1994).

3

The Social and Technological Background for the Patient Self-Determination Act

Like most laws, the Patient Self-Determination Act did not arise merely out of a set of legal circumstances that made it necessary, desirable, or inevitable. On the contrary, the most significant driving force behind the formulation of the law was the social (i.e., medical) situation within the context of our highly developed technological society.[1] The interplay of social forces becomes increasingly complex as new developments in technology emerge. The interactions of individuals are never purely interpersonal. They are always mediated by forces in the society that themselves are the result of human ingenuity. These forces could be, and many times are, social structures that condition the manner of human interaction, such as class divisions, occupational endeavors, or economic stratification.[2] Often, and at times more subtly, technological developments are the factors that condition the quality of human relationships. For example, human interactions were never the same after the development of movable type.[3] In our own age the computer and particularly the personal computer can lay claim to similar alterations in human communication.[4] Perhaps one of the most significant effects of technology on human life is the changing expectations we have for ourselves and others in all facets of our experience. This manifests itself no more dramatically in fields of human activity than in healthcare.

The Expectations of Healthcare

In a less technological society the expectations of the healthcare profession were fairly minimal. In many ways the Hippocratic oath sets the tone for the commitments of physicians and what patients could expect of them. In earlier days there was no healthcare "industry" as we find today. Healthcare began and ended with the relationship between the physician and the patient. The expectations for physicians were fairly clear: they should act for the welfare of their patients, keeping them from harm and injustice.[5] Physicians were expected to rely on the latest developments in the professionals' knowledge of the healing arts and to be prudent in their attempts to extend the lives of their patients. They should not undertake to cure patients when "the disease has already won the day."[6] The oath has set a tone for medical practice and indirectly for the consumption of medical resources.[7]

As the techniques of the medical arts developed through the centuries, society's expectations of those who would aspire to their practice were significantly raised. The sciences underlying medical practice became more and more refined in the area of diagnosis. As case histories were compiled, prognoses became more reliable as well. The knowledge of the etiology of disease became increasingly sophisticated, and with it new preventive, if not curative, measures were instituted.[8] One of the prime examples of this sort of development was the discovery by Dr. Lister of the mechanism for the spread of infection.[9] It took another sixty years for cures to be developed for infectious diseases, but learning to prevent healthcare problems was a major step in revising the expectations that patients had of their physicians. If the physicians could not cure their patients, at least they were expected not to contribute to the causes of their poor health. Relative accuracy in diagnosis and accompanying preventive measures raised the expectations for the application of the principle of nonmaleficence—"do no harm"—to a new level.

With the advent of antibiotics, approaches to curing patients took a radically new turn. No longer were the techniques of the healing arts limited to simply "coaxing" natural processes to cure patients. New substances could be introduced into the patient that would turn natural processes around. Disease-producing entities could actually be destroyed. No longer would physicians have to try only to dispose the human organism in certain ways and hope that the host organ would rally against the invader. They could engage in a full frontal assault on the enemy. The expectations of the healing power of physicians were now raised to an even higher level.

The institutions of medicine, primarily hospitals, took on more prominent roles in the dynamics of healthcare over the last two centuries. With the introduction of effective drug therapies and their supervised administration in healthcare facilities, their role as curative institutions took on increasing importance.[10] The expectations of patients moved from hoping they would not die when they entered the hospital to expecting to be cured in the institution. With the inauguration of antibiotics a new player achieved great and almost revered significance. Those who used the science of chemistry to produce the medication to effect cures had achieved a level of preeminence far beyond that of their predecessors, who could do no more than focus on natural herbal remedies. Pharmacological interventions very quickly took on the role of the treatment of choice. Again, expectations increased as the future success of medicine was often seen as lying in the effective administration of pharmacological remedies that could be provided by physicians and hospitals.

The next significant technological development that raised our expectations of healthcare was the introduction of machines that could replace the function of organs. This technology provided a number of possibilities. It could replace the function of the organ until the organ had healed itself. Or it could replace the function of the organ (or parts of it) indefinitely, allowing the patient to continue to live until either the patient died of another cause or the technology itself failed. In either case the patient's life was extended, and the promise of the technology was that, with better information and more sophisticated equipment the extension of life could be multiplied many times over. This, along with the development of transplant technology, created the perception that there were no limits to addressing disease processes effectively. Currently, patients often reach the point of expecting hospitals and physicians to cure them or maintain them in ways that will allow them to postpone death indefinitely.

The next level of expectations to be embraced by healthcare will probably be the refinement of genetic diagnosis and gene therapy, a technology that is still in its embryonic stage.[11] With this development will come the expectation that all syndromes should be susceptible to diagnosis even before the symptoms emerge. Furthermore, we may soon expect the manipulation of genetic information to allow us to correct all or most disease processes, often before they begin, as well as other forms of disabilities, even the disabilities accompanying aging itself. Genetic diagnosis and gene therapy offer us a great deal of promise, but immortality is probably not one of its outcomes.

Contemporary American culture has created a complex web of features that has made the delivery of healthcare a great problem in our society. The desire to improve the delivery of healthcare seems to know no boundaries.[12] While reaping the benefits of the discoveries of science and its applications to the healing arts, our society has continually raised expectations of medicine and healthcare beyond reason. At the same time each technological innovation seems to add to the belief that there is no unreasonable expectation. Though the frontiers of our expectations of medical technology may be pushed further and our insatiable desire for certainty that medical knowledge will achieve its goals may occasionally be satisfied, there are forces in nature and the human condition that will ultimately cause us to fall short of many of these expectations. Either the achievement of those expectations will be impossible or their accomplishment will require resources far beyond our means to produce them.[13]

In summary, no matter how much we may want medicine to cure syndromes and prevent death and no matter how much we may desire certainty about the successful application of medical technologies, all our desires cannot be satisfied. At best we can hope for some incremental increase in meeting our expectations. But even that increase may actually diminish rather than enlarge as time goes on.

It is not surprising that, in spite of rising expectations in healthcare, a law like the Patient Self-Determination Act would be passed. For the high expectations for what healthcare can deliver on the contemporary scene are often tempered by the fact that these expectations are frequently not met. Their pursuit all too often leads to substantial harm to the patient, a severe compromising of sound medical practice, and a violation of some deeply held beliefs and desires by patients. The Patient Self-Determination Act stands as a witness to the limited ability of medicine to meet the expectations society has for it. It also affirms the patients' right to accept those limitations when they have chosen to do so and act accordingly, thereby escaping from the illusions generated by the general expectations of society.

The Physician-Patient Relationship

The expectations about the promise and accomplishments of health-care have led to a distortion of the basic relationship that permeates the clinical situation. Because much of the recent drama in improving healthcare has centered on developing medical technology, both diagnostic and therapeutic, it seems as though the fundamental relationship in healthcare is now the one between the patient and the technology. The intimacy of the physician-patient relationship has often been replaced by the romance with medical technology.[14] It is important that this primary relationship between the physician and the patient be reaffirmed if the difficult issues facing patients in the clinical setting are going to be properly addressed.[15]

The relationship between patients and their physicians has generally been characterized as a fiduciary one. This means that its primary characteristic is one of virtuous practice grounded in fidelity and motivated by beneficence.[16] The nature of this relationship is traceable to the origins of the Hippocratic tradition.[17]

In a fiduciary relationship the "fiduciary"—in this case the physician—assumes an obligation to act on the patient's behalf and in the patient's interest. On this understanding the physician takes on the role of the patient's advocate.[18] The physician as advocate functions very much like the lawyer as advocate. He or she stands by the patient who is facing a disease or infirmity. The clinician and the patient confront the disease or infirmity as a shared problem. The physician utilizes expert knowledge on behalf of the patient and defends the patient against the disease or infirmity, acting as a guide and support for the patient in the situation. The physician is in a position to compensate for factors that might diminish the patient's autonomy, such as ignorance, confusion, fear, and isolation. In many ways, the physician is in a position to promote the patient's autonomy.

The defining characteristic of the Hippocratic oath was beneficence. The physician was required to act in such a way that the patient would not be harmed but rather would be benefited as a result of the physician's direction of the patient's care. "Beneficence" derives from the two Latin words, "bene" and "facere," meaning to "do good." In the Hippocratic tradition the obligation of the physician to act in such a way that the patient benefited was unconditional. But because of the relatively primitive state of medical practice in the Hippocratic school, the doing of good was relatively easy to identify. First of all, the physician was not supposed to kill the patient. Death was seen as an evil. Second, the physician was supposed to attempt to cure the patient when possible because health was considered a benefit. Finally, beneficence took the form of comforting the patient when curing was impossible.

Unfortunately, in the contemporary world doing good is not as easy to identify. The "good" is not limited to physical goods. There are psychological goods and even moral goods. In thinking that she is keeping the patient from physical harms, the clinician may be imposing on the patient psychological or moral harms that far outweigh the physical good being produced. Unlike Greek society, which had a univocal assessment of what counted as a good, contemporary society is pluralistic and does not have universal agreement on what should count as a good. Thus, death is not always a harm[19] but is often a release from an extraordinarily troublesome existence.

Attempting to cure may not always be the most desirable avenue of intervention. Even if a cure is possible, the means needed to achieve it may impose more burdens on the patient than he or she is willing to endure. Nor does alleviating pain always enjoy universal acceptance as a good. Some patients may view pain as bearing religious significance, perhaps as an act of atonement.[20]

In addition to beneficence the element of trust is an integral part of the traditional notion of the fiduciary relationship. One of the expectations of the patient is that he will trust the physician, listen carefully to the physician, and act on her advice. Sometimes this trust might even take the form of accepting the physician's notion of the good with little questioning. He will minimize noncompliance with the physician and follow orders because the physician, as the expert, is better equipped to know what is in the patient's best interest.

However, this traditional characterization of the patient's role in the relationship is no longer an accurate portrayal. The one-sided view of agency, and the trust that accompanies it, works in a relationship of radical inequality. It works when the *only* element at stake is that of expert knowledge versus ignorance. However, in contemporary healthcare, the relationship between the patient and the physician is no longer radically asymmetrical. Though the physician is the one who continues to have the knowledge of the expert, the patient has access to considerable information either through the physician or through other sources. The requirements of informed consent are designed to ensure that the disparity of knowledge between the parties in the clinical relationship is diminished.

Moreover, the consideration of the patient's values has assumed great importance in healthcare decision making.[21] It is in this area that the patient's expertise takes priority. Physicians can only *assume* that they know what their patients' values are. When clinicians and surrogates make careful inquiries about these values, they often find that their assumptions are wrong.[22] Ideally, the patient is the one who can best identify her values, but, admittedly, assistance in clarifying and articulating those values is often needed.

The structure of the physician-patient relationship in contemporary medical practice now possesses a greater balance of power and authority in the decision-making process. The physician has the power given by expert knowledge and the authority to make recommendations grounded in a wide range of experiences in scientific explanations and clinical judgments. The patient has the expertise in the area of her values. She is the authoritative interpreter of her "value life" as it applies to the clinical setting.[23] Because of this balance of expertise the clinical relationship, as expressed in the dynamics of informed consent, is really an exchange of power. The physician empowers the patient by giving information while the patient empowers the physician by giving consent. Thus, the physician and the patient encounter each other as moral equals whose various assets complement those of the other.

Because of new interpretations of the dynamics of power in the contemporary physician-patient relationship, the concept of trust must also be reinterpreted. Whereas in the traditional view trust was one-sided, in the contemporary view, trust must be seen as a mutual opportunity allowing physicians and patients to reach out to each other as moral friends rather than as moral strangers.[24] The patient must continue to trust the physician, but the physician now must trust the patient. He must trust that the patient has an active interest in what is happening to her in the clinical setting and that she has some knowledge of what is appropriate to her. He must also trust that the patient is ordinarily capable of actively participating in decisions about her healthcare and is willing to assume the risks and consequences of those decisions.[25] Though the grounds for trusting patients may often be deficient in actuality, the physician must begin the relationship *assuming* that the grounds are there.[26]

The nature of the physician-patient relationship and the goals of medicine are most effectively identified in the first edition of the American College of Physicians' *Ethics Manual.*[27] In this document the role of the physician as patient advocate is clearly stated, as is the role of the patient as the one holding final decision-making authority. In addition, the *Ethics Manual* states the goals of medicine in clear and precise terms. The physician is to promote health, relieve suffering, and prevent untimely death while maintaining the dignity of the patient.[28] The first two stipulations are not new, for they have been a constant in the traditions of the healing arts. The prevention of untimely death is an additional element that is given a new dimension because of the way contemporary medicine has advanced the delivery of healthcare. We will discuss this matter shortly.

Maintaining the dignity of the patient is an element of particular interest in discussing the physician-patient relationship and will be explored further in chapter 4. For now it should be noted that a clinician cannot maintain the patient's dignity by ignoring the patient's values and wishes. Nor can the patient's dignity be maintained only in some selective area of medical practice; it must be maintained in all areas. Furthermore, the commitment to patient dignity requires an affirmation of the patient's ability to take risks and accept responsibility for decisions and this will be peculiar to each patient, further individualizing the dignity of each patient. In other words, trust in the patient in spite of decisions with which the clinician might not agree is a pivotal way of maintaining patient dignity.

One aspect of the traditional physician-patient relationship that has commanded an extraordinary amount of attention in the past twenty-five years is the exercise of parentalism (formerly known in more sexist vocabularies as "paternalism") by physicians versus the exercise of autonomy by patients. Parentalism is based on the belief that one individual is in a more privileged position than another individual, either because of a wider range of experience, as in the case of a parent or guardian, or as a result of expert knowledge, as in the case of a physician. The one in the privileged position is presumed to know what is in the best interest of the "subordinate" better than the subordinate herself.[29]

For much of the history of medicine it was believed that disease or injury automatically leaves one unable to make decisions on his or her own behalf.[30] Thus, physicians could exercise different forms of parentalism because they considered decision making on behalf of patients to be one of the privileges of their social position. The expert knowledge of the physician was considered the foundation for this privilege. However, as was noted earlier, the broadening of the knowledge base of the patient has eroded this social position of the physician. The extension of the notion of expertise to the value life of the patient has further contributed to this erosion. Thus the tendency of physicians to adopt a parentalistic posture toward their patients, though historically understandable, now has become ethically inappropriate.[31]

The autonomy of patients is now assumed from the outset.[32] The only form of parentalism generally considered appropriate is that which is exercised when the individual's decisional abilities are permanently compromised or temporarily underdeveloped. Parentalism in this case is ordinarily exercised by the surrogate. When there is a question about a patient's decision-making capacity, parental interventions may be appropriate but they should be limited.[33] It is generally considered inappropriate to override the decision of a functionally autonomous person.[34] Instead the physician is expected to enhance the patient's dignity by promoting the patient's autonomy.[35]

The turn toward patient autonomy in the past twenty-five years, together with all of its accompanying debate, laid the foundation for the Patient Self-Determination Act. If patients are autonomous, then it is appropriate to translate this moral authority into legal protections. Rather than jeopardize the physician-patient relationship, the act strengthens it. For now the patient is viewed as a partner or collaborator with the physician.[36] Each brings strength to the relationship and empowers the other through the dynamics of informed consent. Their communication patterns can reflect and enhance the dignity that both enjoy as persons in a difficult situation facing disease or injury. The respect for autonomy and the use of it as the pivotal point for effective communication emphasize in a dramatic way the central role of the Patient Self-Determination Act in the clinical setting.

The Technological Pressures on Healthcare Delivery

The growth of technology on the American scene has created extraordinary opportunities for individuals. It has made it possible for many to enjoy a quality of life that was unimaginable prior to the Industrial Revolution or even at the turn of the twentieth century. Goods and services have multiplied and become available to an extent unimagined even a few decades ago.[37]

It is little wonder that individuals in industrialized nations tend to equate technology with progress and to consider more technology an unquestioned boon.[38] Nor is it surprising that the advances of industrialized nations should be the envy of less developed countries. The result of the improved quality of life through technology is a vector pointing to more and more technology in the future.

Along with the development of technology is the belief that the employment of technology is required by its very presence. This phenomenon is often referred to as the "technological imperative."[39] The imperative is expressed by the attitude "if the technology is available it must be used." For example, if a fax machine is available in the office, it *must* be used instead of (is not merely preferable to) the postal service. The technological imperative reflects the fact that often technology is viewed as having a life of its own, governed by its own rules[40] and independent of human direction or decisions. The obligation to utilize the technology often seems to be absolute and unquestioned.

However, the technological imperative is an illusion much the same as other illusions that accompany the overpowering presence of technology in our lives. We are seduced into thinking that technology always leads to an improvement in our lives: more is better, faster is better, flashier is better (reflect on rock concerts for a moment), bigger is better.[41] The drive toward developing more technology seems unstoppable (even if stopping it were desirable.[42]) One of the results of these seductions is that we become alienated from many of the fundamental realities of our existence and the natural world around us.[43]

The technological imperative distorts our view of human beings as decision makers. On the one hand, it subverts one of the most fundamental beliefs we have about ourselves—namely, that we have power over ourselves and some of the forces around us, particularly those of our own making. On the other hand, technology often produces the illusion that we have power over all, or most, of the forces of nature merely because we have power over a relatively few natural dispositions.

Nowhere have the opportunities, possibilities, and seductions of technology confronted contemporary human beings more dramatically than in the practice of medicine.[44] As indicated earlier, each new advance in the technologies of diagnosis, prognosis, and therapy has raised the expectations of patients to new heights. And with each triumph of technology over natural barriers, there is an increase in the hope and expectation that additional barriers will fall.

The technological imperative is as prevalent in medical practice as it is in other areas of technological development. The common belief has been that the technological option must be utilized if it is available. For example, if a crash cart is available, the reflex action is to summon it in every case of cardiorespiratory arrest.[45] Human decision making in these cases has been set aside, and utilization of a high-tech intervention becomes automatic. This tendency to employ technology might be characterized as the use of "default" therapy where one simply moves to a preprogrammed system in much the same way a computer functions when a certain stimulus is presented.

It is only in the past two decades or so that this default approach to therapy has been called into question and the role of personal decision making has been reevaluated.[46] Though there is often a continuity from diagnosis to prognosis to therapy, there is no *necessary* connection requiring that therapy flow from a diagnosis and prognosis. Given the diagnosis and prognosis, a decision about therapy must be made on the basis of the values and goals of the patient. Patients do not always see a particular form of therapy, or therapy itself, as a desirable way of addressing the realities of a diagnosis and prognosis. This is why some cancer patients with a particular value framework do not view chemotherapy as an option, while others with a different value framework may wish to utilize it.

Default therapy is often responsible for prolonging the dying process. No matter how bleak the prospect, it almost always seems possible to attempt yet one more variation in therapy, or keep the patient on a ventilator for one more day, or initiate CPR one more time. This often happens because the technological imperative overrides the difficult process of making decisions, and therapeutic interventions are initiated as an automatic response.

Because of this inclination and the attempt to resist the technological imperative, the articulation of "preventing *untimely* death" in the American College of Physicians' *Ethics Manual* takes on great importance in contemporary medicine.[47] Patients or their surrogates are often in the best position to identify when death becomes "timely"— that is, when it is no longer in the patient's interest to resist it by whatever technological means are available. This process involves a particularly reflective decision on the part of the patient or surrogate. They are in the best position to determine whether further technological interventions will fit within the patient's value context and goals.

The Patient Self-Determination Act is an attempt to create an environment in healthcare that directs the patient and the caregiver toward reflective decision making and away from default therapy. Because of the information that must be given to patients at the time of admission to a healthcare facility or a healthcare plan, patients should no longer feel compelled to follow the technological imperative. As healthcare professionals comply with the Patient Self-Determination Act, patients can now see that technological interventions in healthcare are only one of many options to consider as they are coping with their healthcare situations.

The Difficulty of Limiting Technology in Healthcare

We cannot casually assume that patients will forgo technological interventions simply because they know they have the right to do so.

Clinicians often find that many patients still opt for high-tech interventions when facing the ravages of a protracted dying and certain death. Of the many patients who face terminal diseases every year, only about 390,000 in 1995 chose a hospice environment for dealing with their end-of-life decisions.[48] And only about 15% of Americans have an advance directive.[49] There is no way to know how reflective they have been in choosing to sign such documents, or whether the kinds of decisions that an advance directive represents are reflected in the competent decisions they make prior to the onset of decisional incapacity.

Human beings have a very strong desire to live on in spite of our clear understanding that immortality is not a possibility for us. To add a day or a week or a year or ten years to our lives with the possibility of returning to health is a temptation that is difficult to resist. And even if returning to complete health is not in the offing, the avoidance of further deterioration or the development of better means to cope with disease and disability is always an enticement to pursue further interventions.[50] In spite of these strong tendencies in human experience, a counterattitude frequently surfaces. This attitude prompts patients or their surrogates to call an end to measures that extend the dying process. This attitude of acceptance is protected by the Patient Self-Determination Act.

The desire to continue to live is often referred to as hope. Hope and the unwillingness of patients to give up often have very positive therapeutic effects. The mind's ability to set the body on a course of recovery manifests itself anecdotally in every professional's practice. But hope to recover or continue to live is only one form of hope that patients can experience.

There are many forms that hope can take in the process of continued deterioration and dying. Dying patients seem to have three major concerns: (1) pain, (2) isolation, and (3) loss of control.[51] One can always hope that these concerns will be met in a positive way. Comfort care can replace useless aggressive attempts to cure. Companionship on the part of caregivers, family, and friends can reduce the fear of isolation. Ongoing consultation about the direction of the disease, and the interventions addressing it through the process of informed consent, can restore a sense of control to the patient. Technology is not the only answer to the hopes (or fears) patients may have. The human touch is often much more effective in meeting the real needs of the patient.

Patients are in a position to decide which approach to their dying they wish to pursue. But in this simple statement is imbedded one of the greatest difficulties in forgoing technological interventions. A common belief among caregivers, patients, and families is that the refusal or foregoing of medical treatments is tantamount to suicide or homicide.[52] At some point in the dying process all technological interventions will fail. When the patient is moribund, it is the disease that is the cause of death. The causal line leading to death is the etiology of the disease and the inability of the body to shake itself loose from the disease process. Decisions to forgo technological interventions allow the causal forces of the disease or injury to progress uninterrupted. To be sure, any decision contributes to the way in which the progression occurs.[53] However, it does not radically change the outcome of the fundamental causal line. Thus, the stigma against suicide and the prohibition against homicide do not apply to refusing life-sustaining treatments.

Nonetheless, we are still apprehensive about and reluctant to become active participants in our death. We often seem to think that death should be something that overtakes us. "Do not go gentle into that good night/Rage, rage against the dying of the light"[54] is a sentiment that is considered natural and that is extraordinarily difficult to eliminate. Contemporary medical technology has forced us to reassess our responsibilities as persons in the process of dying. It is certainly inconsistent for us to promote and foster the notion of responsibility in our lives only to abandon it when we come to die.

The Patient Self-Determination Act reinforces the need to be responsible decision makers not only in our living but also in our dying. It encourages patients to reflect on the direction of their lives and the extent to which they wish to aggressively resist the dying process. It invites patients to explore the breadth of their courage. It challenges caregivers and families to assist patients in identifying their values and goals and to support them when they make their decisions. For some, going "gentle into that good night" is repulsive, and death must be resisted to the last breath if they are to retain their dignity. For others, death may be a natural outgrowth of the process of living and is another phase to be embraced with a cooperative attitude.

Making end-of-life decisions is, therefore, not a univocal activity.[55] There are many different approaches to this arduous task. They are conditioned by the values patients use to guide their life decisions and the virtues they develop to carry those decisions to completion. In a secular society there is no one preferred range of decisions; that luxury is reserved to moral communities that have articulated religious commitments.[56] The Patient Self-Determination Act does not, in itself, prejudice the direction that patients' decisions should take: whether to elect initiating or continuing treatments or to choose to refuse treatment. For the Patient Self-Determination Act says that patients must be informed that they have the right to "consent to or refuse" treatment. Though there are no limits placed on the refusal of treatments, the same cannot be said for consenting to treatment in the form of demanding treatments that are inappropriate in the sound practice of medicine.[57]

The major decisional advantage of the Patient Self-Determination Act seems to be to reduce societal or professional leanings toward treating or not treating. Instead, the law helps patients realize the options open to them.[58] It helps them to realize that the difficulty in resisting the seductions of technology can be overcome and that default therapy may not be the only way to accomplish our human purposes. Likewise, it allows patients to make therapeutic decisions to initiate or continue treatments, within the range of sound medical practice, that will allow them to achieve the personal goals they have established for their lives.

Healthcare Costs and the Demands of Justice

The cost of the delivery of healthcare in the United States has long been a matter of serious concern to those who fashion public policy. The concern has accelerated along with the rapidly rising cost of the technologies being developed for diagnosis and treatment and the problem of access for many Americans.[59] The expansive paperwork empires of bureaucratic regulations and insurance claims have also contributed to mounting concerns in the public arena. Two of the major issues that have arisen are access to healthcare and controlling healthcare costs.

With large numbers of citizens either without insurance or with less insurance than they need to cover their healthcare needs, the crisis of access has reached alarming proportions.[60] Studies show that for the 14 percent of the gross national product being expended for healthcare in this country, we enjoy no appreciable difference in the overall quality of our public health than in industrialized countries that spend far less of their gross national product.[61] The expenditure of many healthcare dollars for unnecessary testing and ineffective interventions has caused policy makers to surmise that more extensive coverage could be provided to Americans for at least the same expenditure, and probably less, provided better decisions were made about healthcare utilization and the paperwork maze were significantly reduced.

The Patient Self-Determination Act was fundamentally intended to help patients make better decisions about the kind and extent of the healthcare they receive. It can accomplish its purpose because it is based upon the dynamics of informed consent. Theoretically, a renewed emphasis on informed consent could lead patients to better judgments not only about refusing treatment when the treatment will not benefit them, but also about other kinds of healthcare expenditures that can promote their well-being. Access to healthcare is only the first step in healthcare decision making.

One of the fears about universal access to healthcare is that patients will overutilize the healthcare available to them. If properly employed, the Patient Self-Determination Act could provide a measure of defense against this possibility.[62] We noted earlier that one of the major problems in healthcare utilization was the inclination to follow the technological imperative leading to default therapy, that may be unreflectively utilized and provides little or no benefit to the patient. If this tendency were to continue, then no amount of healthcare reform would accomplish its cost-containment goals. The costs would far exceed anticipation in much the same way that Medicare and Medicaid costs have surpassed the expectations of their original authors. Access should not necessarily lead to interventions, particularly ineffective ones. On the other hand, access can lead to interventions that would prevent the more serious (and more expensive) problems that might arise if the interventions were not utilized.[63] The Patient Self-Determination Act can create a climate of reflective decision making within the context of universal access so that patients can make careful decisions about which interventions to pursue and which not to pursue.

The desire for universal access has been prompted by an on-going concern for distributive justice in American society. The ideals of distributive justice are an important part of a democratic society. If democracy is based upon universal participation in political decisions then, by extension, it is appropriate for the goods of society to be distributed in some way that mirrors the common good. Simply stated, the ideals of distributive justice mandate that both the benefits and the burdens of society should be equitably allocated throughout the group.[64] Since it is difficult to disburse benefits and burdens in following this principle, the population must decide through democratic processes which ones should fall within the principles of distributive justice. Not all benefits can be distributed in a free market economy;[65] thus, there is a need for public policy decisions grounded in a democratic process concerned about the ideals of distributive justice.

In making decisions about the benefits to be disbursed in society as entitlements, a frequent criterion is whether the benefit under consideration is essential to the well-being of its citizens. Indeed, this argument has been central to the movement over the years to establish healthcare as a right. The argument for a right to healthcare seems to have gained somewhat wider acceptance among both policy makers and the general citizenry.[66] Certainly this has been prompted by some measure of compassion for the noninsured and underinsured. But it has probably also been fueled by the ever higher costs of healthcare and its insurance, which government intervention holds out the promise of controlling. An additional contributing factor is the volatility of the workplace, where individuals can lose healthcare coverage as a result of the forces of the free market as they are played out in job losses and job changes.

In order to gain these benefits, everyone will have to shoulder certain burdens in the form of higher taxes. The burdens will also take the form of higher prices for goods and services as companies are required to pay a major portion of insurance coverage for their employees, alterations in insurance coverage and premiums, and the necessity of choosing among healthcare plans that might not be to the complete liking of the participants. Whether taxpayers and consumers are willing to shoulder these additional burdens is highly questionable at this time. As in any free market, individuals who can afford to pay for healthcare without recourse to insurance will continue to be able to do so. But even they will bear the burdens of guaranteeing that all will have some level of coverage and access.

It will be impossible to guarantee everything to everyone unless we are willing to invest astronomical sums in the system. To achieve the goals of any effective healthcare reform a great deal of discipline will be required in the delivery of healthcare.[67] The number of tests given to patients will have to be limited. There may be some sacrifice in precision in testing, but after a certain level great expenditures may be required to gain an insignificant level of precision or confirmation.[68] The paper trails for claims will have to be cloaked in the discipline of compromise. Not every insurance company will be able to have all the information it might prefer. Standardization for computer efficiency may lower costs appreciably.

Two problematic issues have been systematically avoided by those espousing healthcare reform. Both involve limiting treatments in order to effect a cost reduction. The easier of the two issues involves limiting treatment when the care being considered is determined to be futile. (This situation will be examined more extensively in chapter 6.) There is no requirement in the traditions of medicine to provide care for patients when it is futile.[69] As a matter of fact, a prohibition against such practices can be inferred from those traditions based upon the principle of beneficence. The problem lies in identifying what it means for care to be futile and when that determination is appropriate.[70] It is estimated that from 40 to 60 percent, and even higher, of the healthcare delivered in the United States is consumed in the last thirty days of life.[71] Even a cursory pass through the ICUs in our hospitals would confirm that much of this care is futile, even allowing for a wide variety of definitions. This means that vast sums of healthcare dollars are spent on care that has no positive return for the patient.[72] Any healthcare reform will ultimately have to address this issue and require the discipline to act with restraint when futile care becomes a part of the clinical determination.[73]

The more difficult of the two issues involving limiting treatments is that of rationing. Rationing generally occurs when the determination is made that a particular intervention, such as multiple transplants, is simply too expensive or when the intervention is not considered costworthy—it is too expensive for the outcome that will be produced.[74] The architects of healthcare reform will have to determine which interventions will not be funded.[75] This may range from drugs that are too expensive to highly technological interventions in tertiary care neonatal units. If we accept the assumption that "everyone cannot have everything", then decisions about such limitations are inevitable.

The second kind of rationing is even more difficult. There are many interventions that are costly, have a questionable effect on the patient, and may be termed "inadvisable."[76] The intervention that received a great deal of attention in 1990 with the Supreme Court decision in *Cruzan* was the continuation of artificial nutrition and hydration for those in a persistent vegetative state. The testimony in the courts was that the cost of Nancy Cruzan's care was $130,000 per year.[77] This went on for seven years with a cost to the taxpayers of Missouri of $910,000. The prognosis was that Cruzan could have lived another thirty years with an additional cost to the Missouri taxpayers of $3.9 million.

This cost may be a bit high because of the kind of facility in which Cruzan was housed, but using this figure for the sake of consistency, we can apply it to the population of those in a persistent vegetative state. Estimates of the number of patients in that condition range from 15,000 to 25,000.[78] This would mean that the annual cost of maintaining such patients would range from $1.9 billion to $3.2 billion per year.[79] The outcome for these patients is that they continue to respire and metabolize. They have no contact with the external environment, nor do they have inner states of consciousness.[80] Their quality of life would be considered zero on virtually any scale. The costworthiness of such an intervention would be considered highly questionable. Whether any meaningful healthcare reform would allow such patients to continue in these states is not clear. This hard question has not been addressed. Nor has it been answered for many other conditions that have a similar lack of positive outcome for a high level of investment. Savings in the area of rationing could be reallocated to forms of healthcare that will have positive outcomes for the quality of life of patients.

Members of an insurance pool and taxpayers at large will have to decide whether they are willing to pay the premiums for such negative outcomes. When the question is asked informally of individuals, the answer is generally no. Most individuals are willing to bear some measure of burden for others' healthcare. But they are not willing to shoulder the burdens if the healthcare is not costworthy or the outcomes result in no, or severely limited, benefit to patients.

The Patient Self-Determination Act could play a decisive role in reaching some of the goals of healthcare reform. If, as was asserted earlier, the intent of the law is to make patients better informed decision makers by applying the principles of informed consent, patients or their surrogates could refuse treatments that consume healthcare dollars with no benefit or could make more careful decisions about treatments that have very limited benefits. It is impossible to draw decisive conclusions about patients' forgoing treatment as a result of the Patient Self-Determination Act. However, there is evidence that, if physicians explain carefully to patients the nature of certain treatments and their effect, a good number of patients will decide to forgo some kinds of treatment.[81] On a microcosmic level, had the healthcare professionals honored the Cruzans' wishes to withdraw the artificial nutrition and hydration from Nancy when her parents first indicated a desire to do so, the taxpayers of Missouri would have saved $520,000. Had they been given more accurate and complete information from the beginning, they could have saved the taxpayers an additional $325,000. If Nancy had had an advance directive, $845,000 in healthcare expenditures could have been saved.

The Patient Self-Determination Act, then, is one of the tools, but only one, that can actually help healthcare reform achieve one of its major goals of cost containment. Patients and surrogates are frequently, but not always, reasonable. Though they desire to recover health and live longer, many will accept that these outcomes are not possible in their situations. Reflection on the goals of medicine by both patients and professionals may assist in this task.[82] Helping them to understand what they can reasonably hope for, assisting them in clarifying their values, and supporting them in the difficult decisions they have to make are aspects of the reforms that we cannot ignore.

NOTES

1. Schneiderman LJ et al. Effect of offering advance directives on medical treatments and costs. Ann Intern Med 1992; 117:599–606.

2. Marx K, Engels F. The German ideology. New York: International Publishers, 1972, page 47.

3. McLuhan M. Understanding media: The extensions of man. New York: NAL-Dutton, 1966, pages 155–162.

4. Gilder G. Microcosm: The quantum revolution in economics and technology. New York: Simon and Schuster, 1989, pages 262–269.

5. The Hippocratic oath. In Lloyd GER (ed). Hippocratic writings. London: Penguin Books, 1983, page 67.

6. The science of medicine. In Lloyd GER (ed). Hippocratic writings. London: Penguin Books, 1983, page 140.

7. Pellegrino ED, Thomasma DC. A philosophical basis of medical practice: Toward a philosophy and ethic of the healing professions. New York: Oxford University Press, 1981, pages 192–193 and 224–225.

8. Hudson RP. The concept of disease. Ann Intern Med 1966; 65:595–601.

9. Nulan SB. Doctors: The biography of medicine. New York: Alfred A Knopf, 1988, pages 366–368.

10. Porter R. Hospital and surgery. In Porter R. The Cambridge illustrated history of medicine. Cambridge: Cambridge University Press, 1996, pages 244–245.

11. Murray TH. Ethical issues in human genome research. FASEB Journal 1991; 5:55–60.

12. Callahan D. Setting limits: Medical goals in an aging society. New York: Simon and Schuster, 1987, pages 61–65.

13. Kassirer JP. Our stubborn quest for diagnostic certainty. N Engl J Med. 1989; 320:1489–1491.

14. May WF. The physician's covenant: Images of the healer in medical ethics. Philadelphia: Westminster Press, 1983, page 97.

15. Pellegrino ED. Humanism and the physician. Knoxville: University of Tennessee Press, 1979, pages 123–124.

16. Pellegrino ED, Thomasma DC. For the patient's good: The restoration of beneficence in health care. New York: Oxford University Press, 1988, page 116.

17. Lloyd GER (ed). Hippocratic writings. London: Penguin Books, 1983, page 9. Some might argue that the Hippocratic characterization of the physician-patient relationship is outdated. In the era of managed care and HMOs it is often considered a mere museum piece that can at best be romanticized in the contemporary practice of medicine. Quite the contrary may be the case. The fiduciary nature of the relationship depends on the character of the physician and the manner in which he or she practices medicine. See Drane JF. Becoming a good doctor. Kansas City, MO: Sheed

& Ward, 1988, pages 23–28 and 89–90. Even in a healthcare environment in which the contact between a physician and a patient may be brief and sporadic, as often happens with specialty practices and HMOs, the attitude of care and focused attention to patients' needs and wishes can still be present. A patient does not have to be cared for by a physician over a long period of time for the patient to realize that the physician is truly functioning as a patient advocate in every sense of that role. And a physician does not have to spend hours with the patient to communicate concern and provide help for the patient to participate in sound decision making. Even in a busy HMO, practice patterns can be designed to reaffirm the Hippocratic view of the physician-patient relationship if the physician and organization are willing to make the effort to do so.

18. American College of Physicians. Ethics manual. 1st edition. Philadelphia: American College of Physicians, 1984, page 13.

19. Thomasma DC, Graber GC. Euthanasia: Toward an ethical social policy. New York: Continuum Publishing Co., 1990, page 3.

20. Engelhardt HT. Bioethics and secular humanism: The search for a common morality. London: SCM Press, 1991, page 39.

21. President's Commission for the Study of Ethical Problems in Medicine and Biomedical and Behavioral Research. Making health care decisions: The ethical and legal implications of informed consent in the patient-practitioner relationship. Washington, D.C.: U.S. Government Printing Office, 1982, page 51.

22. Layde PM et al. Surrogates' predictions of seriously ill patients' resuscitation preferences. Arch Fam Med 1995; 4:518–524.

23. The term "value life" is used to capture the notion of human life as a narrative (see MacIntyre A. After virtue. Notre Dame, IN: University of Notre Dame Press, 1981, pages 202–203) or history that can be explored on many levels. There can be a comprehensive notion of this narrative by recounting the experience of the individual in its most general sense. Or the examination can focus on the actions of the individual giving rise to a virtue narrative of the person. Since human action is permeated with motivating values, whether consciously or unconsciously, it becomes possible to talk about the value life of the individual as the evolving narrative that unfolds as individuals live out their lives and make their decisions based upon what they consider most important to them. The notion of a value life assumes particular importance when talking about advance directives. For the ideal advance directive would be one that reflects the value life of the individual as it has evolved from past experience and as it anticipates future matters of importance.

24. Moral friends are those who share common values and commitments

and respect each other as mutual participants in a moral community. Moral strangers, on the other hand, do not share in the same moral community but may still respect and trust each other across the boundaries that separate them. The trust between moral friends may be easier to achieve than that between moral strangers, but it is nonetheless important in both cases. See Engelhardt HT. The physician-patient relationship in a secular, pluralist society. In Shelp EE (ed). The clinical encounter: The moral fabric of the patient-physician relationship. Dordrecht: D. Reidel Publishing Co., 1983, pages 253–266.

25. President's Commission for the Study of Ethical Problems in Medicine and Biomedical and Behavioral Research. Making health care decisions: The ethical and legal implications of informed consent in the patient-practitioner relationship. Washington, D.C.: U.S. Government Printing Office, 1982, pages 50–51.

26. Ibid., page 62.

27. American College of Physicians. Ethics manual. 1st edition. Philadelphia: American College of Physicians, 1984, pages 7–8.

28. The goals of medicine have recently (1996) been restudied by the international study sponsored by the Hastings Center. (See note 82 in this chapter.)

29. Traditionally family relationships placed wives and children in the "subordinate" role relative to husbands and fathers. Though many Western societies have moved beyond placing wives and mature children in these roles, it is still considered acceptable to maintain immature children as legitimate objects for parentalistic interventions. There is much disagreement about when children move from one social role to the other. In the situation where expert knowledge gives one parentalistic privilege, there is even greater disagreement. How much knowledge, and of what kind, one must have to be free from parentalistic intervention cannot be clearly defined.

Parentalism can take three forms. Parentalistic interventions occur when one overrides the decision of another whose decision-making capabilities are permanently compromised or temporarily underdeveloped. This occurs in many cases of mental retardation, advanced dementia (which frequently occurs in the aging process), and young children, who lack the perspective required for sound decisions. In these cases, the party who is the object of the intervention lacks the fundamental characteristics of being autonomous.

A second form of parentalism is found when the intervention occurs because it is questionable whether the object of the intervention is capable of making decisions about the matter in question. This situation may be found in some cases of mental disorders or when there is suspicion that the individual lacks some key information to make a decision. These interventions are temporary, and they end when it becomes clear that the individual is truly capable of making the decision about the situation.

The final form of parentalism occurs when there is interference with an individual who fulfills the conditions used to describe an autonomous person (see chapter 9). This would occur when one adult intervenes in and overrides the decision of another adult merely because she believes that she is in a better position to judge what is in the other's best interest. This becomes the exercise of power that arbitrarily places the other in a "subordinate" position. This last form of parentalism is the only one that is discouraged by various ethical codes governing physicians. See, for example, Council on Ethical and Judicial Affairs, AMA. Code of medical ethics; current opinions with annotations. Chicago, IL: American Medical Association, 1996, Opinion 8.08.

30. Pellegrino ED, Thomasma DC. A philosophical basis of medical practice: Toward a philosophy and ethic of the healing professions. New York: Oxford University Press, 1981, pages 200–201.

31. American College of Physicians. Ethics manual. 3d edition. Philadelphia: American College of Physicians, 1993, page 8.

32. President's Commission for the Study of Ethical Problems in Medicine and Biomedical and Behavioral Research. Making health care decisions: The ethical and legal implications of informed consent in the patient-practitioner relationship. Washington, D.C.: U.S. Government Printing Office, 1982, page 61. See also American College of Physicians. Ethics manual. 3d edition. Philadelphia: American College of Physicians, 1993, page 8.

33. Greenberg DF. Interference with a suicide attempt. New York University Law Review 1974; 49:227–269.

34. American College of Physicians. Ethics manual. 3d edition. Philadelphia: American College of Physicians, 1993, page 8.

35. Ramsey P. The patient as person. New Haven, CT: Yale University Press, 1970, page 116.

36. Council on Ethical and Judicial Affairs, AMA. Code of medical ethics; current opinions with annotations. Chicago, IL: American Medical Association, 1996, Opinion 8.08.

37. Frank JD. Galloping technology: a new social disease. Journal of Social Issues 1983; 22:1–14.

38. Marx L. Does improved technology mean progress? Technology Review 1987; 71:33–41.

39. Gendron B. Technology and the human condition. New York: St. Martin's Press, 1977, pages 149–156. An excellent application of the problems generated by the technological imperative in the clinical setting can be found in David Eddy's accounts of the end-of-life decisions faced by his

parents. Eddy DM. Cost-effective analysis: A conversation with my father. JAMA 1992; 267:1669–1672, 1674–1675, and Eddy DM. A conversation with my mother. JAMA 1994; 272:179–181.

40. Bazelon DL. Governing technology: Values, choices, and scientific progress. Technology in Society 1983; 5:15–25.

41. Schumacher EF. Small is beautiful: Economics as if people mattered. New York: Harper and Row, 1973, 53–62.

42. Westrum R. Technologies and society: The shaping of people and things. Belmont CA: Wadsworth Publishing Co., 1991.

43. Florman SC. Blaming technology. New York: St. Martin's Press, 1981, pages 90–93.

44. Hellerstein D. Overdosing on medical technology. Technology Review 1983; August–September, pages 13–17.

45. This occurs in spite of the fact that the AMA clearly stated in 1980 that CPR was appropriate only in cases of "sudden and unexpected" death. See Council on Ethical and Judicial Affairs, AMA. Standards and guidelines for cardiopulmonary resuscitation (CPR) and emergency cardiac care (ECC). JAMA 1980; 244:453–509.

46. Personal decision making was brought into focus with the work of the President's Commission for the Study of Ethical Problems in Medicine and Biomedical and Behavioral Research in two of its most significant volumes, Making health care decisions: The ethical and legal implications of informed consent in the patient-practitioner relationship (Washington, D.C.: US Government Printing Office, 1982), and Deciding to forego life-sustaining treatment: Ethical, medical, and legal issues in treatment decisions (Washington, D.C.: US Government Printing Office, 1983). The work of the commission in this matter took into account the expert opinion at the time and the bioethical reflections of the previous decade. Furthermore, it set the course for patient participation in clinical decisions in the following years.

47. American College of Physicians. Ethics manual. 1st edition. Philadelphia: American College of Physicians, 1984, page 7.

48. This number is up from 340,000 in 1994 and 275,000 in 1993. One can easily see the growth in the movement from high-tech medical interventions. These figures were supplied by the National Hospice Organization in response to a telephone inquiry, September 11, 1996.

49. Hanson LC, Rodman E. The use of living wills at the end of life. Arch Intern Med 1996; 156:1018–1022.

50. A recent study sought to investigate the issue of quality of life vs. length of life in the advanced elderly. "On average, patients indicated a fairly strong 'will to live': 40.8 percent were unwilling to exchange any time in their current state of health for a shorter life in excellent health" (page 374). It

would seem, then, that advanced elderly patients would prefer a longer life, even though compromised, rather than refuse treatment when the quality of their health began to deteriorate. This study also confirmed previous studies cited elsewhere in this text (see note 22, above) that indicate a minimal correlation between what surrogates believe to be the preferences of the patient and what the patient himself would wish. See Tsevat J et al. Health values of hospitalized patients 80 years or older. JAMA 1998; 279:371–375.

51. Blues AG, Zerwekh JV. Hospice and palliative nursing care. New York: Grune & Stratton, 1984, pages 29–43.

52. Courts, legislators, and religious groups have all addressed these issues in various ways. The Bouvia case in California (Bouvia v. Superior Court (Glenchur), 179 Cal. App. 3d 1127, 225 Cal. Rptr. 297 (1986)) provided one of the most explicit indications that the refusal of life-sustaining treatments is not suicide. Advance directive legislation in most states explicity defines the refusal of treatments as neither suicide nor homicide. (See Choice in dying. Refusal of treatment legislation. New York: Choice in Dying, 1996, Introduction, page 2.) The latter is underscored by the legal protection given to physicians who honor advance directives. The Roman Catholic Church explicitly states in its Declaration on Euthanasia (Vatican City, 1980), "Such refusal [of treatments that are excessively burdensome without accompanying reasonable benefit] is not the equivalent of suicide; on the contrary, it should be considered as an acceptance of the human condition." Quoted in President's Commission for the Study of Ethical Problems in Medicine and Biomedical and Behavioral Research. Deciding to forego life-sustaining treatment: Ethical and legal issues in treatment decisions. Washington, D.C.: US Government Printing Office, 1983, page 306.

53. Beauchamp TL (ed). Intending death: The ethics of assisted suicide and euthanasia. Upper Saddle River, NJ: Prentice Hall, 1996, pages 5–9.

54. Thomas D. Do not go gentle into that good night. The collected poems of Dylan Thomas. New York: New Directions Books, 1957, page 128.

55. Engelhardt HT. Tractatus bene moriendi vivendique: Choosing styles of living and dying. In Abernathy V (ed). Frontiers in medical ethics: Applications in a medical setting. Cambridge, MA: Ballinger Co. 1980, page 9.

56. Engelhardt HT. Suffering, meaning, and bioethics. Christian Bioethics. 1996; 2:129–153.

57. This issue will be examined in greater detail in chapter 6, where the *demands* for treatment are contrasted with the *refusals* of treatment.

58. The Patient Self-Determination Act does not automatically lead to patients' refusing treatments. The limited use of advance directives and the frequent reluctance of patients and surrogates to forego life-sustaining treatments indicate that patients and surrogates still have an overwhelming ten-

dency to elect treatment, even futile treatment, when faced with healthcare decisions at the end of life. See Tsevat J et al. Health values of hospitalized patients 80 years or older. JAMA 1998; 279:371–375. However, the Patient Self-Determination Act does open the possibility of bringing the option of treatment refusals to the conscious awareness of patients and surrogates. It also provides an incentive for healthcare professionals to develop strategies for helping patients and their surrogates to examine carefully the option of forgoing treatments, which, until recent years, was seldom entertained.

59. Estimates are that 37 million Americans are currently uninsured and a similar number are underinsured. Emanuel EJ, Dubler NN. Preserving the physician-patient relationship in the era of managed care. JAMA 1995; 273:323–329.

60. Engelhardt HT. The foundations of bioethics. 2d edition. New York, Oxford University Press, 1996, pages 381–382.

61. Schieber GJ, Poullier JP, Greenwald LM. Health spending, delivery, and outcomes in OECD countries. Health Affairs. 1993; 12:120–129.

62. Chambers CV et al. Relationship of advance directives to hospital charges in a Medicare population. Arch Intern Med 1994; 154:541–547.

63. Vaccinations are a simple example. Many other forms of preventive medicine and education, while adding to overall healthcare costs, often produce substantial savings by reducing or eliminating serious syndromes before they require more extensive (and substantially more costly) interventions (e.g., medications that address cardiovascular disease).

64. Rescher N. Distributive justice. New York: Bobbs-Merrill Company Inc., 1966, pages 81–83.

65. Allowing the free market alone to regulate the distribution of healthcare would leave many of the most poor and vulnerable in the population unserved or underserved. For many who aspire to moral ideals grounded in a concept of human dignity, such a situation would be intolerable. See The National Conference of Catholic Bishops. Ethical and religious directives for Catholic health care services, 1995, directive 3.

66. President's Commission for the Study of Ethical Problems in Medicine and Biomedical and Behavioral Research. Securing access to health care: The ethical implications of differences in availability of health services. Washington, D.C.: US Government Printing Office, 1983, pages 32–35.

67. One strongly held view is that only some forms of managed care will be able to achieve this goal. See e.g., Kassier JP. Managed care and the morality of the market place. N Engl J Med 1995; 333:50–52. Others hold the opposite opinion—that managed care will ultimately fail in accomplishing this goal. See, e.g., Rodwin MA. Conflicts in managed care. N Engl J Med 1995; 332:604–607.

74   The Patient Self-Determination Act

68. Kassirer JP. Our stubborn quest for diagnostic certainty. N Engl J Med 1989; 320:1489–1491.

69. Council on Ethical and Judicial Affairs. American Medical Association. Guidelines for the appropriate use of do-not-resuscitate orders. JAMA 1991; 265:1868–1871. See also Grant ER. Medical futility: Legal and ethical aspects. Law Med Health Care 1992; 20:330–335.

70. Schneiderman LJ et al. Medical futility: Its meaning and ethical implications. Ann Inter Med 1990; 112:949–954. See also Truog RD et al. The problem of futility. N Engl J Med 1992; 326:1560–1564, and Younger SJ. Who defines futility? JAMA 1988; 260:2094–2095.

71. Callahan D. Setting limits: Medical goals in an aging society. New York: Simon and Schuster, 1987, pages 119–120.

72. A recent study indicates that if futile treatment (called "potentially ineffective care") were forgone for critically ill Medicare patients (a fairly restrictive population), there would be an annual savings of $48 million in California alone. The study suggests that the key to this savings is a more refined use of clinical judgment, which will lead to clearer determinations of futility. Cher DJ, Lenert LA. Method of Medicare reimbursement and the rate of potentially ineffective care of critically ill patients. JAMA 1997; 278:1001–1007.

73. The Patient Self-Determination Act's stipulation that patients and authorized surrogates should be given information about their right to *consent* to treatment is probably moot in this situation.

74. Engelhardt HT, Rie MA. Intensive care units, scarce resources, and conflicting principles of justice. JAMA 1986; 255:1159–1164.

75. Managed care contracts already engage extensively in this practice. See Loewy EH. Guidelines, managed care, and ethics. Arch Intern Med 1996; 156:2038–2040. Managed care groups never say that an intervention may not be done. They only say that they will not pay for it if it falls outside their practice guidelines. See Berger JT, Rosner F. The ethics of practice guidelines. Arch Intern Med 1996; 156:2051–2056.

76. "Inadvisable" treatments are those that are highly unlikely to produce a beneficial outcome for the patient, may be detrimental to the patient's quality of life, or may not meet a patient's or authorized surrogate's reasonable goals. See Ethics Committee of the Society of Critical Care Medicine. Consensus statement of the society of critical care medicine's ethics committee regarding futile and other possibly inadvisable treatments. Crit Care Med 1997; 25:887–891.

77. Cruzan, By Cruzan V. Harmon. 760 S.W.2d 408 (Mo. en banc 1988).

78. Payne K. Physicians' attitudes about the care of patients in the persistent vegetative state: A national survey. Ann Intern Med 1996; 125:104–110.

79. These figures are inflated as a result of the high cost of Cruzan's care in a rehabilitation facility. Had she been cared for in an ordinary extended care facility, the cost of her care would have been substantially reduced (perhaps by as much as 60%). This financial situation will be revisited in chapter 5, note 40.

80. American Academy of Neurology. Position of the American Academy of Neurology on certain aspects of the care and management of the persistent vegetative state patient. Neurology 1988; 39:125–126. See also The Multi-Society Task Force on PVS. Medical aspects of the persistent vegetative state. N Engl J Med 1994; 330:1499–1508, 1572–1579.

81. Murphy DJ et al. The influence of the probability of survival on patients' preferences regarding cadiopulmonary resuscitation. N Engl J Med 1994; 330:545–549. The large majority of elderly patients in this study elected CPR when initially interviewed. After the interview the nature of CPR and the probabilities of survival for those in their age group was carefully explained to them by physicians. After the explanation, the number of those electing DNR status doubled. This indicates that there is a good chance that the Patient Self-Determination Act, if properly implemented with appropriate explanations, could result in some patients' making healthcare decisions with greater restraint. It is, of course, too early to tell just how many patients would take this direction in making such decisions. It may be that many patients would just want very aggressive treatment, no matter the conse-quences. Or it may be that information transfer between patient and caregiver is very inefficient or that less than complete information is still being given to patients who elect highly aggressive treatments.

82. International Project of Hastings Center. The goals of medicine: Setting new priorities. Hast Cent Rep Nov.–Dec. 1996 (Special Supplement); 26:S9–S14. This international study has most recently identified the goals of medicine as: "(1) the prevention of disease and injury and the promotion and maintenance of health; (2) the relief of pain and suffering caused by maladies; (3) the care and cure of those with a malady and the care of those who cannot be cured; (4) the avoidance of premature death and the pursuit of a peaceful death." Among other things that this report counsels regarding the applica-tion of medical interventions is that medicine should be temperate, prudent, just, and equitable. And, very significantly, it should be respectful of human choice and dignity.

4

The Human Context of the Patient Self-Determination Act

Though the social and technological backdrop for the Patient Self-Determination Act is significant for understanding the law, there is a much richer context that must be explored if we are to appreciate the profound issues that the law brings into focus. Patients are the focal point of the law insofar as they confront the essential elements of their humanity. As individuals attempt to carve out their roles in society, they often, and easily, lose sight of the features that define their humanity. The distractions and possibilities that technology presents to us often direct our attention away from the appreciation of our fundamental human realities. We focus instead on the ephemeral and superficial features in our daily lives.[1] It was this tendency that Henry David Thoreau decried in *Walden*. And it was the importance of redirecting his attention to essential human matters that led him to leave Concord for two years and take up residency at Walden Pond. In his words, he did it because "I wished to live deliberately, to front only the essential facts of life, and see if I could not learn what it had to teach, and not, when I came to die, discover that I had not lived."[2]

To reflect upon the fundamental features of our humanity is an essential part of being human. To neglect this reflective process is to lose the ground for all that we are and do.[3] The Patient Self-Determination Act provides the opportunity for patients and caregivers alike to reflect upon the basic elements of the human context. The implementation of the law can provide the impetus for a dialogue between patients and caregivers that will allow patients to make end-of-life decisions with some measure of confidence. At the same time, it can encourage caregivers to assist in those decisions with a minimum of discomfort and even tranquility.

The Recognition of Human Finitude

When we reflect upon our basic humanity, one of the areas that captures our imagination is the power we possess. This is all the more striking as we consider the extraordinary technological achievements we enjoy every day.[4] This ongoing ability to conquer our limitations both captivates and deceives us. For we frequently come face to face with our limitations in spite of our unwillingness to do so. At these times we learn, sometimes dramatically, that "part of the quality of human life, and part of its suffering is the attempt to overcome transcendence of fragmentation while forever remaining confined to it."[5] The ability to recognize the finitude—the boundaries of our human existence—and to integrate its significance into our decisions and actions is the beginning of wisdom and the condition for conducting ourselves in a truly human fashion.[6]

The first and most important feature of our finitude is the reality of our *death*. Martin Heidegger asserts that one of the most distinctive features of human existence is that we are beings-toward-death.[7] He claims that the inauthentic person is one who fails to recognize that death is a reality for her. This individual acknowledges that death is something that happens to others, including relatives and friends. But it is not something that she herself faces. The authentic person, on the other hand, is the one who realizes that death is a real possibility for her and lives her life, and makes decisions, accordingly.[8] The authentic person does not push death off as some shadowy possibility. Nor does she see death as an alien event, something that violates our fundamental reality. Rather, she sees death as a reality that is always there and something that completes our being rather than fragmenting it.[9]

Heidegger's approach, while grounded in an existentialist framework that is not avowedly religious, mirrors many religious traditions. In the religious approach, the reality of death is the result of divine authorship,[10] or perhaps a part of a pantheistic reality. In more naturalistic approaches to religion, death is simply one of the many ways in which human beings are integrated into the whole,[11] a way of maintaining a natural balance that sees reality as larger than an individual's egocentric interests. In these orientations one does not rush toward death but accepts it as a genuine part of one's reality.

These Heideggerian or religious approaches to death are not purely fatalistic. They do not require, nor do they promote, an attitude suggesting that one simply "gives up" when faced with death. There is an appropriate level of resistance to death.[12] Resistance does not, nor should it, deny inevitability. There is a prudential balance required between resistance to death and its acceptance.[13] Each individual will design this balance in a different way. No one way will suit everyone. H. Tristram Engelhardt, Jr. has suggested that, just as there are a variety of lifestyles, there are a variety of deathstyles.[14] There is considerable acceptance in our society for variations in lifestyles. Individuals choose a wide variety of occupations, places to live, priorities in spending their incomes, etc. In a democratic and pluralistic society the virtue of tolerance is the major virtue governing the attitudes toward these variations.[15] Analogously, Engelhardt argues, there ought to be tolerance for a wide variety of deathstyles. Individuals ought to be able to choose to some degree where they will die, whether they will die alone or with someone else, whether they will die in pain or free from it, etc.

The permeating presence of technology in our society introduces a new dimension to the deathstyle issue. Prior to the development of sophisticated medical technology there were basically three choices. (1) One could simply choose to die with no resistance whatsoever. (2) One could choose to resist with the rather undeveloped medical means available, which sometimes worked if the disease was not too severe and the patient's constitution was particularly robust. (3) One could choose to die at one's own hand, "when fortune began to play false with him."[16] Advanced medical technology has vastly enlarged the choices of a deathstyle.

Now one can *decide* the time and manner of one's dying even though one cannot decide whether or not one will die.[17] The latter choice is not granted to us within the context of our finitude. But in terms of time and manner one can decide on a great many deathstyles—for example, at home, in a hospital, in a hospice, or perhaps in one's favorite wooded area. One can decide whether to die in pain (perhaps for some religious reasons), with decently managed pain, or totally free from pain even though this might compromise the ability for conscious interactions or risk an earlier death.[18] One can decide whether to die on a ventilator or not, with CPR or without it, and with or without a whole armamentarium of healthcare interventions. One can decide whether a huge sum of money or a relatively modest sum will be spent on the extension of one's life.

The reflective patient begins with a fundamental acknowledgment of the finitude of her existence by the acceptance of the inevitability of her death. Thus, death is seen as an integral part of the life process.[19] There is a natural process that leads us from birth, through life, toward death. For many individuals there comes a point at which they embark upon a line of causality leading to death.[20] In medical practice this process is called a "terminal condition." A terminal condition is one in which the patient, through either disease or injury, is experiencing a key system or multiple system failure, the failure being part of an irreversible process of deterioration. Death is an inevitable and predictable outcome of this process regardless of whether it will occur in a short period of time or over an extended period.[21]

The choices that one makes within this context of a terminal condition constitute the choices about one's deathstyle. One may decide simply to yield to the natural process and accept death without resistance, or one can accept death and utilize pain medications to make the passage easier even though the medication might shorten the passage.[22] One may choose the maximum level of therapeutic interventions—the Dylan Thomas poetic approach ("Do not go gentle into that good night/Rage, rage against the dying of the light").[23] Finally, one may choose interventions for a period of time and then selectively withdraw them when they no longer meet the patient's goals. Pain medications may be interwoven with other therapeutic interventions to suit the patient's goals for a "good" death.

In each of these alternatives, death occurs inevitably and predictably. The only thing that changes is the time and manner of the patient's dying; for example, the alternative of maximum therapeutic interventions may result in the patient's death at a later time than simply allowing nature to take its course from the outset. To make choices about these alternatives in the process of dying is to assert both the finitude of the human condition and the liberty that individuals enjoy in a democratic society.[24]

But death is not the only limitation that human beings face. What follows is a brief exploration of some additional limiting factors.

An attempt is made below to identify the central features of our human finitude and examine how these features function within the boundaries of our lives. The characteristics explored are disease and injury, decision making, uncertainties, risk taking, helplessness, curiosity, misfortunes, incompleteness, aging, and limitations on resources. They define the landscape of our human existence, and within these boundaries, we must develop appropriate strategies to conduct our lives in a way that will help us to manage them creatively. Many of these strategies will be self-initiated. Other possibilities will be presented by social institutions. Among the latter may be the Patient Self-Determination Act.

The fact that we are all susceptible to *disease* and *injury* is a key element of our condition. One of the many forms that self-determination takes in our lives is the right to refuse treatment even in nonterminal situations. We saw earlier that the right of adults with decisional capacity, and those without decisional capacity speaking through authorized surrogates, to refuse treatment is guaranteed by the Constitution and interpreted by most courts as virtually absolute.[25] Caregivers do not have to agree with the reasonableness of the refusal of treatment. Patients can refuse even on the basis of a whim.

In addition to the boundary condition of death, human existence is fraught with *uncertainties*. This is true in all facets of life but is seldom more dramatically encountered than in the practice of medicine.[26] Medicine is an art and not a science.[27] One can never be completely sure how the practice of the healing arts will carry through in an individual case. For this reason medicine could be characterized as the assessment and management of probabilities. Patients, families, and healthcare professionals alike are continually called upon to make decisions in the face of probabilities rather than certainties. In order to weigh probabilities effectively in healthcare decisions, the development and articulation of the patient's value context is essential. This value context provides the framework for determining the weight to be given to the various factors of uncertainty.

One of the characteristics of human finitude upon we seldom reflect is that human beings are called upon to make *moral decisions,* ascribe reasons for them, and accept the risks inherent in those decisions.[28] Many times we make decisions as a matter of course without realizing that they have a distinctive moral character. Many decisions are considered simply automatic even when they have serious consequences. However, when we are faced with particularly difficult decisions, we pause more than usual before the decision is made. Unfortunately, the positive and negative results of a decision are frequently weighed in a relatively cursory fashion. Rarely do we reflect in detail upon the value framework we have established for ourselves that will allow us to make wise decisions. And yet being aware of our value framework is the most important step in the process of reflectively making our decisions. Making choices is a necessary component for the human situation. And making those choices within a value framework is an inevitable accompaniment, whether or not we are clear about the values underlying our choices.

Refusing treatment, regardless of whether one is in a terminal condition, is a serious decision and one that should not be made automatically. In the struggle to make this decision, patients are made aware of the role of making moral decisions as part of their human condition. They need to think clearly about such decisions and the values framing them. Decisions by surrogates on behalf of patients must be approached in a similarly reflective manner.

Unfortunately, patients are often ill equipped to identify, formulate, and reconsider values upon which they have acted up to the time when they are called upon to make these serious healthcare decisions. Circumstances of daily living do not often encourage reflective behavior and choices. For this reason patients will often need assistance in exploring the decision-making dimension of their finitude. If this occurs, it is frequently done with the help of family or friends, but family and friends are often so deeply affected by the impending decision that they find it difficult to engage in discussions with the patient about these serious matters.

Healthcare professionals are in an ideal position to assist patients in this regard. In providing this assistance it will be helpful if healthcare providers spend some time reflecting on their own finitude and the significant ways in which they have experienced it. By developing the skills required to reflect on their own personal values, individuals have an added advantage in attempting to help others who must engage in the same activity.

As a final consideration in this dimension of finitude regarding making moral decisions, it is necessary to consider the *taking of risks*. The ability to assume risks in our decision making is an important human characteristic. We may weigh the risks inherent in various courses of action and decide on the action that will have the least risk or the action that will yield the greatest good in spite of a high risk factor. Sometimes we run the risk that things will not turn out in the way we anticipate, and even that the eventual outcome might be devastating. All of these possibilities are present in every decision, and our best course may simply be to calculate the probabilities and deal with what happens. These are the decisional struggles that every patient faces, and they become more magnified as the uncertainties and complexities of the clinical setting increase.

There is a strong tendency in those who love another or who accept professional responsibility for the care of another to want to minimize the risks that the other will have to face. This is particularly true with patients who are already rendered seriously vulnerable by disease or injury and who seem to be in need of special protection. When such patients refuse treatment at some risk to themselves, the tendency to override their decisions is intensified.[29] This proclivity for parentalistic interventions has governed healthcare situations as managed both by families and by healthcare professionals all the way back to the dim origins of these relationships.[30] There is little doubt that this disposition is generally benevolent and often can have positive outcomes *if* the patient agrees that it is appropriate in a given situation. However, if parentalistic interventions rob patients of their proper decision-making authority, then they count as a serious assault on the moral decision-making dimension of their finitude, since they are no longer able to participate in decisions that are significant for them and to assume the risks that accompany moral decisions. The result is that patient dignity is seriously undermined.

The right to consent to or to refuse treatment as identified in the Patient Self-Determination Act or the drafting of an advance directive must be taken seriously lest this very important dimension—the assumption of risks—be compromised. Though it is difficult to watch someone assume risks that the observer may determine to be detrimental to that person's well-being, this action is an important element in maintaining the individual's autonomy. Part of the richness of human life is the moral authority to make decisions involving these risks, even if they may be life-threatening.[31]

Another of the dimensions of human finitude that we all experience but are seldom willing to admit is that of *helplessness*. This dimension is often masked by the power we seem to be able to exercise over the conditions in which we live. The mask becomes a part of our daily lives. We seem to be more and more in control when we exercise our decisions to utilize technology. Even the technological imperative contributes to this perception of control because defaulting to the technology *seems* to give us control when, in point of fact, we have very little or none at all. The only control we really have is that manifested in a *conscious* choice regarding the use of the technology. In spite of the mask, overpowering circumstances sometimes cause us to feel helpless.

Often this sense of helplessness is countered by consulting someone who has a particular expertise in our area of vulnerability. For legal problems we go to a lawyer; for spiritual problems we go to a priest, minister, or rabbi; for healthcare problems we go to a physician. Because interventions are so varied in contemporary healthcare and patients' choices of lifestyles are equally multiple, patients now need to explore their values and goals, identify and articulate them, and formulate a plan to achieve them. That plan may involve the discriminating selection of some treatments, the refusal of certain or all approaches to treatment, or the drafting or signing of an advance directive. These many options may introduce decisional gridlock into the experience of patients.[32] This new dimension of vulnerability may require special assistance for patients so that they can achieve the appropriate level of clarity about their values and goals in the face of their healthcare options. Providing this assistance acknowledges this dimension of our finitude and empowers patients to deal contructively with it by reflectively taking command of the direction of their treatment.

One of the most significant dimensions of our lives is our *curiosity* and our tendency to demand explanations for events, especially those with undesirable consequences. This facet of our humanity particularly raises its head when we face the misfortunes of disease or injury. We so often ask why.[33] "Why did this happen to me?" "Why did this happen to me now?" In many ways disease and injury masquerade as unfair events in our lives.[34] We often think that nature should provide for us a fabric of beneficent results and, if it does not, there should be a way to correct the misfortunes we experience. If we cannot correct the misfortunes, we deem ourselves to be treated unfairly in the extreme.

The fact is that *misfortunes* run rampant in our lives and the random forces of nature often touch us in this way. To be sure, there are ways in which we can prevent disease or injury, and if we do not act in preventive ways, we may succumb to them. Thus sometimes the patient is a causal agent rather than a victim of a misfortune. Falling into this category would be situations like heavy smoking, excessive drinking, leading a stressful life, overeating, and choosing a dangerous occupation. But there are many times when none of these explanations fit and the purely natural factors in the etiology of a disease cannot be avoided. Nature's randomness produces a misfortune and, many times, one that cannot be corrected. Our lives are seldom tidy and are often quite messy affairs.

Along with the misfortunes that we find so distasteful is the *incompleteness* we experience in our lives. Human beings have a strong desire to complete the projects they start. The unfortunate fact is, however, that we can never complete all our projects despite our best hopes and intentions. We will never live to see the last weed pulled from our garden. We may never heal all the fractures in our human relationships. To attempt to extend the process of our dying until all our projects are finished stems from the illusion that they will indeed be completed. Reflection on this feature of incompleteness serves to remind us that if we really do want a measure of completeness in our lives, we should work for it while we still have the energy and health to do so.

The only alternative to experiencing the process of *aging* as an essential feature of human finitude is an early death. Since more and more individuals are living longer in our society, aging is becoming a dimension of finitude that demands ever more serious attention. Decline in ability and functioning is an inevitable accompaniment of aging and requires continual readjustments in our expectations about ourselves. Even though healthcare technologies have been able to extend the process of aging substantially and thereby multiply the varieties of deathstyles, the final outcome is certain. Prolonging the process of aging and its accompanying decline may not always be desirable. The values of the patient and the right to self-determination have an important role to play in the extension of the process of aging.

One dimension of our finitude that we are often reluctant to discuss is the *limitation of resources* available to us in the conduct of our lives. Although in a global and abstract way everyone understands that resources are not without end, we frequently behave as though they are infinite in particular instances. For example, the consumption of petroleum and its products occurs without restraint in our society. The use of wood and paper products occurs in the same way. Similarly, we often live with the illusion that healthcare resources in terms of dollars expended, personnel utilized, and technologies developed know no boundaries.

This attitude may have been appropriate two generations ago when the costs of healthcare were still fairly moderate and could be absorbed into most personal and public budgets. However, the development of advanced and highly sophisticated technologies, specialized skills, and multiplying bureaucracies together with an extended life span and a larger population for employing them, has brought into focus the great limitations on resources that are an inevitable part of our human condition.

Just as most individuals cannot afford everything in other facets of their lives, so also there may be limits to what can be afforded in many forms of healthcare. Even if the burden of cost is spread widely over a broad population, there will be limits to what we can spend or what we are willing to spend on healthcare interventions.[35] Healthcare is not the only good that society has an interest in maintaining. Other goods may be just as important as, or even more important than, advanced and highly costly levels of healthcare. And in order to realize those other goods, we will have to act with restraint when it comes to healthcare.[36] Just as other goods, such as education, are not so significant that they may lay claim to unending resources, so also healthcare will have its limits.

At this point two facets of human finitude intersect. On the one hand, the limitation on resources must be acknowledged, and on the other hand, the need to make moral decisions and experience their accompanying risks is ever present. There is no escape from the limitations on our resources in healthcare. There is only left for us the process of identifying where those limits are to be drawn.[37]

The Patient Self-Determination Act provides the occasion for individuals to address many of the issues raised by their finitude as they face choices in healthcare. In order to make self-determining decisions that take the form of treatment consents, refusals, or advance directives when faced with death, disease, uncertainties, risks, etc., individuals must be aware of their values and priorities. That is, they must develop the power of reflection as it relates to their sense of self and the goals they wish to pursue in their lives. Careful attention to the Patient Self-Determination Act can help patients consider and select the time and manner of their death and the strategies to cope with the dying process. It provides a context for understanding the role of disease and injury in patients' lives, particularly when these factors eventuate in death. It can provide perspective on weighing uncertainties and risks as healthcare decisions are being considered. Finally, the Patient Self-Determination Act can help patients realize that they must face limitations in the resources available to them.

But for many patients the awareness that the Patient Self-Determination Act can generate is difficult to attain. They may require assistance in considering their finitude and the place of their values and goals within the context of their limitations. Caregivers can provide the help patients need in understanding their situations and adjusting their values and goals to the healthcare realities they face. Information realistically presented is one important part of this exercise. Equally important is the assistance needed to process the information within the patient's particular circumstances.[38] Providing patients with the assistance and opportunity to consider their healthcare options carefully within the context of their values and goals will be an important strategy for coping with their finitude.

In order for caregivers to be effective in providing this assistance to patients, however, they may have to come to terms with *their own* finitude. They must consider how all the factors that have been identified affect their own lives. Once they have gone through this process of self-reflection they are in a better position to empathically and compassionately help others.

The Assertion of Personal Dignity

Identifying the elements of human finitude tells only part of the story about the human context of the Patient Self-Determination Act. These features can be generalized to all human beings and may be considered abstract and somewhat distant from the particular situation in which individual patients find themselves. But there is another dimension to being a patient, and therefore a citizen of the human context of healthcare, that must be taken into account in the clinical situation: the notion of dignity and its importance in one's life.[39] This notion is multifaceted and constructed of a variety of elements that cannot be ignored if patients are to flourish.

Virtually all codes of ethics that address the care of patients in the clinical setting declare that the dignity of patients must be respected, affirmed, supported, or promoted.[40] However, these codes fail to specify exactly what patient dignity means. Furthermore, few offer detailed instructions on how this dignity is to be nurtured in the clinical setting other than by seeking the "well-being" of patients through a series of specific actions. The presumption seems to be that "respecting dignity" would mean the same thing for each patient. When ethical directives are given, the direct relationship between the directive and patient dignity is seldom articulated. The Patient Self-Determination Act offers us the opportunity to reflect upon the meaning of patient dignity and the many ways in which the spirit of the law can contribute to fostering it.[41]

The word "dignity" comes from the Latin "dignus," meaning "worthy." Thus, to have dignity means to have worth or value. But it carries the connotation of having value of a special sort. When one has dignity, one has worth or value that flows from an inner source. It is not given from the outside but rather is intrinsic to the bearer of dignity. Thus, a painting may have value but it does not have dignity. The value is placed upon it by the members of the artistic community in light of the skill of the artist and the aesthetic priorities of the community. The value does not derive from the painting itself. Persons, on the other hand, can be said to possess dignity as an inner source of worth. If this were not the case, they would simply be the bearers of instrumental value like all other objects in the world. Instead, human beings are set apart and treated in special ways.[42]

Explanations for the source of human dignity vary according to one's belief system, either theological or philosophical. One of the most obvious ways to think about the source of dignity is in terms of a creator-creature relationship.[43] On this view individuals have dignity because they have been created by a divine source that imparts dignity to them as a fundamental constituent of their makeup. This derivation from the divine gives a special significance to the dignity of individuals. It generally carries with it the notion of a providential concern for individuals and a special protection given to them that is accorded to no other creature.[44] For this reason, an affront to the dignity of individuals within this context is also an affront to the divine source. Consequently, special penalties are attached to these transgressions.

Another, and more naturalistic, approach to the derivation of human dignity is the anthropocentric belief that human beings occupy a special place in nature.[45] This belief holds that, in the evolutionary process, human beings have developed a range of intellectual abilities that allow them to lay claim to a superiority among all other species. Human beings are seen as possessing capabilities of such magnitude that they can dominate other species and direct the course of even natural processes to a great extent. This vantage point of control and privilege confers on human beings a dignity and special respect.

An existential approach to human dignity would hold that individuals possess dignity by virtue of their ability to choose.[46] On this view we are the only manifestation of life that can determine itself. All others are totally bound by the exigencies and limitations of nature. Human beings, on the other hand, are undetermined, in major ways, by outside forces. Rather, the assertion is that we make ourselves who we are by the choices we make in our daily lives. As self-makers,[47] we are more self-determining than other species and, as such, individuals can lay claim to a special regard from other human beings. We are required to respect other persons because their being flows from within them through their choices rather than being imposed upon them externally.

Although there may be many other ways of attempting to account for the derivation of human dignity that cannot be explored at this time, one more explanation requires some attention. This view, which is the opposite of the anthropocentric approach, is an undercurrent of many Eastern religions[48] and Native American belief systems.[49] On this view, human dignity depends not on the separation of persons from other species or their superiority vis-à-vis other species. Rather, personal dignity rests on the integration of individual human beings into the larger community of living things and natural processes. Individuals who behave in an independent or "renegade" fashion have no dignity because they have forsaken the ground upon which their being rests—namely, their participation in a process or community larger than themselves. On this view "to be" is "to be related," and to have dignity is to enter consciously into this network of relationships.

Regardless of the explanation for human dignity, there is little disagreement that persons are considered to possess it as a moral claim on the behavior of others.[50] And even if the concept of dignity were to be extended to other living things, human dignity would still remain the foundational model for understanding and laying claim to the notion of intrinsic worth that demands special consideration.

To understand the various ways of deriving human dignity or to subscribe to a particular account is only a small part of exploring the notion of human dignity. For just as there are many dimensions of finitude that must be understood if we are to understand fully its impact on our lives, there are many dimensions or facets of personal dignity that must be explored if we are to have a genuine appreciation of it. To violate one of the facets of dignity is to violate the person's dignity itself. Each individual will emphasize some facets and deemphasize others. Each person will hold tenaciously to some and willingly compromise on others. Each individual will arrange the dimensions in different orders of priority. It is virtually impossible to predict how these personal profiles will be shaped. It is for this reason that caregivers must be sensitive to the various features of their patient's dignity and attempt to discover how each patient's dignity is constituted; for there are as many ways to violate a patient's dignity as there are components of that dignity.

Embodiment is the most obvious but also one of the most neglected facets of personal dignity. Each individual has a special sense of what it means to be a body of a particular type with particular attributes. Often this translates into "body image," but it also can involve the attachment we have to our bodies.

Some individuals require that intrusions into their bodies be kept at an absolute minimum. Such individuals would probably limit surgical interventions and allow them only for the most grave reasons. Some individuals may have developed a view of their bodies as a set of natural processes with great self-healing powers, systems that should not be polluted by foreign substances such as toxic chemicals that others may classify as "therapeutic medications." Some may have aesthetic perceptions of their bodies and resist alterations even as a last resort. For this reason some women will refuse mastectomies even at great risk to their lives. Some will view their bodies as consecrated temples and limit certain kinds of intrusions; Jehovah's Witnesses, for example, refuse blood products. Finally, some individuals may detach themselves from their bodies, particularly in the process of dying, and willingly surrender to bodily deterioration in humbly accepting death as a passage to eternal life.

There is legitimacy in each of these approaches to embodiment, and one cannot respect a patient's dignity without understanding where the patient stands on this issue and how reflectively that stance has been developed. To simply negate a patient's view of embodiment as "foolish" or "unrealistic" is to violate a fundamental feature of that individual's dignity.

Each person has a set of *beliefs* peculiar to that person. And even if individuals have similar beliefs, these often vary in intensity and priority. One may have a strong belief in a divine source guiding her life and destiny. Another may share a similar belief but be eager to take a hand in directing his destiny as well. Some may have certain beliefs about the ability of traditional medicine to act in a healing way while the beliefs of others may point to an alternative direction in the healing arts. Patients have many different beliefs about the benefits of medicine as they approach the ends of their lives.

In all these situations and belief contexts there will be a large variety of alternative treatments possible for selection. For this reason consent to and refusal of treatments are essential, and they must be based not only on relevant information but also on placing that information within the proper belief context. To minimize or disregard a belief system as "inappropriate" violates the patient's dignity because it assaults one of the central forces that allow individuals to orient and manage their lives. In a sense, an individual's beliefs are the gyroscope that guides all the other facets of personal dignity.

Our *attitudes* and *feelings* give texture to our lives in a way that no other facet of dignity can. To truly understand an individual, and ourselves, we must understand the posture we take toward the richness of experience as well as the emotive responses those experiences elicit. These dimensions admit of incalculable levels of intensity. They may make the difference between a cooperative spirit between patients and caregivers and antagonisms that jeopardize any possible healing power. They may make the difference between resisting a disease or surrendering to it. They may cloud our abilities to receive information to make wise decisions or they may enable us to know precisely what we need to know. They may orient us, disorient us, or provide a range of possibilities between those poles, in our attempts to come to terms with our finitude.

As with other facets of dignity, our attitudes and feelings cannot be minimized or disregarded without violating our dignity itself. Caregivers must attempt not only to be aware of the attitudes and feelings of their patients but to be aware of their own as well. Attitudes and feelings are all too seldom communicated in articulated ways. Rather, they are communicated subtly. To be open to this communication is a particular challenge to the healthcare professional. Sensitivity in this area is not easy to develop but may make the difference between following the patient's wishes and doing what the caregiver merely *thinks* the patient wants.[51] The former respects patient dignity; the latter often violates it.

Patients come to the clinical setting with different levels of *cognitive content*—that is, with different knowledge about themselves, the world in which they live, and the healthcare issues they are facing. Our culture has moved far beyond the stage when we could presume that individuals have similar levels of education and intelligence. Similarly, it is unrealistic to assume that patients are totally ignorant of disease processes, symptoms, and therapeutic possibilities. Moreover, many patients frequently desire to overcome any ignorance they may have.

The dynamics of informed consent have been designed to address this facet of patient dignity and others as well. Different patients will have different levels of curiosity about their healthcare conditions and different abilities to understand all that is at stake. If caregivers wish to respect the dignity of their patients, they will be solicitous about the level of understanding their patients wish to achieve.[52] They will speak to their patients in language the patients can comprehend and respect the knowledge patients bring to the clinical setting. To ignore the patients level of knowledge is to subvert the foundation of the patient's power to consent to or refuse treatment.

Another important dimension of personal dignity is the accumulation of the *choices* and *preferences* upon which individuals have acted throughout their lives. Our lives are structured as a result of those choices. The choices we have made and the actions that have resulted from them give texture to our lives; a strong case can be made that the cumulative effect of those choices constitutes our identity.[53] Patients come to the clinical setting with a history of those choices. To deny the impact of those past choices on the present ones would surely constitute an assault on the patient's dignity.

The making of choices in healthcare is another dimension of patient dignity that is protected by informed consent. Just as the "informed" side singles out cognitive content for special attention, so also the "consent" side singles out the process of choosing. Making choices and assuming the accompanying responsibilities for those choices are distinctively human abilities.

The *expectations* and *hopes* individuals have about their lives constitute other areas of personal dignity that are peculiar to each person. Some will have expectations that far exceed reality while others will adjust their expectations to fit within the context they face. In respecting patients' dignity it will be necessary to give them the opportunity to adjust their expectations in light of the healthcare conditions they have encountered. This will be particularly important if their expectations far exceed the reasonable limits of healthcare interventions. It sometimes happens that patients' expectations are at variance with those of their caregivers. Some patients are ready to surrender to a disease process long before their caregivers are. It is important for caregivers to realize that the imposition of their own agenda of expectations on patients may very well constitute a violation of the patient's dignity.

Maintaining hope in a therapeutic relationship is essential for the curative process. However, patients cannot always hope for a cure. The reality of this fact must be made clear to patients when it is appropriate. When this becomes apparent in the disease process, patients can then adjust their hopes according to their own values and the inevitable outcome of the disease process. One need not always have hope for cure in order to have hope. Even in the process of dying one can have hope—for example, hope of being free from pain, hope of not being isolated or abandoned, etc. The direction and intensity of these hopes will be individualized from patient to patient.

One of the most difficult problems caregivers face in their clinical interactions with patients is the tolerance patients have for *taking risks*. We saw in the previous section that it is part of our fundamental humanity to make moral decisions about matters with uncertain outcomes. We continually take risks and generally attempt to minimize them.[54] But each person has a different tolerance level for taking risks. We often find this reflected in ordinary conversation, where it is not unusual to hear comments like: "I would never think of doing something like that" or "It's too risky for me."

Healthcare is an area that expends great efforts to minimize risks. Caregivers are trained in a tradition that urges them to be cautious and to pursue the "safest" course for patients whenever possible. Great risks are undertaken only when there is a concomitant reason for taking them and when the "safer" course is unreliable or ineffective.

However, patients may be willing to take risks where caregivers are not, or vice versa. Patients may wish to pursue experimental treatments or alternative therapies when the caregivers may think such courses of action are foolish. On the other hand, some patients may wish to yield to a disease process and the natural course of events when the caregiver may think that more aggressive efforts may improve the condition of the patient.

Like other facets of patient dignity, risk taking is highly complex and must be regarded with great sensitivity and, often, deference. When patients refuse treatment or particularly when they complete an advance directive, they are assuming risks as a result of their moral decisions. Because of the risks involved, treatment refusals or advance directives are not decisions to be taken lightly or ignored. Instead, the weighing of risks must be carefully undertaken. A discussion of and openness to the risks involved must be an integral part of the clinical relationship.[55]

The nature of the *relationships* individuals have is an area of personal dignity that has received dramatic attention since the onset of the AIDS crisis. Individuals' choices of sexual partners are intensely personal ones. Equally significant are the levels of trust and affection that unite members of families whether they be homosexual or heterosexual families. The variety of the forms families take is a challenge to any caregiver. Caregivers should never hope to mold a patient's relationships into forms that are completely pleasing to the caregiver.

Respecting the dignity of patients means that one respects the network of relationships in which they are involved. This will require caregivers to respect and utilize the patient's relationships when difficult decisions are made about treatment refusals. It will also call for encouraging patients to discuss the details of the wishes expressed in their advance directives with those who are intimate partners of those relationships. Finally, the respect for relationships will require a special respect for the one who is appointed as the attorney-in-fact in a durable power of attorney. Because of the level of trust that exists between the patient and this appointee, it will be necessary for caregivers to extend the same measure of respect to the attorney-in-fact that they extend to the patient. To disregard the wishes of the patient as expressed by the attorney-in-fact is to violate the fundamental dignity of the patient.

One of the features of human dignity upon which we seldom reflect is that of the *activities* that are central to an individual's life. The loss of the voice to a performer, the loss of physical dexterity to the athlete, and the loss of memory to the educator all constitute serious threats to their personal dignity as they have fashioned it. The compromise or loss of mentation is a threat to the dignity of many individuals, a threat that is often considered worse than death itself.

Our personal identity is so bound to some of our activities that we can hardly imagine not being able to participate in them. When the crisis of disease or injury intrudes into our lives, compromising those activities, we may well choose not to maintain our lives in such a compromised condition. For example, the quadriplegic is frequently faced with such a difficult choice. Often, patients in a severely compromised condition would prefer to forgo further treatments that would maintain them in this state. But they are coerced into accepting or receiving the treatments because of the desires of family members or caregivers.[56]

One particular application of this facet of personal dignity applies to the issue of advance directives. Some living will legislation carries the stipulation that patients must be *terminally* ill before the advance directive can be carried out.[57] This stipulation may very well strike at the heart of personal dignity by restricting the exercise of the patient's power of choice. Individuals who anticipate the loss of mentation ought to be able to express such anticipation in their advance directives regardless of the form the directives take.

To maintain personal dignity patients should be able to refuse treatments that will keep them in the state of seriously compromised mentation. These treatments might be antibiotics for infections, tube feedings if they refuse food by mouth, diabetic medications, etc. For such individuals, their dignity lies in their power to choose their lifestyle and in their ability to engage in acts of mentation. To deny them the right to refuse treatment with the loss of mentation would be to violate their dignity on two fronts—namely, the loss of mentation itself and the restriction of choice in the face of this loss.

It is an axiom in healthcare that patients *respond differently to disease and injury as well as to their symptoms and therapies.* Some patients will react with fear and apprehension, some with interest and curiosity, and still others with acceptance and resignation. All these responses make up yet another facet of their personal dignity. Responses in these areas will set the stage for treatment selection or refusals and for an interest (or lack of interest) in advance directives. The responses of patients can be neither ignored nor minimized. Instead, they should be encouraged as yet another expression of dignity.

Although there are many more facets of personal dignity that could be explored, no list would be complete without some discussion of *aging.* Everyone approaches the prospect and the reality of aging differently—some with fear, others with complacency and resignation. Aging is a time of diminishing capabilities and functions, a time when the body begins to break down in significant ways and when an increasing number of healthcare interventions are necessary to maintain some degree of homeostasis. And, of course, the inevitable end of aging is death.

The extent to which one prepares for declining function and disease in the aging process is very much a part of our dignity as human beings. We can be sure that, in the process of aging, there is increased likelihood for a decline in mental functioning. We can also be sure that with increasing decline in physical functioning there will be a greater need for healthcare interventions. And, finally, we can be sure that often interventions in an aging organism might very well not return the organism to a previous level of functioning or a minimally decent quality of life.

The Patient Self-Determination Act affords the opportunity to approach the issue of patient dignity in a comprehensive manner. If taken seriously, the law can encourage a detailed exploration of the components of dignity. Patients can reflect upon them and caregivers can turn their attention to them. In the ensuing dialogue between patients and caregivers, dignity can be both respected and enhanced through a better understanding of patients' beliefs, attitudes, feelings, preferences, hopes, expectations, tolerance of risks, etc. The dignity of the patient lays the foundation for any decision to select or refuse treatment or draft an advance directive. A clear understanding of one's dignity gives direction to the choices one might make.

Of particular interest is the place of advance directives as a manifestation of dignity in an aging population that might suddenly become critically ill. It is not sufficient to simply have an individual sign an advance directive. It is essential that conversations be conducted with such individuals and specific preferences be identified so that the dignity of the critically ill elderly person will be preserved.[58] Situations often develop in which the preservation of the dignity of the elderly and the critically ill is left to the decisions of others. The direction those decisions often take is to make every effort to extend the life of the patient. In fact, however, that approach may be the one that violates the dignity of the patient most forcefully. The only way to avoid this extreme is to enter into carefully crafted conversations with members of the aging population and those who are approaching that time of their lives.[59] These conversations should explore the prospects of aging, health, and decline. They should allow the persons to articulate their wishes by exploring the elements that are most central to their dignity.

The Patient Self-Determination Act provides the perfect opportunity to begin such conversations and to carry them to conclusion and implementation.[60] The law demonstrates that there is a genuine societal attempt to promote dignity at a time in one's life when dignity is so often compromised. The advance directive is, perhaps, one of the most effective tools in addressing the healthcare needs of the elderly. It can enhance the quality of their lives by reducing the fear of what will befall them if they become critically ill, and it can enhance the quality of their dying by guaranteeing that no futile or unwanted interventions will extend their dying beyond the time they themselves specify.

This exploration of personal dignity, has emphasized the dignity of the patient because the Patient Self-Determination Act primarily addresses the interests of patients. However, it must be noted that caregivers and the members of the patient's family are also repositories of dignity, possessing the same features of dignity as patients. Frequently these features will come into conflict. The wishes of the patient are not always the wishes of the family, and often the wishes of patients and families are not the wishes of the caregivers. The foundations of personal dignity underlying those wishes will often not coalesce. The resolution of such conflicts is not always easy, and it may be that some compromises in one or the other facet of dignity will have to be made along the way.

However, the Patient Self-Determination Act gives preference to preserving the dignity of patients when such conflicts occur. There are two reasons for this. The first reason lies in the vulnerability of the patient. Disease and injury make patients particularly vulnerable.[61] When this vulnerability is great, it becomes important to compensate for it by strengthening the patient's position wherever one can. Respecting the dignity of the patient is a very powerful way of limiting patient vulnerability.

The second reason for respecting the patient's dignity above others' is that, in the final analysis, the patient is the one who must most directly bear the burden of the decisions that are made. It is the patient who will linger on in the dying process. It is the patient who will suffer the pain of the disease or injury. It is the patient who will suffer the insult of compromised functioning. It is the patient who will die the death. In respecting patient dignity the sacrifice to families is great and the challenge to the professionalism of caregivers is often extreme. But without meeting these challenges and accepting these sacrifices, the dignity of the patient stands in real jeopardy and its violation seldom enhances the quality of healthcare.

The above analysis does not claim to be an exhaustive list of the facets of individual dignity. Many more features could be explored.

But it does give a reasonable profile of the extraordinary complexity involved when imperatives are formulated about respecting personal or patient dignity.

The process of understanding the dignity of individual patients, and respecting it, is further complicated by the fact that there is a time dimension to each of the facets. There may be a difference in the way patients manifest the various dimensions in the present as compared with their previous encounters with healthcare. Furthermore, there is no guarantee that the present priorities of the facets of their dignity will manifest the same pattern in the future. It is for this reason that advance directives involve some measure of risk. Patients anticipate that their dignity will call for actions in the future that seem to be appropriate in the present. There is only one way to manage this time dimension of personal dignity. It requires that there be ongoing conversations between patients and caregivers that will monitor changes in the way patients view themselves and the demands of their personal dignity. This often involves periodic revisions of one's advance directive.[62]

The Patient Self-Determination Act will not adequately deal with the issues of patient dignity if caregivers and patients rely only on pieces of paper to fulfill the spirit of the law. A signature on a consent form or a refusal of treatment form does little to reveal the personal issues with which an individual has dealt in reaching the conclusion documented by the form. The signature does not even guarantee that the patient has addressed the issues at all with any measure of reflection. Similarly, a signature on an advance directive may not demonstrate the facets of personal dignity that lie behind it. Without the interpersonal exchange through conversations between caregivers and patients, the Patient Self-Determination Act will remain a fundamentally sterile exercise, and any respect for patient dignity that results from it will be accidental at best.

The Role of the Virtues in Conducting the Moral Life

The kinds of activities in which individuals engage comprise a significant part of their dignity. One special way to think about these activities is as the practice of the virtues. Particular attention needs to be paid to this area of personal dignity if we are to appreciate fully the human context for the Patient Self-Determination Act and its role in the clinical setting. What will be undertaken in this section is an exploration of the role of the virtues in general and an identification of some of the specific virtues that play a central role in the clinical setting. These specific virtues will be examined in light of the opportunities the Patient Self-Determination Act presents for their practice.

Virtues represent states of character and habits of behavior possessed by a moral agent.[63] In combination, these two features of virtue offer a powerful portrait of individuals as they interact with others. These states or habits do not come by chance to individuals. Rather, they are chosen as dispositions toward actions as a result of personal deliberations. Individuals choose the virtues they plan to practice.[64] The choice takes place over a period of time. Just as one does not "fall into" a virtuous life, so also one action does not constitute a virtuous disposition.[65]

Individuals choose the virtues they will practice within a context of the human goods they wish to pursue and the ends or purposes they wish to accomplish. The virtues are always directed toward some end.[66] Since the ends of human life are multiple in a pluralistic society, the virtues to be practiced and the priorities among them will vary widely. It is difficult to identify one virtue or set of virtues or priority of virtues that will or should be practiced in a pluralistic society.[67] As opposed to a society in which all individuals agree about the ends to be achieved, in a pluralistic society there is no general agreement on ends.[68] If there is no agreement about the ends, there can be no agreement about the means to achieve the ends.

In order to develop a society that will allow individuals to interact with a reasonable degree of tranquility, individuals must develop attitudes and practices that will allow others to achieve their goals with some measure of latitude. The attitude fundamental to a democratic pluralistic society is that of tolerance, and this may be the only candidate for a common virtue in such a society.[69] Though not everything is possible in such a society, nonetheless many variations in goals and purposes are possible. When disagreements between individuals arise as to the ends to be accomplished or the virtues to be practiced to achieve those ends, then the process of negotiation becomes the fundamental practice.[70] In negotiating differences, some compromises will need to be made about goals as well as the manner of achieving them. Individuals engaged in virtuous practices will not always be able to practice their virtues to the maximum extent they wish. Negotiation becomes the standard behavior rather than a forceful imposition of one person's will on another.

The right to self-determination is a good example of the dynamics of the practice of virtue in a society that promotes tolerance of differences. There can never be total self-determination for individuals who must live in a social context.[71] There will always be limits on one's behaviors for the general good of all, but there remain spheres of actions where it is appropriate for individuals to exercise their self-determination.[72] The boundaries between the self-determination of individuals and the general good of society or the welfare of others are continually shifting. The virtues come upon the scene as the good of self-determination and the good of society are being tested.

The virtues, then, represent a dynamic flow of personal dignity according to which individuals carve out their places in the world as they encounter a variety of circumstances. Aristotle viewed a virtue as a mean between two extremes.[73] The virtuous person will find herself in a diversity of circumstances that could all be approached from different extremes. Since the extremes shift, the mean will shift. Each individual must figure out how the virtues are to be practiced in different situations.[74] Thus the practice of the virtues is not just a matter of negotiating with others who may see the situation and the appropriate virtuous practice differently. There must be an inner dialogue and negotiation that occurs in each moral agent to determine the precise practice pattern for the virtue in various situations.

Because of the wide variety of practices possible for individuals in a pluralistic society, the Patient Self-Determination Act can never apply automatically and nonreflectively. A simple signature on a piece of paper will never suffice. Any decision, whether or not it is symbolized by a signature, must be made against a backdrop of the virtues that individuals have chosen to practice. Though the virtue narrative of patients is often tacit and seemingly casual,[75] it still represents, in a significant way, the background a patient brings to any individual decision. This background must be explored with a patient before any decision exhibiting self-determination can be made with any degree of credibility. Decisions cannot be made without some reflection on their historical background and the choices leading to the practice of the virtues that direct patients to their desired goals.

Thus far we have identified and explored several facets of the life of virtue in the human condition as it applies in the clinical setting. (1) Virtues are states of character or habits that guide us toward the accomplishment of the goals we have chosen to pursue.[76] (2) The virtue history or narrative constitutes a major part of what makes us individuals.[77] (3) Negotiation is often necessary as different individuals choose to practice different sets of virtues or similar virtues but in substantially different ways.[78] (4) The Patient Self-Determination Act brings into focus the importance of understanding the role of the virtues in the clinical setting.

No presentation of the human context of the Patient Self-Determination Act would be complete without some detailed study of the virtues that surface in the clinical setting and the way they interface with the Patient Self-Determination Act. The following analyses should provide some guidance for identifying these virtues and ways of addressing the issues they raise. Since the Patient Self-Determination Act is primarily patient-centered, the virtues to be practiced by patients are the focal point of this discussion. However, we will explore the virtues of the professional as well, insofar as they directly affect patients' decisions to consent to or refuse treatment and to draft advance directives.

Patients come to the clinical setting with a history of the virtues they have consciously or unconsciously chosen to practice. This history provides a significant backdrop for understanding the patient. Clinicians who ignore this virtue history do so at great risk to the clinical encounter. To disregard the virtue history of the patient is tantamount to saying that what the patient has done up to the point of the clinical encounter is of no value. But clinicians know this is not the case. The medical history of the patient is one of the most important factors to consider in attempting to address the patient's healthcare problem. But this only reveals clues to the symptomatology of the patient's presentation; it does not give a picture of the *whole* patient. The virtue history of the patient adds significant information for the clinician if she is to treat the patient as a capable decision maker rather than simply a bundle of symptoms.

A few tactical observations may be helpful in addressing the practice of the virtues in the clinical setting. Sometimes patients will come to the clinical encounter with a full range of virtues already in place.

In these instances the clinician needs to do three things: (1) identify the virtues the patient possesses, (2) foster the virtues already present, and (3) create no obstacles to the practice of the virtues. Sometimes patients will be somewhat tentative in suggesting they might want to practice some of the virtues. In this case the practice should be encouraged so that the patient will be able to be an active participant in decision making.[79] In other situations patients may not have the prerequisite virtues for collaborating in clinical decisions and may therefore be pointed in the direction of those virtues they may have failed to develop prior to the clinical encounter.[80] They should be given the opportunity, encouragement, and assistance to develop those virtues. However, they cannot be forced to do so because such coercion could violate their liberty and, hence, their dignity.[81]

When patients make it clear that they simply do not want to practice a particular virtue, they should probably be let alone unless they later send clues to the caregivers that they might be interested in developing a particular virtue. Caregivers should always be sensitive to the clues patients might send to them in a variety of disguises. This responsibility is implicit in the codes of ethics that identify an obligation for caregivers to respect the dignity of patients.[82] For, as we have seen, developing and practicing virtues is an essential component of personal dignity.

Caregivers and patients are not immune from the many ways the virtues can be practiced and the priorities among the virtues, which are common features of the human context. Not only will they have to negotiate about which virtue is appropriate in a particular circumstance, but they will often have to negotiate about the manner in which individual virtues are to be practiced. We have seen how this disparity calls for negotiation with particular virtues. As they encounter each other in the conversations attendant to the implementation of the Patient Self-Determination Act, curiosity, responsibility, acceptance, and detachment may require special attention on the part of patients, while the virtues of tolerance, compassion, integrity, and empathy will have special significance for the professional.[83]

Among the virtues that first surface in the clinical setting is the virtue of *curiosity*. This virtue allows us to make our way in the world, where we are constantly bombarded by a variety of stimuli. It allows us to gain understanding of stimuli and facts and lays the foundation for selecting courses of action that will enable us to accomplish our goals. Curiosity functions in a similar way in the clinical setting. It is a virtue that enables patients to acquire the information and understanding necessary to make their decisions about approaches to treatment.[84] It is this virtue that informed consent attempts to address and that the Patient Self-Determination Act can foster.

Unfortunately, some patients do not utilize this virtue in the clinical setting. Though they may bring it to the encounter, they may think that it is inappropriate to make inquiries of their caregivers. If the Patient Self-Determination Act is to be effective, patients will have to be encouraged to practice this virtue. Curiosity is a good example of a virtue that may be practiced in different ways by the patient and the clinician. The patient may be so curious that the clinician might become uncomfortable in providing all the information requested. In cases such as these, the interested parties will have to negotiate the limits of the practice of curiosity so that both can work effectively in the decisional process.

Hope is a virtue that is generally considered essential in the clinical setting. It is the virtue that leaves us open to possibilities and propels us to pursue goals when they become difficult to accomplish. It is hope that causes individuals to fight a disease even when the odds for victory seem to be quite small. But in the clinical setting hope must be grounded in a realistic assessment of one's situation. False hope—a hope that has no chance of being realized—only creates an illusion for the patient and ultimately creates great harm without producing significant benefits.

Though it is true that everyone has something for which to hope, the parameters of hope are continually readjusting themselves in our lives. Persons cannot hope for the same things in old age that they could hope for when they were young. Those embarked upon a process of disease with accompanying inevitable deterioration and disability cannot have the same hopes as one who may be facing an acute episode but is otherwise vigorously healthy. Our hopes must be adapted to the real, rather than simply desirable, boundaries of our circumstances. But there are no circumstances without some measure of hope, even if the hope is limited to a "gentle" death, care and comfort from one's caregivers, family, and friends, and the companionship needed to overcome the feelings of isolation that so often accompany the process of dying.[85]

The Patient Self-Determination Act presents the possibility of practicing this virtue by allowing the patient to make the relevant inquiries about the boundary conditions regarding her healthcare situation, and whether those conditions can be adjusted. She can clearly define her reasonable hopes within the confines of her situation and make healthcare decisions accordingly, even to the point of refusing treatments.

Pressure from caregivers to continue aggressive treatments when cure, decent recovery, or reasonable management is not possible often indicates that they are uncomfortable with patients who seem to have abandoned hope for a cure. But patients may be well aware that though it may be unreasonable to hope for a cure, it is not unreasonable to hope for a comfortable passage through the dying process. In this instance, as in many others, the patient and the caregiver will have to negotiate the parameters of hope. However, the patient's practice of the virtues will be the deciding factor because it is primarily the patient's virtues that will help her with the reality of dying and preserve her dignity.

Courage and *risk taking* are virtues that play an important role in making decisions about treatment refusals and advance directives. It is often easy to surrender to fear and simply say "do everything" even though "everything" may be totally inappropriate. It is an act of courage to discriminate among healthcare alternatives when one has to weigh medical probabilities and burdens against benefits. Moreover, courage and the acceptance of risks are essential to anticipating the future and giving directions for healthcare interventions when one may not be in the position to make decisions at the time.

Some patients are simply better risk takers than others, and often they are better risk takers than their caregivers. Frequently caregivers would like patients to pursue treatments with low probabilities even though the patients may not be disposed to do so. This attitude on the part of caregivers often leads to the utilization of futile care.[86] Acknowledgment of the legitimacy of risk taking may be an important approach to avoiding the initiation or continuation of futile care. The Patient Self-Determination Act acknowledges the moral integrity of patients by giving them the opportunity to exercise these important virtues of courage and risk taking, which lie at the very heart of their personal dignity.

Responsibility is a key virtue in human life and lies at the foundation of all moral behavior. Without the practice of this virtue all of our moral imperatives would be hollow. Actions would be undertaken simply because they are required by some external source and not because they flow from some internal conviction. They would be "*an* action" rather than "*my* action."

There is a strong tendency in human life to attempt to escape responsibility.[87] When undesirable consequences result from our actions, we frequently attribute them to someone else's behaviors or other circumstances beyond our control. This phenomenon occurs particularly in healthcare settings, where patients already feel overwhelmed by the disease process. It is a recurrent theme to blame healthcare professionals for therapeutic outcomes resulting from therapies that should not have been chosen in the first place but were chosen because patients evaded their responsibility to take an active part in the decision-making process.

The Patient Self-Determination Act reinforces the virtue of responsibility in patients. It clearly places the responsibility for healthcare decisions on the patient's shoulders.[88] It is the patient who can and should make the decisions to consent to or refuse treatment and to anticipate his healthcare needs in the future by considering an advance directive.[89]

Some caregivers may wish to derail the patient's practice of the virtue of responsibility. This has the effect of producing a compliant patient who follows directions and causes no friction in the clinical setting. Unfortunately, this approach also takes responsibility away from the one who must bear the consequences of the decisions that have been made.[90] Compliance frequently violates rather than affirms the personal dignity of the patient. If the outcomes are ultimately seen as undesirable, the patient has every right to complain and may do so with grave consequences for the caregiver and the healthcare facility.

By encouraging the practice of the virtue of responsibility, caregivers not only protect themselves but help their patients develop their distinctively human side. This may be one of the most positive outcomes of the clinical encounter. But before the patient can act responsibly, she must be given all the tools for the practice of the virtue. She must have appropriate information and be clear about her values and goals. Then the necessary connections can be made and the appropriate therapeutic pathways chosen. But even with all of these precautions, undesirable outcomes may still result. Such are the contingencies and uncertainties that are an inevitable part of exercising the virtue of responsibility.

Prudence is an important virtue to be fostered in the life of all individuals, particularly patients. This virtue encourages them to weigh the various elements of a situation and to approach creatively the uncertainties and probabilities of life in general, and medical practice in particular. Weighing the role of each intervention against the condition it attempts to address and assessing its possible risks, as well as benefits, require a great deal of practical wisdom on the part of the patient.

The practice of prudence requires not only careful judgments on the part of the patient but considerable tolerance on the part of the caregiver. For it is practically certain that the patient will weigh the various elements in the clinical situation somewhat differently than the caregivers do. Negotiation between caregivers and patients in the practice of this virtue is essential. Both will have to be open in their conversations about what they see as the benefits and risks or burdens of particular approaches to treatment. They will also have to communicate about how those possible clinical outcomes may fit into their own value priorities. Finally, each will have to acknowledge the legitimacy and integrity of the value priorities of the other, and generally deference will have to be given to the patient because he will bear the consequences of the prudential judgments.[91]

The conversations that can result from the implementation of the Patient Self-Determination Act will certainly afford ample opportunity for patients to practice prudence. Acquiring relevant information as well as determining how it fits into the total healthcare picture and the patient's value life will make it possible for patients to practice this virtue as a central part of their decision-making power.

Trust is the virtue that lies at the heart of the clinical fiduciary relationship. Without trust the relationship would always be open to suspicion. But this virtue enables both caregiver and patient to have confidence in each other's ability to fulfill an appropriate role in the clinical encounter. Trust also allows the parties in the relationship to view each other as moral equals who are both worthy of respect. It protects both the autonomy of the patient and the integrity of the caregiver.

The Patient Self-Determination Act casts a new light on the virtue of trust. It encourages conversations in the clinical relationship that go far beyond the discussion of symptoms and treatments. It allows individuals to penetrate behind the wall of decisions to the reasons underlying them and the values that drive them. In the case of advance directives, it also encourages discussions about the contingencies of human life that are most difficult to confront.

Both caregivers and patients must practice this virtue and set the groundwork for it early in the relationship.[92] If there is a lack of trust, the relationship is bound to deteriorate. Negotiations about the parameters and expectations of trust will be necessary.[93] Without the understanding that can result from these discussions, the autonomy of the patient will be placed in jeopardy, and the integrity of the caregiver will be severely compromised.

Assertiveness, communicativeness, and *decisiveness* are virtues directly related to the process of entering into conversations with caregivers, resisting coercion in the discussions, and making clear and unambiguous decisions.[94] If patients do not actively enter into the exchange with their caregivers and provide clear messages about their wishes, the patients and caregivers will be at a great disadvantage. The caregivers will have to either guess about what patients want or do everything possible for the patients in order to protect themselves from liability exposure.

Because of the legal requirements of the Patient Self-Determination Act, patients can communicate openly with caregivers and receive enough information to begin the process of making clear decisions. For patients who find it difficult to begin these conversations and practice these virtues, the law provides the impetus. Even if the practice of these virtues by patients disturbs some caregivers, they will nevertheless have a better chance of benefitting from the advantages for informed consent along with the practice of the virtue of responsibility of the part of patients. Adjustments in the quality of their conversations will have many positive outcomes for the quality of patient care.

Acceptance is an important virtue in our daily lives when we encounter obstacles or situations we cannot change. It helps us to define the boundaries for our activities and keeps us from expending our energies in fruitless behaviors that often produce great anxiety with no change in the problems we face.

In the healthcare setting we most dramatically face the limitations of our finitude, which require acceptance. Because of the frequent success of medical interventions we are often seduced into thinking that healthcare interventions will always be successful. It is important for patients to realize that this is not the case. Because the Patient Self-Determination Act opens the door to an enriched discussion involving the communication of information leading to consent or refusal of treatment, patients can acquire a more complete understanding of their healthcare conditions and what realistic possibilities of treatment are available for them. Once patients accept their conditions, they can reject futile treatments.

Frequently there will be a disparity between caregivers, patients, and families around the practice of acceptance. Sometimes the caregivers are more prone to its practice than patients. Many times patients understand their situations very readily and wish to practice the virtue long before caregivers or family members. This is one of the most striking examples of a situation where negotiation about the practice of the virtues needs to occur in an open and honest fashion. The reality, however harsh, of the clinical situation must be outlined and the practice of the virtue that most closely reflects that situation must be pursued. The conversations prompted by the Patient Self-Determination Act and subsequent conversations within that context will promote the practice of acceptance to enhance the well-being of the patient.

Finally, the virtue of *detachment*, which has the virtue of acceptance as its foundation, plays a major role in the lives of patients. This virtue allows us to enjoy our lives and special events in them without clinging to them in some dysfunctional fashion. Detachment allows us to let go when that is the appropriate and prudent thing to do. This virtue keeps patients from attempting every possible intervention no matter how remote the probability of success merely to extract out of life its last possible moment. Detachment is the virtue that allows us to surrender to natural processes, or to a greater wisdom.

The Patient Self-Determination Act provides the arena for patients to play out the virtue of detachment. It confirms the legitimacy of the virtue by calling to patients' attention that they have the right to refuse treatment, the right to designate an end to the use of therapies when they are no longer capable of making those decisions, and the right to authorize someone else to make those decisions for them if they cannot do it for themselves. This law indicates that it is no longer the role of caregivers to impose their view of the clinical setting on the patient's circumstances. It legitimizes, in a very significant way, the ability of patients to yield to the forces struggling within them.

There are many other virtues that patients can practice, but the above seem to play the most significant roles in healthcare decision making and to underscore the new role for the Patient Self-Determination Act in that process. It is apparent that these virtues also apply to the broad spectrum of human life beyond healthcare.

For this reason it must be emphasized that patients are not the only individuals in the clinical setting who have an interest in practicing the virtues. Caregivers have an equal claim to a virtuous life.[95] Caregivers have their own set of virtues and priorities.[96] This feature of the clinical encounter must also be respected. Caregivers cannot be asked to surrender the practice of the virtues they have cultivated throughout their lives simply to satisfy the whim of patients or social forces.[97] But their professional lives must also be driven by a set of virtues that reflect their professional commitments.

Though the healthcare professional may possess and practice all the above virtues on a personal level when dealing with the patient, there are additional virtues that he should possess and practice as a professional. As in the case of patients, professionals may cluster their virtues in different configurations and with different priorities. The Patient Self-Determination Act provides professionals with the opportunity to reemphasize and discover enhanced ways of practicing virtues. The following professional virtues complement the patient virtues that are an integral part of the human context of the Patient Self-Determination Act.

Professionals are expected to be *benevolent* toward their patients. This is the most comprehensive of the virtues of the professional. Benevolence propels the professional to perform acts of beneficence that are directed to the best interests of the patient. Often benevolence takes the form of *self-effacement*—placing the good of the patient above the preferences the professional espouses.[98] Thus, in consenting to or refusing treatment, patients may move in a direction that the caregiver may not prefer but that the patient considers in her best interest. Such decisions by patients may call upon the professional to behave with self-restraint.

As a comprehensive virtue, benevolence can take various forms in medical practice. *Fidelity* is the virtue professionals practice in keeping their promises to their patients as they carry out their mutual obligations in the fiduciary relationship.[99] This involves both an element of mutual *trust* and the dedication to be faithful to the professional obligations to which one is committed. Thus, if the professional is committed to patient self-determination, fidelity requires actions in the decisional process that will enhance this aspect of the patient's value life.

Compassion is another form of benevolence. The Latin roots of the word means "to suffer with." This virtue calls upon the professional to view disease, injury, disability, and pain as the patient views it, rather than as a disinterested observer. Compassion helps the professional to see the world through the value eyes of the patient and to enter into that world as a "friend" rather than as a total "stranger."[100] Compassion also moves the professional to do everything possible to reduce the distress of the patient's malady. In being compassionate, the caregiver will attempt to understand the values that prompt patients to select or refuse treatment or decide to develop advance directives.

The virtue of *respect* is another form of benevolence. In practicing this virtue, the professional recognizes that the patient is her own center of valuing. The patient is seen not as an object to be used to satisfy the selfish aims of the professional but rather as a subject who has ultimate worth in herself. Respect is directed toward preserving the dignity of the patient in its most profound sense. This virtue will prompt the professional to honor the patient's agenda for healthcare, whenever this can be done within the boundaries of acceptable medical practice, rather than impose the professional's agenda on the patient.

Caregivers who exercise benevolence are also going to practice the virtue of *honesty*. They will give to patients the information necessary for patients to make wise decisions in directing their healthcare. They will also provide candid assessments of the patient's condition, including the prognosis and the probabilities for successful therapies. Honest caregivers will not distort information to make it easier to converse with patients, nor will they hold out false hopes. It requires *courage* to face patients with grim news about the future they may face. Honesty is the foundation for helping patients make sound decisions regarding consents to and refusals of treatments. It will also help patients reflect effectively on any advance directive project in which they might wish to engage.

In the process of interacting with patients, caregivers must exercise their *integrity*. They must be true to themselves and their professional duties as well as to the patients for whom they care. Patients may make demands on caregivers that require them to go beyond yielding to the patient to respect the patient's autonomy. Some demands may require caregivers to betray their fundamental professional obligations or their deeply held moral convictions.[101] Integrity requires the practice of *courage* because of the difficulty required in telling patients that the caregiver cannot accede to their demands. The practice of courage in pursuing personal and professional integrity may be particularly difficult when patients select futile treatments or refuse life-saving treatments. These virtues also manifest themselves in particularly poignant ways when the caregiver is required to honor an advance directive when the patient's family may demand otherwise.

The person with integrity will also exercise *prudence* in making recommendations to patients and in sharing the decision-making process with them. Since there are so many ways in which the art of medicine can be practiced in applying scientific information to a particular patient's condition, there can be no strict algorithms that can be applied to a particular clinical situation. The variables are often different from patient to patient, and each variable must be weighed against the others. All these judgments are matters of prudence or "practical wisdom."[102] The person of prudence will not only make prudential recommendations and decisions but will also communicate to the patient that the judgment is a prudential one. Prudence comes strongly into play when discussing decisions to consent to or refuse treatments. But it may be even more necessary when patients set down stipulations in their advance directives.[103]

"*Tolerance* is the primary cardinal virtue in the morality of mutual respect."[104] In our secular society, which admits of a plethora of views of the good life, no one person is recognized as having a special claim to wisdom about how the good life should be led. For this reason, we bear the burden of allowing many different views to flourish and of tolerating a great many that are at variance with our own. To respect another is to tolerate behaviors that may be viewed as disadvantageous, deviant, and even bizarre. Of course, society draws some limits around these behaviors when they harm another.[105] But in a democratic society that values liberty, a great many behaviors are tolerated.

Consequently, healthcare professionals are often required to tolerate and implement patients' decisions with which they do not agree. This can take the form of ordering treatments that patients desire but that go against the better judgment of the practitioner or ending treatments at the request of the patient or authorized surrogate when the practitioner thinks that the treatments might benefit the patient. The same issues may surface in conversations about advance directives. Caregivers will always have to balance the practice of tolerance against the practice of integrity and respect. The only guidance upon which they can rely is the practice of a reflectively structured virtue of benevolence.

Because the intersection of the personal virtues of the patient and the personal and professional virtues of the caregiver is extraordinarily complex, negotiation is essential in the clinical setting. Ideally, the outcome of the negotiation would be a respect for the virtue life of all the parties involved, keeping in mind the goals and purposes of the clinical encounter.

When disagreements occur, one overriding consideration should be kept in mind. The clinical encounter is designed for the welfare of the patient and it is generally the patients who are the best judges of what is in their best interests. Additionally, patients have probably developed a set of virtues that have allowed them to cope with the various exigencies of life. The caregiver's role as clinician does not generally give her selection of virtues and the forms of their practice any privileged position in the clinical setting. Therefore, the caregiver at most should make recommendations and provide guidance. In the final analysis, however, the caregiver very often must defer to the patient because it is the patient's virtue life that is primarily at stake in coping with disease, injury, or disability. If things go awry in the clinical setting, it is the patient who must bear the consequences of his own decision.

If patients and caregivers view themselves, and are viewed by others in the clinical setting, as virtue narratives that are unfolding in time and interacting in space, the richness of their lives as they have practiced their virtues will take on ever increasing significance in healthcare decision making. Not only will the well-being of patients be promoted but the integrity of caregivers will be optimized because they will look at patients not as clusters of symptoms but as integrated wholes worthy of respect as moral equals.

The practice of the virtues provides an insightful and transparent approach to understanding the dignity of the patient. To know the virtues a patient has chosen to practice, and to understand the virtues to which the professional is committed, is to come a long way to understanding the foundations of the patient's dignity and how it presents itself in the clinical setting. To appreciate those foundations will inevitably prompt respect for the patient. In the patients' desire to select and practice a cluster of virtues to achieve their goals, reflective caregivers will unavoidably see a mirror image of their own struggles in practicing virtues and developing aspirations for the good life.

NOTES

1. McGinn RE. Science, technology, and society. Englewood Cliffs, NJ: Prentice Hall, 1991, pages 113–115.

2. Thoreau HD. Walden. New York: Harper & Row Publishers, Inc. 1965, page 67.

3. Heidegger M. Being and time. Macquarrie J, Robinson E (trans). New York: Harper & Row, 1962, pages 36–40.

4. Hellerstein D. Overdosing on medical technology. Technology Review 1983; August–September, pages 13–17.

5. Fackenheim EL. The religious dimension of Hegel's thought. Bloomington, IN: Indiana University Press, 1967, page 13.

6. Engelhardt HT. The counsels of finitude. Hast Cent Rep 1975; 5:29–36. See also McCue JD. The naturalness of dying. JAMA 1955; 273:1039–1043, and Jonas H. The burden and blessing of mortality. Hast Cent Rep 1992; 22:34–40.

7. Heidegger M. Being and time. Macquarrie J, Robinson E (trans). New York: Harper & Row, 1962, pages 296–304. Martin Heidegger spends a

great portion of this investigation reflecting on the nature of the human reality as we are "beings-toward-death."

8. For "authentic" read "reflective." Only the reflective person is truly human. The history of this notion goes all the way back to Socrates, who said "the unexamined life is not worth living." Plato, The apology. Grube GMA (trans). Indianapolis, IN: Hackett Publishing Co. Inc., 1975, page 39.

9. Levine S. Meetings at the edge. New York: Anchor Press/Doubleday, 1984, pages, 130–131.

10. John Paul II. The gospel of life. Washington, D.C.: National Conference of Catholic Bishops, 1995, part 2.

11. Rinpoche S. The Tibetan book of living and dying. San Francisco: Harper San Francisco, 1992, pages 340–341.

12. The Roman Catholic Church has captured this notion by admonishing its faithful that they have the obligation to pursue forms of medical treatment that are considered ordinary or proportionate in producing a positive or beneficial effect for the patient without undue burdens. Catechism of the Catholic church. Washington, D.C.: United States Catholic Conference, 1994; ## 2278–2279.

13. Sacred Congregation for the Doctrine of the Faith. Declaration on euthanasia. Vatican City, 1980. See President's Commission for the Study of Ethical Problems in Medicine and Biomedical and Behavioral Research. Deciding to forego life-sustaining treatment: Ethical, medical, and legal issues in treatment decisions. Washington, D.C.: U.S. Government Printing Office, 1983, page 306.

14. Engelhardt HT. Tractatus artis bene moriendi vivendique: Choosing styles of dying and living. In Abernathy V (ed). Frontiers in medical ethics: Applications in a medical setting. Cambridge, MA: Ballinger Publishing Co., 1980, pages 10–11.

15. Engelhardt HT. The foundation of bioethics. 2d edition. New York: Oxford University Press, 1996, pages 340–347.

16. Seneca. On the proper time to slip the cable. In Epistola morales. Vol. 2. Gumere RM (trans). The Loeb Classical Library. Cambridge: Harvard University Press, 1920, page 59.

17. This feature of contemporary human existence was directly and forcefully expressed in the decision of the Ninth Circuit Court of Appeals on physician-assisted suicide. Compassion in Dying v. Washington. 79 F.3d 790 (9th Cir. 1996). Its importance was further acknowledged by Justice Stevens in his concurring opinion in Washington v. Glucksberg, 117 S. Ct. 2302 (1997), even though the process of adjusting the time and manner of one's dying does not result in a constitutionally protected right to physician-assisted suicide.

18. Truog RD et al. Barbiturates in the care of the terminally ill. N Engl J Med 1992; 327:1678–1682. See also Quill TE et al. Palliative options of last resort: A comparison of voluntarily stopping eating and drinking, terminal sedation, physician-assisted suicide, and voluntary active euthanasia. JAMA 1997; 278:2099–2104.

19. Levine S. Who dies: An investigation of conscious living and conscious dying. New York: Anchor Press/Doubleday, 1982, pages 268–271.

20. Some individuals avoid this process because their deaths are sudden and unexpected, as in the case of a fatal accident. However, for those who experience the process of a terminal condition the concerns for patient participation in healthcare decision making that underlie the Patient Self-Determination Act come into sharp focus.

21. The definition of a terminal condition is often a key issue in the utilization of advance directive documents. [The controversial decisions of both the Ninth and Second Circuit Courts of Appeals on physician-assisted suicide identify the problems generated by the lack of a clear, precise, and consistent definition. See Compassion in Dying v. Washington. 79 F.3d 790 (9th Cir. 1996), and Quill v. Vacco. 80 F.3d 716 (2d Cir. 1996). Some state laws require that the patient be in a terminal condition as one of the prerequisites for implementing the living will form of an advance directive. If there is such a condition, many state laws (e.g., Indiana and Ohio) stipulate that there is a time element (e.g., "death within a short period of time," "death within a relatively brief period of time," etc.) that is necessary for a condition to be considered terminal. However, some states (e.g., Texas) have no such time limitation. (See Choice in dying. Refusal of treatment legislation. New York: Choice in Dying, 1996. This compilation of the laws in the fifty states allows one to determine the nuances of the various states in this matter.) Many states enlarge the condition for implementing an advance directive by including the condition known as a "persistent vegetative state." See King NMP. Making sense of advance directives. Revised edition. Washington, D.C.: Georgetown University Press, 1996, page 10. There is some modification of the "terminal condition" requirement when employing the healthcare proxy form of an advance directive. But there is no consistent pattern to this practice. For example, Ohio requires that the patient be in a terminal condition if the decision is about refusing life-sustaining treatments (Senate Bill 1, 1991), whereas New York does not (New York Public Health Law, par. 2980–2994 (McKinney 1994 and Supp. 1997)).

This author takes the view that the stipulation of a time period is misguided because it is an arbitrary designation. Medical indicators are the only reliable signs of a terminal condition and these are system failure, irreversibility, and deterioration. How long it will take a person to go though this process is irrelevant for calling the condition "terminal," although it may have some bearing on the extent of treatment the patient or her surrogate may wish to authorize while the patient is dying.

22. One might even wish to go to the extreme of utilizing terminal sedation, a practice suggested as a possibility for patients who are suffering from intense levels of pain that are difficult to control. See Rousseau P. Terminal sedation in the care of dying patients. Arch Intern Med 1996; 156:1785–1786.

23. Thomas D. The collected poems of Dylan Thomas. New York: New Directions Books, 1957, page 128.

24. Vacco v. Quill. 117 S. Ct. 2293 (1997).

25. See the discussion of *Bartling v. Superior Court* in chapter 2.

26. Kassirer JP. Our stubborn quest for diagnostic certainty. N Engl J Med 1989; 320:1489–1491.

27. Pellegrino ED, Thomasma DC. A philosophical basis of medical practice: Toward a philosophy and ethic of the healing professions. New York: Oxford University Press, 1981, page 60.

28. Rachels J. The elements of moral philosophy. 2d edition. New York: McGraw-Hill, Inc., 1993, page 182.

29. In re Osborne. 294 A. 2d 372 (1972).

30. Veatch RM. Models for ethical medicine in a revolutionary age. Hast Cent Rep 1972; 2:5–7.

31. It is surely a recognition of this moral feature of human experience that caused Justice Warren Burger to underscore "the right to be let alone," which was previously identified by Justice Louis Brandeis. Justice Burger eloquently spoke to the matter of taking risks when he wrote in commenting on Justice Brandeis: "Nothing in [his] utterance suggests that Justice Brandeis thought an individual possessed these rights only as to *sensible* beliefs, *valid* thoughts, *reasonable* emotions, or *well-founded* sensations. I suggest he intended to include a great many foolish, unreasonable, and even absurd ideas which do not conform, such as refusing medical treatment even at great risk." [emphasis in original]. Application of President and Directors of Georgetown College, 331 F. 2d 1010 (D.C. Cir.) (1964).

32. This dimension of excessive choices is not a new phenomenon, nor is it exclusive to medical practice. It can be observed in all facets of our lives. See Toffler A. Future shock. New York: Bantam Books, 1971, pages 343–367.

33. Levine S. Meetings at the edge: Dialogues with the grieving and the dying, the healing and the healed. New York: Anchor Press/Doubleday 1984, page 109.

34. Engelhardt HT. The bad, the ugly, and the unfortunate. In Spicker SF et al (eds). Ethical dimensions of geriatric care. Dordrecht-Holland: D. Reidel Publishing Co., 1987, pages 263–270.

35. There is an important difference between what we *can* spend as a society on healthcare and what we are *willing* to spend. Though we can spend a great deal more than we currently do, there seems to be a generalized unwillingness to increase spending on healthcare beyond current levels. If this attitude remains, then societal or self-imposed limits are inevitable. The curious feature that accompanies this phenomenon is that individuals are quite willing to accept these limitations when they apply to strangers but not when they apply to them or those they love.

36. Callahan D. Setting limits: Medical goals in an aging society. New York: Simon and Schuster, 1987, pages 141–153.

37. Whether the Patient Self-Determination Act will be instrumental in helping us draw those limits will have to remain an open question for the moment. However, some clues to this issue will be found in chapter 3, the section on technological pressures, and in chapter 5, note 40.

38. Lidz CW et al. Two models of implementing informed consent. Arch Intern Med 1988; 148:1385–1389.

39. Garrett TM et al. Health care ethics: Principles and problems. 3d edition. Upper Saddle River, NJ: Prentice Hall, 1998, page 7.

40. A sample of these codes would include the Code of Ethics of the American Medical Association (item # 1), the American Nurses' Association Code for Nurses (item # 1), and The Patients' Bill of Right developed by the American Hospital Association (item # 12).

41. Because the Patient Self-Determination Act places such emphasis on informing patients that they have the right to consent to or refuse treatments, and because such decisions can be made effectively only against the backdrop of patients' values and many other elements that are intensely personal to them, the Patient Self-Determination Act invites us to explore and understand the range of those elements that comprise the dignity of the patients who are making the decisions.

42. Immanuel Kant best articulated this approach to the issue of dignity with his basic moral principle that "persons are to be treated as ends and not merely as means." Kant I. Critique of practical reason. New York: Bobbs-Merrill Company Inc., 1956, pages 114–115. See also Kant I. Metaphysical foundations of morals. In Friedrich CJ (ed). The philosophy of Kant. New York: Modern Library, 1949, page 176.

43. National Conference of Catholic Bishops. Ethical and religious directives for Catholic health care services. Washington, D.C.: National Conference of Catholic Bishops, 1995, page 5.

44. Catechism of the Catholic church. Washington, D.C.: United States Catholic Conference, 1994, # 321.

45. Gould SJ. Ever since Darwin: Reflections in natural history. New York: W. W. Norton & Co., 1977, pages 113–114. See also Teilhard de Chardin P. Human energy. Cohen JM (trans). New York: Harcourt, Brace, Jovanovich, Inc., 1969, page 115.

46. Sartre JP. Being and nothingness. Barnes HE (trans). New York: The Citadel Press, 1965, pages 529–532.

47. Fackenheim EL. Metaphysics and historicity. Milwaukee, WI: Marquette University Press, 1961, pages 28–34.

48. Crawford C. The Buddhist response to health and disease in environmental perspective. In Fu CW, Wawrytho SA. Buddhist ethics and modern society. New York: Greenwood Press, 1991, pages 185–193.

49. Waters F. Book of the Hopi. New York: Penguin Books, 1963, pages 7–11.

50. Engelhardt HT. Medicine and the concept of person. In Beauchamp TL, Walters L. Contemporary issues in bioethics. 2d edition. 1982, page 95.

51. It is instructive to note that caregivers often misunderstand patients' attitudes toward healthcare interventions, presuming that patients would want an intervention when, in point of fact, they do not. Caregivers seem to be wrong as least as many times as they are right. (See Seckler AB. Substituted judgment: How accurate are proxy predictions? Ann Intern Med 1991; 115:92–98.) Thus, it is important for caregivers to explore the attitudes of patients about healthcare interventions. Moreover, the suggestion has been made that when patients or surrogates demand "futile" therapies, the proper response is to explore the patients' and/or surrogates' attitudes and feelings that prompt the demand rather than automatically comply with their wishes. See Ruark JE et al. Initiating and withdrawing life support. N Engl J Med 1998; 318:25–30. This approach to communication with patients and surrogates underscores the importance of this facet of personal dignity.

52. President's Commission for the Study of Ethical Problems in Medicine and Biomedical and Behavioral Research. Making health care decisions: The ethical and legal implications of informed consent in the patient-practitioner relationship. Washington, D.C.: U.S. Government Printing Office, 1982, pages 57–60.

53. MacIntyre, A. After virtue. Notre Dame, IN: University of Notre Dame Press, 1981, pages 202–204.

54. Fischhoff B. Acceptable risk. New York: Cambridge University Press, 1981, pages 2–7.

55. Allowing risk-taking choices is not only a matter of respecting one's moral integrity but a feature of our humanity protected by the law in the

classical notion of the right to be let alone. This right comes particularly into play when there are conflicts between patients and caregivers regarding appropriate risks. Justice Warren Burger put the matter very clearly when he wrote: "Nothing in [his] utterance suggests that Justice Brandeis thought an individual possessed these rights only as to *sensible* beliefs, *valid* thoughts, *reasonable* emotions, or *well-founded* sensations. I suggest he intended to include a great many foolish, unreasonable, and even absurd ideas which do not conform, such as refusing medical treatment even at great risk." [emphasis in original]. Application of President and Directors of Georgetown College, 331 F.2d 1010 (D.C. Cir.) (1964).

56. The four cases examined in chapter 2 are good examples of this phenomenon.

57. There may be more latitude accorded to an attorney-in-fact when appointed in a durable power of attorney for healthcare. See note 21, above.

58. The need for these conversations *and their implementation* has been made clear because of the inconsistency with which specific instructions from patients were followed in the SUPPORT study. See Teno JM et al. Do advance directives provide instructions that provide care? JAGS 1997; 45:508–512.

59. Walker RM. Living wills and resuscitation preferences in an elderly population. Arch Intern Med 1995; 155:171–175.

60. Carney MT, Morrison RS. Advance directives: When, why, and how to start talking. Geriatrics 1997; 52:65–73.

61. Pellegrino E. Altruism, self-interest, and medical ethics. JAMA 1987; 258:1939–40.

62. Carney MT, Morrison RS. Advance directives: When, why, and how to start talking. Geriatrics 1997; 52:65–73.

63. Aristotle. Nichomachean ethics. Irwin T (trans). Indianapolis, IN: Hackett Publishing Co., Inc. 1985, page 33.

64. Pellegrino ED, Thomasma DC. The virtues in medical practice. New York: Oxford University Press, 1993, page 5.

65. Aristotle puts this feature in a more poetic way when he says that "one swallow does not make a spring time." Aristotle. Nichomachean ethics. Irwin T (trans). Indianapolis, IN: Hackett Publishing Co., Inc. 1985, page 7.

66. Aristotle identifies this overall end as "happiness . . . that which all men seek." Ibid., page 1.

67. Engelhardt HT. The foundation of bioethics. 2d edition. New York: Oxford University Press, 1996, pages 74–83.

68. Ibid.

69. Ibid., pages 80–81. This, however, does not mean to imply that tolerance is a common "human" virtue. For there may be many societies

where tolerance is neither a regulative ideal to guide behavior nor a commonly practiced virtue.

70. Engelhardt HT. Bioethics and secular humanism: The search for a common morality. London: SCM Press, 1991, page 121.

71. Thomas Hobbes understood this in the seventeenth century and devoted much of his major treatise, *Leviathan,* to the major issues involved in the limitation of self-determination. Hobbes T. Leviathan. London: J. M. Dent and Sons, 1937, pages 66–74.

72. John Stuart Mill identified these special spheres of action as "self-regarding," actions that have an impact only upon the agent or have only a remote impact on others. Mill JS. *On liberty.* Buffalo, NY: Prometheus Books, 1986, page 18. What counts as "remote" is often in need of reflective discussion.

73. Aristotle. Nichomachean ethics. Irwin T (trans). Indianapolis, IN: Hackett Publishing Co., Inc. 1985, pages 42–43.

74. Drane JF. Becoming a good doctor: The place of virtue and character in medical ethics. Kansas City, MO: Sheed & Ward, 1988, page 157.

75. Polanyi M. Personal knowledge: Towards a post-critical philosophy. New York: Harper and Row, 1964, pages 299–303.

76. Pellegrino ED, Thomasma DC. The virtues in medical practice. New York: Oxford University Press, 1993, page 21.

77. Brody BA, Engelhardt HT. Bioethics: Readings and cases. Englewood Cliffs, NJ: Prentice-Hall, Inc., 1987, page 27.

78. Engelhardt HT. The foundations of bioethics. 2d edition. New York: Oxford University Press, 1996, page 289.

79. For example, a patient may hesitate to be decisive in determining the course of treatment. But this virtue is often essential and must be encouraged and supported if the patient is to empower the caregiver to practice her art. It may also be necessary if the patient is to stay the course of therapy, especially if the therapy is lengthy.

80. For example, a patient may come to the clinical setting without the virtue of curiosity because he had been previously encouraged to play only a passive role in his healthcare encounters. The importance of curiosity can be pointed out to him as an essential ingredient for the gathering of information to empower him to make treatment decisions that will help him accomplish his goals.

81. John Stuart Mill may have put this matter best when he said: "[T]he only purpose for which power can be rightfully exercised over any member of a civilized community, against his will, is to prevent harm to others. His own good, either physical or moral, is not a sufficient warrant. He cannot rightfully be compelled to do or forbear because it will be better for him to

do so, because it will make him happier, because, in the opinions of others, to do so would be wise, or even right. These are good reasons for remonstrating with him, or reasoning with him, or persuading him, or entreating him, but not for compelling him, or visiting him with any evil, in case he do otherwise. Mill JS. *On liberty*. Buffalo, NY: Prometheus Books, 1986, page 16.

82. American College of Physicians. Ethics manual. 3d edition. Philadelphia, PA: American College of Physicians, 1993, page 4. See also Council on Ethical and Judicial Affairs, AMA. Code of medical ethics: Current opinions with annotations. Chicago: American Medical Association, 1996, page xiv.

83. Engelhardt HT. The foundations of bioethics. 2d edition. New York: Oxford University Press, 1996, pages 419–420.

84. President's Commission for the Study of Ethical Problems in Medicine and Biomedical and Behavioral Research. Making health care decisions: The ethical and legal implications of informed consent in the patient-practitioner relationship. Washington, D.C.: U.S. Government Printing Office, 1982, pages 70–77.

85. Levine S. Healing into life and death. New York: Anchor Press/Doubleday, 1987, pages 252–255.

86. This matter will be discussed in detail in chapter 6.

87. Yalom ID. Existential psychotherapy. New York: Basic Books, 1980, pages 276–280.

88. This is not to say that the observations of the President's Commission related to "shared decision-making" as the ideal structure for informed consent have been nullified by the Patient Self-Determination Act. See President's Commission for the Study of Ethical Problems in Medicine and Biomedical and Behavioral Research. Making health care decisions: The ethical and legal implications of informed consent in the patient-practitioner relationship. Washington, D.C.: U.S. Government Printing Office, 1982, pages 15–39. The Patient Self-Determination Act reinforces the patient's role in participating in this process and stipulates some significant signposts for the physician-patient interaction.

89. The issue of patient responsibility will be extensively explored in chapter 9.

90. President's Commission for the Study of Ethical Problems in Medicine and Biomedical and Behavioral Research. Making health care decisions: The ethical and legal implications of informed consent in the patient-practitioner relationship. Washington, D.C.: US Government Printing Office, 1982. The commission takes the position that compliance is not truly an exercise of patient autonomy and, by implication, responsibility. In the view of the commission, true autonomy is exercised only when the patient has received

information and made a conscious and deliberate choice based upon that information.

91. At least one notable exception has been extensively debated in contemporary medical practice—physician-assisted suicide. The medical community has strongly asserted that they should not defer to patients' wishes for physician-assisted suicide no matter how grounded in virtue those wishes may be. See Callahan D. When self-determination runs amok. Hast Cent Rep March/April 1992; 22:52–55. These voices have been reinforced by the decision of the U.S. Supreme Court in Vacco v. Quill. 117 S. Ct. 2293 (1997).

92. Carney MT, Morrison RS. Advance directives: When, why, and how to start talking. Geriatrics 1997; 52:65–73.

93. Lidz CW et al. Two models of implementing informed consent. Arch Intern Med 1988; 148:1385–1389. The authors here address this matter by talking about the necessity for both patients and physicians to clarify their role expectations of each other early in the clinical encounter.

94. Loewy EH. Changing one's mind: When is Odysseus to be believed. J Gen Intern Med 1988; 3:54–58.

95. Pellegrino ED. Toward a reconstruction of medical morality: The primacy of the act of profession and the fact of illness. J Med Phil 1979; 4:32–56.

96. Drane JE. Becoming a good doctor: The place of virtue and character in medical ethics. Kansas City MO: Sheed & Ward, 1988, pages 14–19. Throughout this work there is a catalog of what the author considers the major virtues to be practiced by physicians: benevolence, truthfulness, respect, friendliness, justice, and religion. Another such catalog is found in Pellegrino ED, Thomasma DC. The virtues in medical practice. New York: Oxford University Press, 1993, pages 65–164. Their catalog includes trust, fidelity, compassion, phronesis (prudence), justice, fortitude, temperance, integrity, and self-effacement. A similar, but shorter, catalog is found in Brody BA, Engelhardt HT. Bioethics: Readings and cases. Englewood Cliffs, NJ: Prentice-Hall, Inc., 1987; pages 23–27. They identify compassion, courage, honesty, and integrity.

97. Pellegrino ED. The virtuous physician and the ethics of medicine. In Shelp EE (ed). Virtue and medicine: Explorations in the character of medicine. Dordrecht-Holland: D. Reidel Publishing Co., 1985, pages 243–255.

98. Pellegrino ED, Thomasma DC. The virtues in medical practice. New York: Oxford University Press, 1993, page 144.

99. See chapter 3 for an examination of this relationship.

100. Engelhardt, HT. The foundations of bioethics. 2d edition. New York: Oxford University Press, 1996, pages 74–78.

101. President's Commission for the Study of Ethical Problems in Medicine and Biomedical and Behavioral Research. Making health care decisions: The ethical and legal implications of informed consent in the patient-practitioner relationship. Washington, D.C.: U.S. Government Printing Office, 1982, page 3. "Patients are not entitled to insist that health care practitioners furnish them services when to do so would violate either the bounds of acceptable practice or a professional's own deeply held moral beliefs or would draw on a limited resource on which the patient has no binding claim." The most recently debated public issue that falls into these restricted areas is physician-assisted suicide.

102. Aristotle. Nichomachean ethics. Irwin T (trans). Indianapolis, IN: Hackett Publishing Co., Inc. 1985, page 44.

103. The difficulty in making these stipulations and exercising prudence in this process will be closely examined in chapter 7.

104. Engelhardt HT. The foundations of bioethics. 2d edition. New York: Oxford University Press, 1996, page 419.

105. Mill JS. On liberty. Buffalo, NY: Prometheus Books, 1986, page 16. "[T]he sole end for which mankind is warranted, individually or collectively in interfering with the liberty of action of any of their number, is self-protection. . . . [T]he only purpose for which power can be rightfully exercised over any member of a civilized community, against his will, is to prevent harm to others."

5

The Institutional Context of the Patient Self-Determination Act

As medical practice became institutionalized in the modern world, it became customary for institutions to provide a place where physicians could care for their patients in a closely supervised setting.[1] At the same time institutions were careful to avoid any interference in the physician-patient relationship.[2] The physician has been viewed as a primary caregiver.[3] Physicians were responsible for communicating with their patients and giving them information about their conditions and their treatments, provided the physician thought the patient should have such information. The physician determined the course of treatment and decided when the treatment should commence and stop.

Thus it is strange that the Patient Self-Determination Act applies only to healthcare *facilities* while exempting physicians from its requirements. It might seem that requiring healthcare institutions to discuss the issues covered by the Patient Self-Determination Act would be an inappropriate intrusion into the physician's fiduciary relationship with the patient. Additionally, the institutional requirement could be construed as an undue burden on healthcare institutions already overburdened by bureaucratic regulations and reporting requirements. Regardless of the concerns that could be raised about the place where conversations about the Patient Self-Determination

Act belong, institutions were given a new role. In many ways this was a role that was unfamiliar to them and one for which many were ill prepared. And yet it is not an unnatural role. It is one that, if fulfilled with diligence, can significantly improve the quality of the decision-making process in the clinical setting because it can encourage patients to begin reflecting on approaches to treatment before the immediacy of decisions is upon them.[4]

The Social Obligations of Institutions

The institutions identified by the Patient Self-Determination Act as having obligations under the law are all those healthcare institutions that are supported in any way by Medicare or Medicaid funding.[5] This stipulation includes hospitals, extended care facilities, HMOs, hospices, and home health services. If these organizations receive government payment for their services to their patients, they fall under the restrictions of the law. The proper information has to be given to the patient or the patient's authorized surrogate upon admission to the facility or upon enrollment in the health maintenance organization.

The institutions are required to inform patients of their right to consent to or refuse treatment, their rights under their state's laws regarding advance directives, and the policies of the institution regarding the withholding or withdrawing of life-sustaining treatments.[6] This information is required to be in written form so that there can be some assurance that patients have received it. There must also be documentation that the information has been given and the status of the patient's advance directive, if any. Institutions are also obligated to conduct ongoing educational forums for employees and the local community about the stipulations of the Patient Self-Determination Act.

Healthcare institutions now have obligations imposed upon them based upon the (positive) right of the patient to have certain information.[7] No longer can these institutions either say that the obligation to convey the information belongs to the physician or hold themselves free from negligence if the patient does not receive the information.[8] Accordingly, the law may create a new and serious area of liability for institutions that can now be held accountable in court for failure to

provide the designated information.[9] Furthermore, it could be inferred that the liability extends to the delivery of any care that is
contrary to the information the patient has received.[10] These institutions now have become powerful social agents, not only for the
delivery of healthcare but also for the quality of the decision making
which occurs within their confines.

Informing patients (or surrogates) of hospital policies regarding the
withholding and withdrawing of life-sustaining treatments and removing treatment from critically ill patients emerged as a significant issue in
the case of Karen Quinlan. Until *Quinlan* in 1976,[11] decisions about
withholding treatment or withdrawing it from patients who could not
benefit from it were made at the bedside.[12] The decision was made as
the result of discussions among the physician, the patient (if he or she
possessed decisional capacity), and the patient's family. Indeed, if the
Quinlan court had had its way, this pattern would have continued and
the court would not have become involved. Its opinion clearly stated
that the preferred place for making such decisions was at the patient's
bedside and not in the courtroom,[13] but since the matter had been
brought to the court, it had no alternative but to enter into the decision.

Many of these decisions remain at the bedside in the healthcare
setting today. As a matter of fact, since *Quinlan* and until 1988 only
about seventy-five cases of withholding or withdrawing treatment
have gone to court.[14] Healthcare practices indicate that there have
been and continue to be many more such decisions every day in
healthcare institutions. But even though the practice has continued,
healthcare professionals and institutions have become increasingly
nervous about making such decisions independently of the courts.
This became a particular problem when some courts, such as the one
in *Superintendent of Belchertown State School v. Sakewicz,* said that
every such decision should be made by the courts.[15] In contrast, *In re
Colyer* set up a procedure for making these end-of-life decisions for
incompetents and explicitly indicated that recourse to the courts was
unnecessary.[16]

The *Quinlan* court attempted to suggest procedural avenues that
could ensure the quality of the decision-making process in withholding or withdrawing treatment. It suggested the establishment of ethics
committees in healthcare institutions that would review such cases
and determine the appropriateness of the decision. Ethics committees

began to be formed in significant numbers after *Quinlan*,[17] but few institutions mandated a review of *all* cases involving the withholding or withdrawing of life-sustaining treatments. Instead, they reviewed cases that were brought to them and discharged the role of *adviser* rather than *adjudicator*.[18] But even this was not sufficient to make institutions and healthcare professionals feel comfortable about making such serious decisions, particularly when the possibility of appeals to the courts was still very strong.

Institutions turned to the task of formulating policies addressing end-of-life decisions, often through the efforts of their ethics committees.[19] The policies thus designed are largely procedural in character rather than substantive. That is, the policies point out the considerations that have to be made, the individuals to be consulted, and the documentation that must be provided. They have seldom, if ever, stipulated that in a particular case, treatment is to be withheld or withdrawn. Current concerns about futile care and healthcare economics have led some institutions to develop policies that govern the withholding or withdrawing of treatment with certain well-defined criteria that are still primarily procedural in character.[20]

Prior to the passage of the Patient Self-Determination Act many institutions had developed policies that addressed DNR (Do Not Resuscitate) orders.[21] Some had developed policies about the removal of ventilator support.[22] A few had policies about artificial nutrition and hydration.[23] And in extended care facilities even fewer had policies about transferring patients to the hospital.[24] There is no doubt that many more policies on these matters have been developed than are reported. There was a flurry of activity in this area as the Cruzan case was moving through the courts. Activity increased after the Supreme Court decision and after the Patient Self-Determination Act was passed.[25]

Even though the policies were in effect at the institutions providing their care, patients frequently did not know of the existence or content of the policies. They became aware of them only when caregivers brought them to the patient's or surrogate's attention with the aim of utilizing them in the patient's case. Patients or surrogates had no way of initiating the implementation of the policy in their own right or of checking to be sure that the policy was being followed correctly when its implementation was suggested. Thus, information about a very significant piece of the patients' care was withheld from them. The resulting lack of power adversely affected the patient's or surrogate's ability to participate in the full range of clinical decisions.

Since information about the policies of healthcare facilities is now required by the Patient Self-Determination Act, patients have gained two significant advantages. First of all, they can decide at the time of admission whether they wish to be in facilities with certain policies. Second, they are now empowered to begin discussions about withholding or withdrawing treatment when they think it is appropriate. They do not have to wait for others—that is, caregivers—to decide when it might be appropriate to begin thinking about applying a particular policy in a particular patient's case. Thus patients have the liberty to follow their own value agenda rather than being submissive to the value agenda of another.[26]

Moreover, patients or surrogates can check to be sure that the healthcare facility or their caregivers are following the policy that governs the institutional behavior in a particular area. Sometimes policies are not followed correctly and patients suffer considerably because of it. Some physicians who may practice at an institution only on rare occasions, or who seldom have critical cases in an institution, may be unfamiliar with the institution's policies or simply ignore them.

Finally, there is a great advantage to knowing a facility's policies on withholding and withdrawing treatments before submitting oneself to its services. A patient or surrogate may not like a particular policy of a healthcare facility and would like to look for a facility whose policies are more suitable. For example, some extended care facilities may have policies requiring a certain calorie intake by residents and, if necessary, will deliver those calories by artificial nutrition and hydration. Or a facility might have certain stipulations about DNR orders that do not fit into the patient's views on her quality of life.[27] It is best to know these policies at the beginning rather than become involved in treatment that will make transfer to another facility difficult, if not impossible.

This knowledge of policies is particularly important when it comes to the matter of advance directives. Most advance directive legislation contains a "conscience" clause that allows a physician or a facility to refuse to honor advance directives in some cases.[28] Patients who feel strongly about their advance directives would surely want to know about the scope of a conscience clause before entering into treatment with those physicians or facilities.[29]

Most healthcare facilities are "public" institutions or resources insofar as they are available to provide service to the general public. As such they are accountable to those whom they serve. Their obligations extend not only to providing the highest-quality technical care possible but also to discharging their duties of respect for the personal dignity for those whom they serve. This means that they must maximize the ability of individuals to make careful choices about the direction of their care and see to it that their patients receive all the information necessary for them to make choices that fit within their value life. They would do well to reduce and even eliminate the possibility that their patients will become victims of an institutional atmosphere at odds with the patients' views of their own best interest.

Institutions that provide statements of the required policies to their patients demonstrate that they take their social obligations seriously. They approach their services from a holistic perspective ("holistic" extends to ethical concerns) and provide the atmosphere that allows their patients to thrive as good decision makers and to receive cures for their syndromes or relief of their symptoms. Making this decision-making opportunity possible with full disclosure of information about institutional policies that directly affect both the life and death of their patients demonstrates both institutional respect for patients and institutional integrity.

The Mission of the Institution

Most institutions have mission statements that express the fundamental beliefs and commitments the institutions have made to those whom they serve and to the community at large.[30] Whether simple or elaborate, healthcare mission statements generally have one thing in common—namely, a commitment to respect the dignity of the patient. It is important now to outline some of the extraordinary challenges that the Patient Self-Determination Act presents for the mission of healthcare institutions.

The law requires that *notification* be given to patients or their authorized surrogates about the stipulations of the law. In many ways this requirement is not particularly burdensome because it requires only that the notifications be written. State Departments of Health are encouraged to develop some of the written material on advance directives so they will be uniform across the state. Of course, written institutional policies have to be generated by the institutions themselves. But a serious question arises as to whether this approach is sufficient to guard the patient's right to know the information required by the law.

When patients are admitted to a healthcare facility, they are met with an avalanche of papers; some are to be signed, some are to be read at the time of admission, some may be read during the patient's stay at the facility, and some are to be read when the patient prepares to leave the institution. The apprehension caused by a stay in a healthcare facility is such that many times the papers are only read in a cursory fashion, if at all. For this reason, written information alone will not work effectively to discharge the obligation of the law. There is a significant need for conversations to be held with the patient at some point during the patient's stay in the institution.[31] The earlier the conversation is held, the better it will be for the patient because the patient can begin to reflect upon the information before the immediate moment of decision arises and while caregivers are available for the discussions. It will also be important that some monitoring of the patient be conducted to determine whether more than one conversation should be held about the issues contained in the Patient Self-Determination Act.[32]

An institution that takes seriously its mission commitment of respecting the dignity of patients will expend extra effort to be sure that its patients are able to benefit from the information involved in the Patient Self-Determination Act. Such an institution needs to provide a mechanism to *assist* patients in understanding and processing the stipulations of the law within the context of the patient's own beliefs and value commitments.[33] From the outset of this phase of our discussion it must be noted that conflicts of interests may be a matter of concern. If employees act as agents of a healthcare institution, it is conceivable that they may try to persuade a patient to make certain types of decisions that would benefit the institution rather than the patient. It is precisely because of possible conflicts of interest that communicators must be well trained to elicit from patients and surrogates decisions that flow from *their* life experiences and values rather than from the agenda of the institution. For an institution to take a minimalist stand and provide only the bare essentials required by the law without assistance in processing that information in the interests of "neutrality" will leave the patient disempowered and without the skill necessary to make extremely important healthcare decisions.

Assistance becomes an institutional issue if the institution wishes both to promote the best decision-making atmosphere for its patients and to minimize its liability in the face of the law. Patients can hold institutions both morally and legally accountable for not providing them with information they need in making decisions about their care or for not helping them understand the information. Malpractice litigation considers both features when dealing with informed consent.[34]

The mission commitments of an institution to uphold patient dignity go beyond the minimum required to avoid malpractice claims. They should encompass attempts to make patients better decision makers. This requires them to help patients understand what it means to refuse treatments, what matters need to be considered, and how they should be weighed. Patients need to get a clear sense of the role advance directives can play in their healthcare—both the positive aspects and the shortcomings. In other words, patients must have a solid understanding of the choices that may affect their lives and deaths. These are major issues to consider if patients are to have power over their futures in the decision-making process.[35]

A healthcare institution must consider hiring the necessary personnel or retraining those already employed to work with patients to help them understand the range of decisions opened to them by the Patient Self-Determination Act.[36] This ability does not occur automatically, nor is everyone capable of providing the necessary assistance. A variety of approaches can be utilized, but it is essential to avoid the fallacious belief that understanding of these matters will occur with a mere shuffling of papers. We know that is not the case with traditional informed consents.[37] Why would we think any differently about the Patient Self-Determination Act?

Institutions have a predictable economic concern when a new need for personnel is suggested. Immediately, new expenditures of limited healthcare dollars are visualized. Whether the use of advance directives or treatment refusals in terminal cases will save a great deal of money in overall healthcare resource allocation has not been definitively determined. There are conflicting studies on this matter. Emanuel and Emanuel indicate that, at best, 3.3 percent of national expenditures may be saved; this is translated into $29.7 billion of $900 billion in total expenditures.[38] On the other hand, Chambers et al. indicate that a substantial sum of money (65%) could be saved in the Medicare population they studied.[39] At any rate, in individual cases the savings might amount to a substantial sum.[40]

But only a cursory reflection on the experience of healthcare professionals with critically ill patients may reveal that new personnel expenditures are appropriate. In fact, the effective implementation of the Patient Self-Determination Act may well result in respectable savings in healthcare dollars. For example, at the end of a patient's long, tedious, and fruitless stay in an intensive care unit many families of patients are heard to remark: "Was this really necessary?" "Why did we do this?" "I wish we could have stopped this treatment when it was clear that it wasn't doing any good." "The patient would never have wanted this!" "The patient told me not to let this sort of thing happen!" A combination of advance directives, utilization of futile-care policies, treatment refusals, and effective palliative care would not only result in cost savings but provide better care by addressing the patient's needs and wishes in the context of the Patient Self-Determination Act.[41]

The law is criticized by healthcare professionals who think that such conversations or exchanges of information are inappropriate at the time of admission.[42] At this time patients are already nervous and fearful about what they may be facing when they come to a healthcare facility. To suggest that they might want to consider refusing treatments, or that there might be a need for an advance directive in case they should lose decisional capacity during their stay, could have serious adverse reactions for their mental health at a time when they may need all the composure they can muster.

Though it may be questioned, there is some legitimacy in this criticism.[43] While anxiety may focus the attention of some individuals in making decisions, for other patients it can result in anxiety and fear that distort the ability to think clearly.[44] For this reason great care must be taken in developing communication processes that make patients comfortable while, at the same time, giving the necessary information.[45] Here again the mission of the institution plays a major role in respecting patient's fears while, at the same time, empowering them as decision makers.

Expectations should not be too high that the conversations with patients about the Patient Self-Determination Act will be fruitful.[46] It may take time for patients and families to assimilate all the necessary information and respond accordingly. This is partly why the conversations have to be conducted with each admission for each patient. Ultimately the information will permeate the patient population and, though the Patient Self-Determination Act may not be particularly effective on the first admission, it may gradually affect patients and their families at a future time.[47]

The edge can be taken off the concerns about the conversations being conducted upon admission by preparing patients for these conversations *prior to* admission to the healthcare facility. One way to prepare patients would be to conduct the required educational programs in the community. We shall examine these in the next section. Another way would be to encourage physicians to begin a discussion with their patients about these matters in their offices.[48] Physicians can have a powerful influence on patients by their suggestions alone.[49] Healthcare facilities can promote these conversations by generating literature about the issues covered in the Patient Self-Determination Act that can be made available to patients in their physician's offices. Physicians can call this material to the attention of their patients and begin the conversations where patients may be more comfortable and where they can discuss these difficult issues with a person in whom they have already expressed their confidence.

By utilizing the existing resources of the offices of physicians who practice in their institutions, healthcare facilities make another important step in delivering on their mission commitments to respect and promote the dignity of their patients. This approach can make patients much better decision makers by helping them to appreciate that they and their physicians constitute a collaborative team. Patients will not come to the healthcare institution for admission thinking that their physicians might have told the institution something they did not confide in the patient directly simply because they hear for the first time about refusing treatment and about signing or drafting an advance directive.

The Patient Self-Determination Act provides an opportunity for institutions to rededicate themselves to their mission commitments in tangible ways.[50] The mission of a healthcare institution is a very significant part of its operation, but it is not often as visibly presented as the Patient Self-Determination Act encourages it to be. Whether it is driven by religious beliefs or commitments or by simply humanitarian concerns, the mission tells patients that the institution is willing to go beyond minimal requirements to meet the needs of its patients. It tells patients that their welfare as total persons is important and that it will take the extra steps necessary to ensure their well-being. Patients can tell whether an institution has such commitments and takes them seriously. They can feel when their dignity is an object of respect, and they can have trust and confidence in such a facility.

Healthcare Institutions as Centers of Education

One of the most far-reaching stipulations of the Patient Self-Determination Act is the requirement that healthcare institutions that are governed by the law must conduct ongoing educational programs for their employees and the community on the stipulations of the law. At the time the law went into effect and for about a year or so thereafter many institutions conducted such programs. However, with the passage of time the programs have dwindled in frequency. Healthcare institutions will have to remain vigilant about conducting the programs. Turnover in personnel in the institution and the need to continually bring before the public eye the decision-making factors of the law necessitate some frequency in the programs to be offered. The patient population in need of information related to the Patient Self-Determination Act is always changing as individuals develop healthcare concerns and as the population ages.

It is appropriate that institutions educate their employees for a number of reasons. The most obvious is that if the institution is to discharge its obligations under the law in the context of its mission commitments, the staff members entering into conversations with patients or their surrogates must be skilled communicators who are knowledgeable about both the law and the ethical issues it raises. This requires some in-depth understanding of patient concerns and the ability to help patients bring them to the surface for examination and action. Comprehensive training programs ensure that staff members acquire such knowledge and skills, including the skill of avoiding elements in their conversations that might be interpreted as conflicts of interest.

There is another group of employees who would profit greatly from education about the Patient Self-Determination Act. Those who may not be directly implementing the law still have a direct interest in any alterations in the climate of healthcare delivery that the institution may experience as a result of the law. For example, if patients have made certain decisions about treatment refusals, there must be a continuity between these decisions and the care they receive throughout their association with the institution. Not only the decisions patients make but the attitude of caregivers toward them must be carefully monitored. It would clearly be a violation of patients' dignity if they had discussed information in the context of the Patient Self-Determination Act at the time of admission only to find that subsequently caregivers either did not understand the basis for the patients' decisions or attempted to undermine the rights the patients were exercising.

Another reason for educating all employees is that they are a ready audience for learning about becoming more reflective participants in healthcare decisions for themselves. They, too, may be patients one day and to understand their rights within a healthcare context will give them an important advantage. Beginning to think about their own healthcare situations and the decisions they may face in the future should help them to develop greater empathy for their patients who are facing those difficult decisions at the present time. It would be paradoxical for employees of healthcare institutions to be expected to enter into reflection and dialogue with patients about the important and sensitive matters required by the Patient Self-Determination Act without having addressed those issues for themselves. The learning acquired through the self-examination fostered by a sound educational program will put employees at a decided advantage in dealing effectively with patients.

Educational programs in the community can provide considerable assistance to potential patients in understanding what they will be told at the time they are admitted to the healthcare facilities. This may reduce their fear and make the exchange of information at the time of admission more effective. Advance directives need considerable thought before they are signed or drafted. Educational programs can set that thought process in motion. And since not all individuals will be ready to address the issue of advance directives at the same time, periodic programs need to be made available to individuals who are beginning to consider their value.

Community education is an ideal method to begin conveying the information relevant to the Patient Self-Determination Act. As was pointed out in the previous section, patients seeking the services of a healthcare institution often experience considerable anxiety and preoccupation with the cause of their admission. As a result, they may block the information presented to them, avoid making decisions that need to be made, or make decisions that are not appropriate for their conditions.

Community education is one of the most useful tools to address the difficulties of having conversations about the Patient Self-Determination Act at the time of admission. When individuals come to community educational programs, they are not experiencing the same vulnerability that they would at the time of admission to a healthcare institution. They are normally not facing a healthcare crisis. They are in familiar surroundings, and they know that after the program is finished they can go home, where they can forget about all they were told if the information is too burdensome for them.[51] The matters can be discussed in a calm and congenial atmosphere rather than in the emotionally charged atmosphere of admitting rooms or elsewhere in the clinical setting. They can discuss the issues with others who have similar concerns and reflect upon them without feeling the pressure to come to immediate decisions.

Some sort of follow-up is essential for these programs to be successful. Often questions occur to individuals after the initial educational program has concluded, and there should be some way to address the questions when they arise. Either a second informal opportunity for the group attending the educational setting can be provided or a contact person or persons at the healthcare facility can be identified. Additional questions could be addressed to these individuals. If the subsequent questions are not addressed in a timely fashion, they may be forgotten or neglected until it is too late to deal with them in a calm and nonthreatening atmosphere. The next time they may be addressed may very well be when the individual is admitted to the facility or is in crisis. And this may be too late to give them reflective consideration.

Healthcare institutions have several options for conducting the mandated educational programs. They can conduct them on their own premises, which will likely result in a less than optimal response. Potential patients are often reluctant to come to hospitals or other healthcare facilities for reasons other than treatment interventions. Or they can make programs available to local organizations that can provide a ready audience. For example, programs can be conducted under the sponsorship of local churches. Many individuals find this to be the place for the discussion of serious issues about the meaning of life and death. An atmosphere of trust probably already permeates such gatherings, and the features of the Patient Self-Determination Act will receive careful consideration.

Service clubs could also provide an important venue for such programs. Here the companionship of the club members would help to dispel anxiety and provide the atmosphere for an open and honest sharing of the concerns of the members. Health maintenance organizations may wish to have periodic group meetings to help their members understand the stipulations of the law and use it to their advantage.

Finally, employers may wish to cooperate with healthcare institutions in presenting programs for their employees. To help employees become wiser and more reflective consumers of healthcare not only will benefit the employees directly but may also have a positive impact on the rising costs of healthcare about which employers are so deeply concerned.

One creative approach has been for healthcare facilities to make their meeting rooms available to physicians' groups, who can conduct programs in cooperation with the institution's personnel.[52] These programs are conducted for the patients of a particular group practice. Such programs have the advantages of getting the information to patients, letting them talk to their physicians about their concerns in a group setting, and reducing the time needed to talk about these matters in their physician's office.

In summary, then, healthcare institutions have important choices to make about implementing the Patient Self-Determination Act. They can follow the easier path of giving "Miranda" type information to patients, such as "You have the right to refuse treatment and your rights in this state regarding advance directives are . . . and, furthermore, the policies in this institution regarding withholding and withdrawing treatment are. . . . " They can add to that minimal compliance perfunctory and infrequent educational programs that few people will attend.

Or they can take the more challenging approach, consistent with their mission commitments, of going beyond notification to embellishing the information with appropriate value content and massaging it into the patients' beliefs, value preferences, and life goals so that they can make reflective decisions that will have a significant impact on their healthcare decisions and their lives. They can design truly effective educational programs, providing a comprehensive view of the issues, which will extend the spirit of the Patient Self-Determination Act throughout the population, thereby becoming dynamic contributors to the life of the community. The social obligations of healthcare institutions as centers of education as well as centers of medical practice and their mission commitments would seem to dictate the latter approach.

NOTES

1. Mechanic D. The growth of bureaucratic medicine: An inquiry into the dynamics of patient behavior and the organization of medical care. New York: John Wiley & Sons, 1976, pages 9–13.

2. Pellegrino ED. Humanism and the physician. Knoxville TN: University of Tennessee Press, 1979, pages 147–150.

3. May WF. The physician's covenant: Images of the healer in medical ethics. Philadelphia PA: Westminster Press, 1983, pages 29–31.

4. Oleson KJ. A quality improvement focus for patient rights: Advance directives. J Nurs Care Qual 1994; 8:52–67.

5. Patient Self-Determination Act of 1990, sections 4206 and 4751 of Omnibus Reconciliation Act of 1990, Pub L No. 101–508 (November 5, 1990). See chapter 1, note 1.

6. Ibid.

7. The right is a positive one requiring institutions to engage in an activity

to accomplish the good implicit in the law. This is in contrast to a negative right, which would require an institution only to refrain from behavior that might interfere with an individual's exercise of a right. See Facione PA et al. Ethics and society. 2d edition. Upper Saddle River, N.J.: Prentice Hall, 1991, pages 108–110. For example, the First Amendment to the U.S. Constitution identifies negative rights: "Congress shall make no law. . . . " In the Patient Self-Determination Act the healthcare organization has to do something —give information—rather than refrain from doing something.

8. If the healthcare facility has a moral responsibility, it may be said that, in this case, it has an accompanying legal responsibility as well. See De George RT. The moral responsibility of the hospital. J Med Phil 1982; 7:87–100.

9. Paridy N. Complying with the Patient Self-Determination Act: Legal, ethical, and practical challenges for hospitals. Hosp & Health Servs Admin 1993; 38:287–296.

10. Mulholland KC. Protecting the right to die: The Patient Self-Determination Act of 1990. Harvard J on Legis 1991; 28:609–630.

11. In re Quinlan. 70 N.J. 10, 355 A.2d 647 (1976).

12. Weir RF, Gostin L. Decisions to abate life-sustaining treatment for nonautonomous patients: Ethical standards and legal liability for physicians after *Cruzan*. JAMA 1990; 264:1846–1853.

13. In re Quinlan. 70 N.J. 10, 355 A.2d 647 (1976), page 668.

14. Emanuel EJ. A review of the ethical and legal aspects of terminating medical care. Am J Med 1988; 84:291–301. Since *Cruzan* the number has abated significantly.

15. Superintendent of Belchertown State School v. Sakewicz. 373 Mass. 728, 370 N.E.2d 417 (1977).

16. In re Colyer. 660 P.2d 738 (Wash. 1983)

17. This is not to say that there were no ethics committees before *Quinlan*. There were, but their number was very small.

18. Craig RP et al. Ethics committees: A practical approach. St. Louis MO: Catholic Health Association of the United States, 1986, page 4.

19. To 1996 approximately sixty institutions have reported their policies on withholding and withdrawing treatment. These policies can be found in Monagle JF, Thomasma DC (eds). Medical ethics: Policies, protocols, guidelines & programs. Gaithersburg MD: Aspen Publishers, Inc., 1996, sections 5 and 6. No doubt many more institutions have such policies. This compilation provides only a sample of the wide range of approaches to this matter.

20. Dayton, OH: Grandview Hospital and Medical Center, 1998. Columbus, OH: Mount Carmel Health, 1996. Anderson, IN: Saint John's Health System, 1995. Kokomo, IN: Saint Joseph Hospital and Health Center, 1995.

Santa Monica, CA: Santa Monica-UCLA Medical Center, 1991. See also Halevy A, Brody BA. A multi-institution collaborative policy on medical futility. JAMA 1996; 276:571–574.

21. Seventeen such policies are reported in Monagle JF, Thomasma DC (eds). Medical ethics: Policies, protocols, guidelines & programs. Gaithersburg MD: Aspen Publishers, Inc. 1996, section 5.

22. Sixteen such policies are reported in Monagle & Thomasma (eds.), ibid.

23. Two are reported in ibid.

24. Only one such policy is reported in ibid.: South Bend IN: Holy Cross Care Services, 1989.

25. After the Patient Self-Determination Act the activity focused on policies regarding advance directives. Only eleven such policies are reported in Monagle and Thomasma (eds), ibid., as samples of these policies, but it would probably be safe to say that a large majority of healthcare facilities have some form of advance directive policy at this time.

26. This issue becomes particularly significant if a patient is being admitted into an institution that has religious sponsorship and thus some particular religious values it wishes to uphold. An example would be the prohibition against sterilization, which occurs as a result of Roman Catholic sponsorship. See National Conference of Catholic Bishops. Ethical and religious directives for Catholic health care services. Washington, D.C.: United States Catholic Conference, 1995, directive 53. This matter could also be a concern in institutions that might have some particular beliefs about the role of nutrition and hydration in the care of terminal patients. See Committee on Ethical Responsibility. The role of medically administered nutrition and hydration. Kokomo, IN: Saint Joseph Hospital and Health Center, 1990.

27. Dorff EN. A Jewish approach to end-stage medical care. Conservative Judaism 1991; 43:3–51. In the Orthodox Jewish approach to end-of-life decisions (particularly in post-Holocaust theology), a poor quality of life is not sufficient to warrant withholding or withdrawing life-sustaining treatments.

28. King NMP. Making sense of advance directives. Revised edition. Washington, D.C.: Georgetown University Press, 1996, pages 153 and 251. "The federal regulations that implement the PSDA also require providers to give patients 'a clear and precise statement' describing how services will be limited according to any conscience clause policy regarding advance directives" (page 251). This issue will be examined in more detail in chapters 7 and 8. But a quick overview of advance directive legislation reveals that the conscience clause is often found. There should be good reason, of course, to employ it. A simple disagreement with a patient would not suffice.

29. Kapp MB. State statutes limiting advance directives: Death warrants or life sentences? JAGS 1992; 40:722–726.

30. Reiser SJ. The ethical life of health care organizations. Hast Cent Rep 1994; 24:28–35.

31. Informed consent about any healthcare issue is seldom satisfied without some discussion with a caregiver. Katz J. The silent world of doctor and patient. New York: Free Press, 1984, pages 59–80. The more serious the matter, the more extensive the conversation needs to be. Few matters are more serious than when to withhold or withdraw treatment in cases of critical illness.

32. The rationale, dynamics, and advantages of this ongoing monitoring will be more fully explored in the discussion on informed consent in chapter 6. See Lidz CW et al. Two models of implementing informed consent. Arch Intern Med 1988; 148:1385–89. The goal of this monitoring is to move beyond the passing of information to genuine comprehension on the part of the patient.

33. To provide this assistance, individuals trained in discussing healthcare matters are essential. The least desirable alternative would be the utilization of the admitting clerk to reflect on some of these issues with patients. Admission personnel are ordinarily trained neither in discussing healthcare alternatives nor in communication processes. See Wolf SM et al. Sources of concern about the Patient Self-Determination Act. N Engl J Med 1991; 325:1666–1671.

34. Veatch RM. The patient-physician relationship: The patient as partner, part 2. Bloomington, IN: Indiana University Press, 1991, pages 86–91. See also Hickson GB et al. Factors that prompted families to file medical malpractice claims following perinatal injuries. JAMA 1992; 267:1359–1363.

35. The SUPPORT study, published in 1995, raises serious questions about the ability of caregivers to improve patient decision making. There are many ways to interpret this study, one of which is simply to say that improvement cannot be accomplished. Another way is to say that current methods are not working, so more innovative approaches may need to be tried. The authors themselves suggest that we must try "more creative efforts at shaping the treatment process, and, perhaps, more proactive and forceful attempts at change" (page 1597). It is this challenge that this book is attempting to meet. See Connors AF et al. (the SUPPORT principal investigators). A controlled trial to improve care for seriously ill hospitalized patients: The study to understand prognoses and preferences for outcomes and risks of treatments (SUPPORT). JAMA 1995; 274:1591–1598.

36. The SUPPORT study, ibid., claims that this move may be of no advantage. Unfortunately, that was certainly the case in the study, but it does

not mean, as the authors conclude, that redoubled efforts would not have been more successful. Though it may not be appropriate to set one's educational goals too high, it is certainly possible to improve on current practice.

37. Weston WW, Lipkin M. Doctors learning communication skills: Developmental issues. In Stewart M, Roter D (eds). Communicating with medical patients. Newbury Park, CA: Sage Publications, 1989, pages 43–57.

38. Emanuel EJ, Emanuel LL. The economics of dying: The illusion of cost savings at the end of life. N Engl J Med 1994; 330:540–544.

39. Chambers CV et al. Relationship of advance directives to hospital charges in a Medicare population. Arch Intern Med 1994; 154:541–547. The reality of significant savings in the Medicare population is confirmed in Cher DJ, Lenert LA. Method of Medicare reimbursement and the rate of potentially ineffective care of critically ill patients. JAMA 1997; 278:1001–1007. This latter study projects an annual savings of $48 million in California alone, if more careful attention is paid to clinical judgments and the futility of treatments. Similar savings might analogously be realized by the effective use of advance directives.

40. One need only consider the costs of Nancy Cruzan's care after it was clear that she was in a persistent vegetative state. Those costs can be estimated from court documents, based on a cost of $130,000 per year, to be approximately $850,000. Cruzan v. Harmon. 760 S.W. 2d 408 (Mo. 1988) (en banc). If the estimate is correct that 15,000 to 25,000 patients in the United States are in a persistent vegetative state, with a conservative estimate of $40,000 per year per patient in extended-care facility costs (rather than rehabilitation center costs like those for Nancy Cruzan), the figure of $600 million to $1 billion gives some idea of costs in one disease category. See Payne K. Physicians' attitudes about the care of patients in the persistent vegetative state: A national survey. Ann Intern Med 1996; 125:104–110. Payne's estimate is $1 to $7 billion in healthcare costs. Full use of advance directives could be significant. However, if only 15 percent (the figure usually quoted for advance directive usage in the general population: see Lapuma J et al. Advance directives on admission: Clinical implications and analysis of the Patient Self-Determination Act. JAMA 1991; 266:402–405) of those patients had advance directives, then only $90 to $150 million would be saved by advance directives. (Payne's figures would come to $150 million to $1 billion.) Though these costs (and possible savings) may not be substantial in the large scale of expenditures in the United States, they cannot be ignored. And increased use of advance directives will certainly improve the savings.

41. Of course, not all patients in end-of-life situations will choose the option of refusing treatments. See Tsevat J et al. Health values of hospitalized patients 80 years or older. JAMA 1998; 279:371–375. They may exercise

their right of self-determination by choosing to pursue treatments. This is not inappropriate and may actually help patients achieve some of their goals. However, when the treatment chosen is futile, then self-determination may be limited. One can only hope that if the Patient Self-Determination Act is fully discussed with patients, the discussion of futility will be much easier. The issue of futility is more fully explored in chapter 6.

42. Wolf SM et al. Sources of concern about the Patient Self-Determination Act. N Engl J Med 1991; 325:1666–1671.

43. Edinger W, Smucker DR. Outpatients' attitudes regarding advance directives. J Fam Prac 1992; 35:650–653.

44. Yalom ID. Existential psychotherapy. New York: Basic Books, Inc. 1980, pages 41–54.

45. Strategies in the various professions for addressing these communication opportunities will be explored in chapter 8.

46. Siegert EA et al. Impact of advance directive videotape on patient comprehension and treatment preferences. Arch Fam Med 1996; 5:207–212. This study found no impact on patients' comprehension of resuscitation preferences or advance directives. Of course, this could be the result of a poorly designed videotape or a lack of conversations with the patients after they viewed the tape.

47. Danis M. A prospective study of advance directives for life-sustaining care. N Engl J Med 1991; 324:882–888.

48. Carney MT, Morrison RS. Advance directives: When, why, and how to start talking. Geriatrics 1997; 52:65–73.

49. Murphy DJ et al. The influence of the probability of survival on patients' preferences regarding cardiopulmonary resuscitation. N Engl J Med 1994; 330:545–549. In this study the number of elderly patients who elected DNR doubled after a conversation with their physicians about the likely outcome of CPR. This study indicates both the effectiveness of the physician's role and the value of appropriate informed consent.

50. Lo B. Improving care near the end of life: Why is it so hard? JAMA 1995; 274:1634–1636.

51. This can be an important defense mechanism exercised by individuals who are not ready to integrate this information into their life choices. Much the same phenomenon occurs when patients are given information about their healthcare condition when they are not ready to hear it. They simply ignore the information or deny its truth. This is a defense mechanism that gives them the time to gather their inner resources and then deal properly with the situation. See Bok S. Lying: Moral choice in public and private life. New York: Pantheon Books, 1978, pages 241–242. Unfortunately, it is not uncommon to interpret this phenomenon as a sign that patients do not want

information. Instead, what it often means is that the patient does not want the information *at this time.*

52. Cardiology, Inc. Patient's rights, opportunities, and advance directives. Columbus, OH: June, 1992.

6

The Ethical Foundations of the Patient Self-Determination Act

The Patient Self-Determination Act challenges caregivers, institutions, and patients alike to clarify and develop an ethical context for implementing the law. Many of the issues that have been discussed in bioethics in the last generation come to bear directly on the law. All these issues have been discussed extensively over the years and a good bit of agreement has been generated about them. But to interconnect them in such a fundamental way with direct focus is a major contribution of the Patient Self-Determination Act.

This chapter will attempt to delineate the ethical foundations that support the implementation of the law in both its letter and its spirit. Furthermore, some of the key ethical issues will be discussed that relate directly to the law or produce substantial challenges to the law. This examination should reveal that a violation of the law or its casual implementation means disregarding a number of ethical principles and issues that lie at the heart of the provider-patient relationship. Furthermore, an awareness of some of the ethical issues related to the law should provide an incentive to meet not only the letter of the law but its spirit as well. Attempts to assist patients in making decisions within the context of the law will both respect and promote their dignity and well-being.[1]

The Supporting Principles of Bioethics

There are many entry points for examining the ethical foundations of the Patient Self-Determination Act, but perhaps the most logical one is an identification and elaboration of the general principles of bioethics. The Patient Self-Determination Act reinforces the significance of the principles of bioethics, which have become a major part of the fabric of ethical decision making.[2] A few general observations about ethical principles will set the stage for a more detailed presentation and application to the Patient Self-Determination Act.

Ethical principles can be a part of any ethical system. They will always be formulated within the context of the ethical goods and values that are identified in the particular system. Their rankings relative to each other may also be determined by the ethical system. These systems are grounded in the beliefs of a moral community that subscribes to a particular ranking of goods and values.[3] One system that is used as a context for ethical principles is natural law ethics.[4] This system contextualizes its principles within an understanding of individual moral agents as parts of a larger order, a belief of dependence on a creator, and/or the importance of fulfilling human potential. Another system that is often used is the deontological approach.[5] This system focuses on a belief in the intrinsic rightness of actions and the obligation to follow rules that promote such actions. Out of this system has grown a strong emphasis on autonomy. The utilitarian system with its emphasis on consequences is a system frequently used in democratic, secular societies, which are often called upon to settle competing claims.[6] It uses the approach of assessing and weighing desirable consequences against undesirable ones and making a decision based upon the results of the comparison. Regardless of the systems (and there are many variations), the major principles of bioethics will find some application.

Ethical principles take the form of statements of obligation. Thus they always contain the word "should" or some equivalent of it. Concepts are not principles. Thus, "personal dignity" is a concept rather than a principle. "One should respect the personal dignity of patients" would be the statement of a principle. The function of principles in moral discourse is to promote a particular value or feature of a person (such as dignity) or thing (such as aesthetic significance of a work of art) and thereby promote its well-being and allow it to flourish or be preserved.

In the clinical situation a number of ethical principles often intersect. On occasion they will conflict. When conflict occurs, it is necessary to examine each principle to determine how it arises in the particular set of circumstances and to balance the principles against each other so that a decision can ultimately be made about which principle(s) governs the case. Healthcare situations are not always governed by a single principle. Often several principles will govern the decision to be made by providing mutual support.[7]

The Principle of Autonomy

The principle of *autonomy* has come to occupy a preeminent position in healthcare in only the last two generations. This principle, which is most directly operative in the Patient Self-Determination Act, may be formulated in the following way: **A person should be free to perform whatever action he/she wishes, regardless of risks or foolishness as perceived by others, provided it does not impinge on the autonomy of others by intentionally harming them.** This principle gives ultimate control (self-governance or self-determination) for the action to the agent who is making the decision to perform the action. It is a moral principle of empowerment and places the responsibility for the consequences of the action on moral agents themselves. Someone acting on the principle of autonomy cannot legitimately blame another for adverse consequences.

The mere perceptions of others (independent of harms that might result to others as the result of an action) are not sufficient to stop an autonomous action. If the agent is competent or possesses decisional capacity, then the possibility of risk to the agent that might impress an observer does not give the observer the right to override the decision of the agent.[8] Even if the observer considers the action foolish as well as risky, the agent still has final control over the action.[9] Of course, the observer is in no way obliged to assist the agent in performing the action unless there is a clear professional obligation to do so.[10]

The claim that individuals act completely autonomously is a difficult one to make.[11] Their behaviors are frequently conditioned and they may lack some information that, if known, might cause them to behave otherwise. However, others can maximize the autonomy of moral agents by assisting them in reflecting on their proposed actions and by providing appropriate information so that the agent can have a more refined perspective on the anticipated action.[12] Assisting patients to be more autonomous may be one of the most important roles of the healthcare professional.[13]

In healthcare, the emphasis on the principle of autonomy is a strong reaction to the overemphasis on the principles of parentalism and beneficence throughout the traditions of medicine.[14] As medical information became "user-friendly," patients came to understand more about their healthcare conditions and their therapeutic possibilities. They also became clearer about their values and goals relative to healthcare practices.[15] This led to a diminishing reliance on the judgment of clinicians alone. In the current healthcare situation, clinicians frequently take on the roles of sources of information and healthcare advisers.[16] In the last analysis, however, the patient makes the necessary healthcare decisions according to the principle of autonomy.[17]

In spite of its centrality in healthcare, the principle of autonomy is not absolute. It functions contextually and its exercise frequently depends upon other values, priorities, and social conditions that are part of the patient's healthcare setting.[18] The principle clearly states that decisions cannot be made that impinge on the autonomy of others. Actions cannot be justified under the principle of autonomy if they cause unconsented to harm to others. Determining exactly how much harm, or what kind of harm, must be done to override the principle of autonomy requires extensive analysis and discussion in particular circumstances.

In healthcare, the following stipulations have been considered legitimate reasons for overriding patient autonomy in making healthcare decisions.[19] (1) Patients lacking decisional capacity cannot be protected by the principle of autonomy because they are not autonomous.[20] But it must be noted that a negative determination about decisional capacity may not apply to all decisions by patients. Patients may lack capacity in one area while retaining capacity in other areas.[21] (2) Patients cannot require a clinician to provide a treatment that lies outside the bounds of acceptable medical practice. What counts as "acceptable" medical practice sometimes has fuzzy edges, as is illustrated by the debates about medical futility.[22] (3) Patients cannot demand a treatment that provides no benefit. This raises, once again, the issue of medical futility, which will sometimes override patients' autonomous choices as a matter of beneficence.[23] (4) Patients cannot demand a treatment that violates the *deeply held* beliefs of the clinician. Thus, patients cannot require a physician to perform an abortion or to assist them in committing suicide if the physician has strong beliefs to the contrary.[24] (5) Patients cannot legitimately demand a treatment that is a limited resource or a resource for which they cannot pay.[25] In this case autonomous choices are overridden by considerations of justice. At the moment, some organ transplants are an example of such treatments, although this limitation may be modified depending upon specific provisions in healthcare reimbursement contracts.

The importance of the principle of autonomy, especially when exercised within a structured set of beliefs, values, and goals,[26] cannot be overemphasized. As the foundation of the Patient Self-Determination Act, it underlies such important decisions in healthcare as consenting to treatments, the refusal of treatments (whether or not they are life-sustaining), the drafting or signing of advance directives, and the selection of treatments according to the patient's values and goals.

The Principle of Beneficence

The principle of *beneficence* is a long-standing principle in the tradition of Hippocratic medicine.[27] The Hippocratic oath requires that practitioners of the medical arts keep their patients from harm and injustice.[28] In some versions of the oath the notion of avoiding harm is coupled with an expression of the requirement to benefit the patient.[29] The principle of beneficence can be stated in the following way: **One should render positive assistance to others (and *abstain from harm*) by helping them to further their important and legitimate interests.** In the Hippocratic context it was probably easier to identify harm (e.g., death or further injury) than it was to identify what might benefit the patient. Of course, the Hippocratic physician should not kill his patient. Thus, the earlier versions of the principle of beneficence generally took the minimalist form of the principle of nonmaleficence (*primum non nocere*—first do no harm).[30] Today, however, the concept of harm is much more complex. We can identify physical harms, psychological harms, social harms, and moral harms. In order to apply properly even the principle of nonmaleficence (i.e., **one should abstain from harming another**), a detailed account of the possible harms to the patient is required.

When the focus is promoting benefit to the patient, the matter becomes even more complex. There is an enormous variety of possibilities for benefiting patients. For example, patients can be benefited by surgery, by pharmacological interventions, by minimally invasive procedures such as meditation, or by electing to allow a disease to run its course. Added to the variety is the fact that patients may have their own ideas about what benefits them—ideas that may be at variance with those of the clinician. This principle requires both patients and caregivers to be clear about what they consider beneficial as they enter into a dialogue. The exercise of this principle is central to fulfilling the expectations of the Patient Self-Determination Act. For the spirit of the law, coupled with the exercise of beneficence, directs caregivers to assist patients in achieving clarity about their values and goals in order to make sound decisions about refusing treatment and drafting advance directives.

Clinicians not only have an obligation to follow the principle of beneficence; they also have a professional interest in behaving beneficently.[31] Their professional commitments should always dispose them to behave beneficently. However, there are some restrictions on the employment of the principle of beneficence. (1) Beneficence can be overridden by the patient's desire to follow her own value agenda and priorities (according to the principle of autonomy) when that value agenda might be at variance with the treatment preferences of the clinician.[32] On the other hand, a case might be made that the clinician is acting beneficently if he respects the patient's value agenda and promotes it through the course of therapy. (2) Clinicians are not acting beneficently if they are pursuing a course of treatment for the patient that is futile or if the burdens disproportionately outweigh the benefits for the patient.[33] Thus, beneficence often takes the form of acting with restraint: not intervening or following a less invasive course is often the beneficent thing to do.[34] (3) Clinicians are not required to act beneficently toward patients by providing interventions that are scarce resources (e.g., certain kinds of transplant surgeries).[35] In this situation, considerations of justice may override beneficence, particularly if the organs for transplant are a scarce resource.

The principle of beneficence is largely responsible for keeping the practice of medicine humane through the centuries.[36] It should not be disregarded simply because the principle of autonomy has grown in importance. It still has an important place in healthcare practices in its own right as well as providing a valuable support for the principle of autonomy. It plays an especially vital role in therapeutic efforts on behalf of the incompetent and those who have no surrogate. It is central to the determination of futile therapies and recommendations made to patients who are facing the possibility of futile therapies.[37] Its most significant role may be in guiding clinicians as they accompany terminal patients along the pathway to death.

The Principle of Justice

If there is a candidate for an overriding principle of bioethics, it may very well be the principle of *justice*. This principle cuts a very broad path across ethical situations, and the other principles are often applied within the context of justice. The principle is a complex one, and its brief statement requires elaboration. **One should give to persons what they are owed, what they deserve, or what they can legitimately claim, treating equals equally unless there is a morally relevant difference requiring persons to be treated unequally; consideration must often be given to a proper allocation of benefits and burdens within the social context.**

What individuals are owed or deserve can be determined in a variety of ways. (1) The claim could be made that this arises from the nature of the person. (2) It may be revealed by particular factors in an individual's condition that warrant a specific response. (3) It may be determined by decisions made by social institutions.

In the first instance, the fundamental dignity of the person may require a measure of respect calling for certain actions.[38] For example, persons may be said to possess an intrinsic value, and the maintenance or restoration of health is one of the primary ways of helping individuals fulfill their natural potentials. Furthermore, to be able to exercise full moral agency, as an expression of one's nature, requires that the individual be an active participant in a decisional process in which significant information is available to her and her value preferences are seriously considered.[39] Thus, *informed* consent becomes a matter of justice in healthcare. If individuals have the right to consent to treatment as is stipulated in the Patient Self-Determination Act, and if competent consent requires adequate information upon which to base one's consent,[40] it can be inferred that patients have the right to the means required to give consent in a proper manner. Information is considered an indispensable component of the giving of consent. Thus, patients are owed information as a matter of justice based upon the nature of the consenting person.[41]

In the second instance, the individual's situation may be the factor that warrants a particular response.[42] In healthcare, the types of pathology from which patients are suffering often call for different responses. Psychological problems are not always treated in the same way as purely physical problems. Diseases are frequently treated differently from injuries. Terminal diseases should probably be treated differently from chronic diseases. Diseases from which patients can recover elicit therapeutic responses that are different from those used in the final stages of a terminal disease.[43] Justice, as an appropriate response to one's condition, requires different approaches to pathologies. In a similar way, patients who are not able to make decisions for themselves should be treated differently than competent adults.[44] The requirements of justice can be met in this situation by having someone designated to make decisions that will reflect the patient's own wishes or best interests.

In the last instance, public policy decisions may provide certain kinds of healthcare for individuals (e.g., dialysis). It becomes, then, a matter of justice to provide such treatments. Distributive justice—the fair allocation of benefits and burdens in society—is frequently codified on the basis of society's assessment of human needs and the resources available to meet those needs. In distributive justice there is an identification of the goods or benefits that should be available to individuals in society; the principle requires that the benefits be available to individuals in some equitable way and that the burdens (e.g., cost) for providing these benefits should also be distributed in an equitable manner across the population. Generally speaking, no one person or group of persons should bear a substantially greater burden than another unless there are relevant moral reasons for imposing the burdens in this way.[45]

The application of this principle lies at the heart of the healthcare reform movement. Initially, it seemed desirable to determine that some measure of healthcare is a benefit that should be enjoyed by everyone. How much healthcare should be incorporated in a base package and the manner of its distribution to everyone are matters of social policy. The financing of this benefit (the burden for making it available) would also have to be determined by social policy. Within the basic package no one would get more or less than he deserves (determined by social policy decisions) or pay more or less than he should. Since a base package would very likely not satisfy everyone's needs or wants, a second tier of care could be added to allow patients to get more healthcare provided they were willing to bear the burden of additional cost on an individual bases. In a laissez-faire economic system, this would work.[46] However, those who are more inclined to egalitarian approaches to justice would find a two-tiered system fundamentally unjust.[47]

On the surface it would seem that healthcare professionals acting in a clinical setting should not have to worry about the principle of distributive justice. This seems to be a social policy matter. But as a practical matter distributive justice often becomes an issue.[48] It arises when questions are asked about whether a particular approach to treatment is costworthy, particularly when someone besides the patient is paying the cost.[49] It arises in rationing decisions—for example, determining whether a particular patient is a good candidate for an ICU bed.[50] It arises in cost-shifting practices, as in charging higher prices to those patients who can afford to pay in order to compensate for those who cannot afford to pay.

Treating equals as equals and unequals as unequals lies at the heart of the principle of justice as its formal principle.[51] In a democratic society we begin with the assumption that there is a basic equality that runs through the population.[52] The ethical mandate based upon this assumption is that equals are to be treated equally. Thus, if a right is recognized—for example, the right to self-determination—then each person should be able to act on such a right and expect duties entailed by the right to be honored; hence the passage of the Patient Self-Determination Act. The right cannot be arbitrarily given to some and not to others. However, individuals are not equal in every respect. They are sometimes unequal because of a morally relevant difference between them. For example, individuals above age sixteen in most states can obtain a driver's license, and those below sixteen may not.

In attempting to apply the principle of justice in any particular situation, a determination must be made as to whether there is a morally relevant difference separating the individuals involved.[53] For example, disease often counts as a morally relevant difference in our society. Those who are sick are often excused from their work obligations while they are sick. What counts as a morally relevant difference in healthcare is often open to debate. The type of disease,[54] the age of the patient,[55] the decisional capacity of the patient,[56] the ability of the patient to pay for services,[57] and the presence of an advance directive[58] are all discussed in terms of whether they are morally relevant differences.

Of particular significance in identifying morally relevant differences is the ability of an individual to engage in mature decisions of self-determination. The Patient Self-Determination Act is grounded in the ability of individuals who are of legal age and possess decisional capacity to become active and legally determinative participants in the decisions that govern their healthcare.[59] This ability constitutes a fundamental morally relevant difference for determining applications of the principle of justice. The concept of a morally relevant difference also extends to whether or not a patient has an advance directive. Thus, the exercise of autonomy in both consents to and refusals of treatment as well as its application to drafting advance directives is an essential component in governing the manner in which caregivers must behave toward patients in the clinical setting. To conform to the stipulations of the Patient Self-Determination Act is to promote the patient's well-being. To violate the Patient Self-Determination Act is to violate the principle of justice, which strikes at the heart of patient dignity.[60]

Another application of the notion of equality (or lack thereof) in the principle of justice that is of particular concern is the issue of terminal illness. The question is whether terminal illness counts as a morally relevant difference in treating a patient: should those who are terminally ill be treated as aggressively as those who are chronically ill or recoverable?[61] In other words, does the kind of pathology with which a patient presents provide a sufficient warrant to place different values on the overall way in which the patient should be treated? A terminal condition is different from others, and to treat patients contrary to their conditions can be considered a violation of the principle of justice. It would be just as wrong to treat terminal patients as if they were recoverable as it would be to treat recoverable patients as if they were terminal.[62] Thus, those patients who are terminally ill and wish to exercise their rights under the Patient Self-Determination Act have a double claim to exercising their judgment to refuse treatment; they have a right to refuse treatment for any reason, and in this case a terminal condition is their reason.

Futile care may be yet another application of the principle of justice and the notion of identifying a morally relevant difference.[63] Treatments that can lead to recovery or a decent quality of life may be assessed as substantially different from treatments that are not beneficial for patients and do not accomplish the goals of therapy. As a morally relevant difference, futile treatments and their pursuit constitute a violation of the principle of justice because they do not properly reflect the patient's condition and respond to it appropriately.[64] For example, a patient in the end stage of metastatic cancer will not survive a CPR attempt.[65] Her condition is such that the attempt will accomplish none of the goals of CPR. CPR is, then, futile. Thus, the utilization of futile treatments constitutes a violation of the principles of both beneficence and justice: beneficence because the patient does not benefit, justice because the treatment approach does not properly address the patient's condition. In addition, if the patient wishes to refuse, or is denied the opportunity to refuse, futile treatment, then the additional principle of autonomy is violated. Futile treatment has become such an important issue because it lies at the intersection of all the recognized principles of bioethics and carries the potential of violating all of them as well as violating the basic canons of acceptable medical practice.[66]

The issue of resource allocation cannot be ignored in the context of futility and justice. Highly aggressive treatments of those in terminal conditions may not represent the best expenditure of limited healthcare dollars.[67] The same issue of equality has been raised about the matter of age in elderly patients who may be candidates for CPR.[68] The question is whether age should count as a morally relevant difference to the extent that CPR would not be given to patients of advanced age or, minimally, the bias would change in the elderly population, with CPR being given only when there are clearly positive indications that the patient will benefit from it in significant ways.[69]

The Patient Self-Determination Act can contribute in a major way to addressing the issue of restricting futile treatments, particularly through the promotion of advance directives.[70] Information about the conditions individuals may face with the onset of a terminal condition or of advanced age gives patients and potential patients a realistic perspective on what they may be facing in the future. The advance directive, then, presents them with the opportunity to maintain some measure of control over the direction of their care. Many patients who consider these issues will often refuse to pursue treatments that would prolong their dying[71] and thus violate the principle of justice by failing to treat them in accordance with their terminal condition. This approach, fostered by the Patient Self-Determination Act, not only will reduce the suffering of patients but may save resources in healthcare.[72]

It may be difficult to conceive of restrictions on the application of the principle of justice. However, there may be some modifications to it. One can go beyond the principle of justice. (1) Compassion may prompt one to provide services to a patient even though justice does not require it. A practitioner may provide treatments even though there is a very low level of probability for their success in a particular healthcare situation. This may occur even in situations of scarce resources. (2) If there are abundant resources, or resources allocated for certain extreme situations, one may provide services for which payment may not be received. (3) An institution may have special mission considerations that go beyond the strict requirements of justice—for example, the practice of never turning a patient away when care is needed.[73]

In chapter 5 we examined the importance of institutions in going beyond the letter of the law by assisting patients in considering the stipulations of the Patient Self-Determination Act and their application to their particular situations. This assistance, as an example of a mission commitment, complements the broad principle of justice (rather than following its more restrictive distributive sense.) For, strictly speaking, the law itself does not require such assistance. On the other hand, a case could be made that such assistance fits into the requirements of the broadly stated principle of justice. If the principle of justice requires that responses be made to patients as warranted by their conditions, then patients who are confused, uncertain, or simply in need of greater help in addressing the stipulations of the Patient Self-Determination Act require an appropriate response. This response comes in the form of assistance in helping patients become clear about their values and goals as the context for consenting to or refusing treatments as well as addressing concerns they may have in drafting or signing an advance directive. Thus, the Patient Self-Determination Act can be interpreted as cutting a broad path through the expectations of the principle of justice.

From the above considerations it can be seen that the clinical situation is so complex that no one single material principle of justice can be identified. That is, there is no single feature that serves as a morally relevant difference to determine when equality or inequality should govern a clinical decision. The kind of disease the patient exhibits is certainly one factor. But others include financial need, self-determination, decisional ability, and advance directives, to name only a few. The lesson is that clinicians should always be sensitive to the particularities in the clinical situation, identify them clearly, understand their role in the situation, and employ them carefully to be sure that the formal demands of justice are met when dealing with patients.

Thus far we have seen three principles: autonomy, beneficence, and justice. Though sometimes the principles may conflict, they are often complementary. One behaves justly toward another by respecting her autonomy. Autonomy counts as a morally relevant difference requiring equal treatment based upon self-determination. When one behaves beneficently toward another in cases where beneficence is required, one is also behaving justly because the patient is given what she deserves. On the other hand, if a patient is autonomous and is legitimately exercising her autonomy, a violation of the principle of autonomy also entails a violation of the principle of justice. In a similar way, a violation of the legitimate exercise of beneficence entails a violation of the principle of justice.

The Principle of Parentalism

Another guiding principle for healthcare practice throughout its tradition is *parentalism*.[74] It is only within the last two generations that the principle has been largely supplanted by the growing emphasis on the principle of autonomy. This principle can be stated in the following way: **One should restrict an individual's action against his/her consent in order to prevent that individual from self-harm or to secure for that individual a good that he/she might not otherwise achieve.** The principle of parentalism is based on one fundamental assumption—namely, that the one acting parentalistically has a privileged position allowing him to know what is best for the moral agent being restricted. The restricted agent is presumed to be in such an inferior position that she cannot determine what is in her best interest.

Sometimes the privileged position of the intervener is due to age and/or relationship. For example, parents intervene in the lives of their small children because they have the experience that comes with age as well as the special responsibilities of parents. For those who lack decisional capacity, guardians intervene because of their special social role. Throughout the history of medicine physicians were seen as occupying a privileged position due to their special knowledge and experience. Thus, physicians were generally viewed as knowing what was best for their patients to a higher degree than patients who might be tempted to make the judgment for themselves.[75]

The principle of parentalism was employed to protect moral agents from their own errors in judgment. This was applied particularly to patients. There was fear that patients from their limited perspective might make a decision that would bring harm to them. For example, the refusal of a treatment might result in the continuance or increased severity of a disease, the selection of a particular form of treatment by the patient might not lead to recovery.

There are two basic forms of parentalism, weak and strong.[76] In healthcare, weak parentalism is exercised in three situations. (1) Patients may have severely and permanently diminished capacity. Such patients may still be able to make decisions but have no way of calculating the consequences of the decisions. The application of parentalism to situations of this type is generally recognized as appropriate. (2) There are situations when patients are temporarily incapable of exercising proper decisional capacity. Examples would be patients suffering from a psychotic break or children who have not reached their majority. Interventions are considered appropriate here until the patient recovers or the child comes of age. (3) Weak parentalism is also exercised through interventions that are undertaken when it is unclear whether or not the agent is autonomous. To be appropriate this intervention must be time-limited. If the agent is ultimately considered to lack decisional capacity, continuing parentalism is appropriate. If the agent is ultimately considered to possess decisional capacity, then the parentalism should cease in deference to the principle of autonomy.[77]

Strong parentalism occurs when the liberty of a moral agent who is functionally autonomous is restricted in order to prevent self-harm and/or to secure a benefit for that individual. Current ethical thinking judges parentalism to be inappropriate in this case.[78] Most codes of medical ethics support this judgement and favor the principle of autonomy in this case.[79]

Two principal reasons for restricting the application of the principle of parentalism in medical practice may be identified. (1) The privileged position of the physician due to the possession of special knowledge has been eroded. Medical information is currently available that patients can understand, and the canons of informed consent require that such information be made available to them in a balanced way prior to decisions about treatment. (2) Healthcare decisions are not made simply on the basis of information. Information must be situated within a value context. Since the decision falls most squarely on the patient, the patient's value framework must provide the context for the decision. The patient is the one who is in the privileged position of knowing her own value priorities. Thus, the principle of autonomy overrides the principle of parentalism in the case of patients with decisional capacity.

The major restriction, therefore, on the principle of parentalism is the principle of autonomy. In any conflict between the two principles where a competent patient is concerned, the principle of parentalism must yield.[80] One can never act parentalistically and respect the principle of autonomy. On the other hand, one can act both beneficently and parentalistically at the same time—for example, when a patient lacks both decisional capacity and a legitimate surrogate to speak for her. However, in cases where the patient is autonomous, one does not act beneficently by using the principle of parentalism. When a nonautonomous patient is involved, then the warrant for a response according to the principle of justice may very well prompt a parentalistic intervention. On the other hand, to behave in a parentalistic manner toward a patient who is autonomous is a serious violation of the principle of justice because the patient's condition warrants respect for her autonomy.

The principle of parentalism has often served patients well in the practice of medicine over the years. But as patients have become empowered by increased knowledge, the ability to have the knowledge communicated effectively,[81] and a more empowered sense of their role as patients, the principle has been largely transcended. The result is a very positive one for both patients and physicians. For they can now function as partners or collaborators in healthcare decision making, sharing both power and responsibility.[82]

It should be clear that the Patient Self-Determination Act can be characterized as a codification of this move away from exercising the principle of parentalism as a matter of course. As an antiparentalistic law, the act acknowledges the power of patients with decisional capacity to make healthcare decisions on their own behalf. For patients who may be making decisions that are questionable in the judgment of caregivers, the correct approach is not to initiate a parentalistic intervention. Rather, such patients should be given the opportunity to reflect upon their decisions in light of the values underlying them and the goals that might, or might not, be achieved by pursuing the decision in question. The Patient Self-Determination Act is a guard against inappropriate parentalistic interventions and at the same time calls the patient to be a responsible and reflective decision maker. When this role is effectively exercised, parentalism ceases to be an issue.

The Role of the Virtues in Clinical Decisions

Chapter 4 explored the role of the virtues in expressing personal dignity. In that context we saw that virtues are states of character or habits that guide us toward the accomplishment of the goals we have chosen to pursue.[83] We saw that the virtue history or narrative constitutes a major part of what makes us individuals.[84] We also saw the inescapable role of negotiation, which is necessary as different individuals choose to practice different sets of virtues or similar virtues but in substantially different ways.[85] We asserted that the

Patient Self-Determination Act brings into focus the importance of understanding the role of the virtues in the clinical setting.

In chapter 4, a number of virtues were identified and examined insofar as they are expressions of personal dignity within the context of the human situation. It was noted that virtues are practiced in many different ways by individuals as they encounter one another in various situations. Virtues, then, are a concrete, situational presentation of one's individuality. They are historically developed and conditioned by the experience and choices of the individual who practices them. At one time, a patient may practice the virtue of assertiveness, attempting to take control of every feature of her life. At a later time, the same patient may act with humility, accepting circumstances and yielding to outside forces.[86]

It is the richness and variability of human experience that the acknowledgment and practice of the virtues reflect. And it is this dimension of human experience that the ethical principles examined in the previous section may not fully capture. For the principles, with their abstract formulations, may present us with sterile guides for our behavior. They look at human actions as discrete events that must be judged against the principle that purports to govern them. Thus, the historical and situational context of the action is often ignored. Aristotle captured the situational variability of the practice of the virtues in his doctrine of the mean.[87] For the mean can shift as the moral agent assesses his obligations differently in light of varying circumstances in his situation.

Just as principles are often of great assistance in guiding judgements about actions, considerations of the virtues that guide moral agents can also be of great value.[88] This may be particularly the case when there is an ethical dispute. Suppose a patient were in the last stages of a devastating disease process. It is clear to the clinicians that the patient has deteriorated to the point where CPR would be medically ineffective. And yet the patient wants resuscitation to be attempted. This dispute involves a classic conflict between the principles of autonomy and beneficence. On this level of analysis the case would probably be resolved in favor of beneficence overriding autonomy. But if we look at this confrontation from the level of the virtues operating in the situation, a substantially different conclusion might result. The patient may have exhibited the virtues of courage and hope throughout the history of the disease and even before its onset. While accepting the inevitable outcome of the disease, the patient may see resistance to the very end to be central to his personal dignity. On the other hand, the clinicians may wish to practice the virtues of efficiency and benevolence by utilizing only effective remedies and not putting the patient through any additional suffering. But the virtue of compassion is also in their armamentarium and may very well place them in a position that is compatible with the virtue life of the patient. Thus, considering the existential situations and richness of the virtue lives of all the parties involved in the decisional process may allow for a more flexible resolution.

The Patient Self-Determination Act opens the door to an even more comprehensive examination of clinical decisions—from the vantage point of virtues. Consenting to and refusing treatment by a particular patient may be viewed in a way much stronger than the principle of autonomy. Consents and refusals can be seen against a backdrop of the virtue life of the patient, whose virtue history yields valuable clues to the foundation for the consent or refusal. Similarly, when drafting an advance directive or assisting a patient in doing so, the exercise may be sterile when viewed from the vantage point of autonomy but will be immeasurably enriched by signing or formulating the advance directive in view of the virtue history of the patient.

Furthermore, since the selection of virtues and their practice are matters of choice, as was pointed out in chapter 4, the virtue approach to the Patient Self-Determination Act serves to underscore the dimension of responsibility in patients.[89] Since virtues are practiced by both healthcare professionals and patients, a consideration of the virtues of the professionals will add an important dimension to the stipulation of the Patient Self-Determination Act. For professionals can bring their own virtue lives to bear on any assistance they might render to patients who wish to utilize fully the various powers identified in the law. In addition, taking seriously the virtue life of healthcare professionals may add a much needed dimension of self-reflection in their encounters with patients. Considerations of virtue in those who are participants in the clinical encounter both reflect the human experience and add to its richness and uniqueness in ways that abstract considerations of laws and principles simply cannot achieve.

Informed Consent

If there is one single issue besides the patient's right to self-determination upon which the Patient Self-Determination Act is built it is informed consent. The notion of informed consent has come a long way from the Hippocratic notion of keeping patients ignorant of their conditions and allowing physicians to make all decisions on their behalf.[90] When informed consent finally became an issue in healthcare ethics, the physician was still the one who determined its conditions. Prior to *Canterbury v. Spence* the criterion was that patients were to be informed about matters that the "reasonable *physician*" thought they should know.[91] After *Canterbury* the criterion shifted to giving patients information that a "reasonable patient" would want to know.[92] Currently, approximately half the states in the United States use the former criterion and half use the latter.[93]

The historical shifts in the informed consent dynamics have very likely occurred as a result of better information being available about healthcare conditions and the accessibility of the information to patients in forms they can understand. Another likely reason for the shifts may very well lie in an increased awareness that the principle of self-determination, so essential to a democracy, ought to operate in the healthcare setting as well as in the political arena.[94] Adequate information to make choices lies at the heart of self-determination.

The President's Commission, in setting the parameters for informed consent, identified two basic values underlying it: personal well-being and self-determination.[95] These two values are the foundations for the Patient Self-Determination Act, as well as for informed consent in the healthcare setting. Patients are in the best position to make decisions that affect them and to determine what will contribute to their well-being. The use of the term "personal" to qualify "well-being" conveys the intimate character of such judgments. No one can make such judgments about an individual's well-being as well as she. But the judgments cannot be made without adequate information, thus underlining the "informed" part of informed consent.

The commission goes on to affirm that there is a dimension of mutuality in the informed consent exchange that cannot be ignored. At first glance it would seem that informed consent is directed only to the patient. In some ways this is the case. For the *Ethics Manual* of the American College of Physicians clearly states that the patient who is entitled to complete explanations about her healthcare condition possesses full decision-making authority with regard to her medical care.[96] But the President's Commission sees a more participatory model in informed consent. Both the physician/caregiver and the patient have a stake in the outcome of the therapeutic relationship under consideration.[97] The patient's stake clearly results from the fact that the patient is the one to bear, in the most personal way, the outcomes of the decision. The caregiver has a stake insofar as he has a keen interest in engaging in the best form of healthcare practice possible according to the standards of the profession.

As suggested in chapter 3, the dynamics of informed consent constitute a relationship of mutual empowerment because the mutuality of informed consent gives true power to each of its participants.[98] The patient does not have the power to make a proper healthcare decision and consent to a course of treatment without having the information necessary as a resource for giving consent. By giving the patient information adequate for making a sound decision, the physician is empowering the patient. One of the greatest areas of patient vulnerability is that of ignorance.[99] Patients often come to the healthcare setting ignorant of the problem they are facing and of the measures that will help them overcome that problem. In giving the patient appropriate information, that vulnerability is reduced. If pertinent information is withheld, the patient's vulnerability is perpetuated and often magnified.

The other side of the relationship is equally important. The initial power of the physician lies in his expertise. The knowledge the physician brings to the clinical setting gives him the power to diagnose, render a prognosis, and recommend treatments. But this all remains distant from the patient until the patient gives consent because the physician may not engage in any nonconsensual touching of the patient.[100] Thus, though the physician has power and some measure of authority granted by society, he cannot exercise that power and authority without the patient's consent to do so. Thus, the patient empowers the physician by giving consent, in much the same way as the physician empowers the patient by giving information.

There are many components to the information package that patients must know if they are to be truly empowered to make wise decisions about their healthcare.[101] The most obvious element is that they should know the nature of the problem they are facing and the outcome of the problem if it is left untreated. The practice of fully disclosing this sort of information, particularly in cases of critical illness, became common only in the last two generations of medical practice.[102] Prior to this practice many practitioners thought that it was more beneficial to patients to keep them ignorant of their problem, because knowledge would only exacerbate their plight and create additional problems of depression, despair, and inappropriate refusals of treatment.[103] This silence has come to be known as "therapeutic privilege."[104] Though some patients still may wish to remain ignorant of their problem, the suppression of information is often now the result of the patient's conscious desire rather than a default to the clinician's judgment.

The next component of the information package is the nature of the recommended treatment. The patient will have to know what the treatment can accomplish—that is, its benefits and the likelihood of its success.[105] The patient will also need to know the detrimental effects that may accompany the treatment.[106] None of these elements can be communicated to the patient with absolute certainty, which is not possible in the art of medicine.[107] The patient will need to know about this limitation in medical knowledge. The information will have to be couched in the language of probabilities, for medicine is largely the management of probabilities in the design and administration of treatments.

Finally, patients need to know a reasonable range of alternatives to the recommended treatment. They do not always find a recommended course of treatment to their liking because its side effects might interfere with their lifestyles. Or they might weigh the risks and benefits of a course of treatment differently than their clinicians do.

Giving patients information is not as simple as it may sound. It involves a complex dynamic that has as its base the use of language the patient can understand.[108] It is easy for practitioners to fall into the trap of using professional jargon in communicating with patients because it is their language of everyday use. Unfortunately, essential information often escapes the comprehension of the patient because of the use of technical language. A case can be made that the use of technical language may actually violate the patient's dignity by keeping this critical information from her.[109]

Beyond the use of understandable language, three levels of working with information can be identified in the dynamics of informed consent.[110] The first level is the communication of mere facts.[111] At this rudimentary level the patient is merely acquainted with a body of factual knowledge, the parts of which may be fairly discrete and unrelated. For example: "There is a cancer. Cancer of such and such a type often responds to chemotherapy in the following way. Radiation therapy is sometimes an alternative to chemotherapy." At this level the patient has information but the elements are generally disconnected from one another, floating independent of the patient.

The next level beyond simple communication of facts is the level of understanding. Here the patient possesses mastery of the facts and is able to establish some meaningful connections. For example: "There is a cancer and it is responsive to this form of therapy in the following way. The therapy has the following benefits but also poses the following risks. If the therapy is pursued the results for the cancer in six months will be significant remission of the growth of the tumor or shrinkage of the tumor. The therapy even has X percent probability of actually destroying the tumor." Here the patient can clearly see the relationship between the various pieces of information. The causal relationship of the elements has been understood and the outcomes explicitly projected. But there is still a significant dimension lacking, which becomes possible only at the next level.

The final level of managing information in informed consent can be called the level of "processing" information, in which both patient and physician may share.[112] The emphasis here is on the patient's integrating everything she knows at the first two levels into her own value framework. She personalizes it. For example, the cancer is no longer "a" cancer but "my" cancer. The therapy is no longer a therapy for "the cancer" but a therapy for "me." "My therapy" no longer affects the cancer in such and such a way; "my therapy" affects "me." And it does not affect "me" as an abstraction but "me as a living, breathing subject with a particular lifestyle and particular goals I wish to accomplish and particular values I wish to pursue. I may or may not wish to consent to this regimen." Thus, the patient has seen the disease as an intimate part of herself about which she must make some significant decisions. Thus, the disconnected information communicated in the first level is finally integrated with the patient's innermost values and preferences. Processing information in this way is not the result of an automatic decision to have therapy (the technological imperative). Rather, it requires considerable reflection on the part of the patient and often some extensive assistance on the part of the caregiver who shares in the processing of information.

Three authors, Lidz, Appelbaum, and Meisel, have structured the issues of informed consent a bit differently but with similar results for understanding the implementation issues related to the Patient Self-Determination Act.[113] An examination of their analysis would be most helpful. They point out that the standard way of approaching informed consent in the clinical setting follows what they call the "event" model. Here the communication between clinician and patient occurs as a discrete act in their relationship. The information is given and is seldom revisited. The patient signs a consent form as a symbol of the "communication event."[114] Though this transaction may satisfy the legal requirements for informed consent, there are two lingering questions: How much does the patient truly understand and how can the patient open a discussion about reconsidering her decisions?

The authors suggest an alternative approach—the "process" model of informed consent.[115] In this model, information is exchanged and consent reconsidered and reaffirmed over the entire course of treatment. Whereas the event model allows the patient to be passive about consent after the consent form has been signed, the process model is structured around continuing conversations between the clinician and the patient about both the patient's condition and the possible treatment.[116] The process model is predicated on the active participation of the patient in decision making, thereby emphasizing the patient's responsibility. The patient's personal and value history are viewed as important backdrops for the dialogue between the parties in the clinical setting. Both patients and physicians articulate their expectations of their own roles as well as those of each other. This allows them to negotiate any differences as they arise and resolve them quickly.

One of the most significant features of the process model is the continuous dialogue that takes place. Nothing is considered automatic and everything is open for reappraisal. A mutual monitoring between the partners in the clinical relationship involves ongoing reflection on, and reordering of, knowledge, both new and old, in light of further information and experience. This approach opens the pathways of discussion about the patient's feelings about what is being faced and the processing of those feelings throughout the experience.[117]

The strategies that reinforce the process model help to define more carefully the parameters of the problems the patient faces and help the patient select the appropriate approach to treatment. By using the strategy of soliciting the patient's reflections, caregivers can more immediately address the patient's concerns before they become overwhelming and an additional obstacle in the therapeutic relationship.

The major advantage of the process model of informed consent is that it enhances both the patient's autonomy and responsibility. The patient is not considered a spectator but rather an active participant in the therapeutic process and a primary source in decision making. And this is precisely the objective of the Patient Self-Determination Act. For the law intends to place some measure of control in the hands of patients by letting them know some broad features of their rights in the therapeutic relationship. The Patient Self-Determination Act confers on patients a cluster of interrelated rights flowing from the dynamics of informed consent in medical situations: (1) the right to be informed upon admission to a healthcare facility or organization of their right to consent to or refuse treatment; (2) the right to know the policies of the institution regarding the withholding or withdrawing of life-sustaining treatments; and (3) their rights under current state laws regarding advance directives. Failure to implement fully the Patient Self-Determination Act means that an institution is neglecting its obligation to patients under the canons of informed consent as well as federal law.

The advantages of informed consent have become increasingly obvious over the past generation. The first, and perhaps most important, advantage is that informed consent creates a bond of trust between the patient and the caregiver by opening avenues of communication between them.[118] Without the expectations and dynamics of informed consent, there could be a measure of mistrust between the patient and the caregiver. There could be a suspicion that even though the caregiver is giving the patient some information, other important information might remain hidden. There could also be a suspicion that the information might be weighted in such a way that consent could be the result of manipulation or coercion rather than free choice. The bond of trust has always been central to the physician-patient relationship. But for a large part of the history of medicine it has been asymmetrical—that is, the patient was supposed to trust the physician. Informed consent adds a measure of symmetry to the relationship that it never before possessed by challenging the physician to trust the patient.

The second advantage of informed consent can be found in the way it opens the possibility for patients to take greater responsibility in the course of their treatment. Thus, informed consent is intimately connected to the practice of autonomy.[119] If patients do not have information about their healthcare conditions, they will be at the mercy of others in the decision-making process. The responsibility for what happens to the patient will fall upon those who have the information and who make the decision on that basis. If it is desirable for patients to be responsible for their healthcare, it will be necessary for them to have the information that will act as a foundation for their decisions.[120]

But patients are not the only ones to be benefited by the dynamics of informed consent. Physicians and other caregivers also benefit. And the third advantage of informed consent can be significant for them. Physicians can be more effective in the care they give to their patients if they spend time discussing the patients' healthcare conditions with them. This dialogue will allow the patient to reveal the value basis that underlies her decisions and sets particular decisions within the context of those values. Beneficence is well served by any strategy that gives patients a significant advantage in participating in decisions about their healthcare. In this case, physicians are being beneficent by cultivating this advantage in patients through the process model of informed consent.

A special advantage of this exchange is that it averts a very significant conflict in the physician-patient relationship. All too often, when a conversation is brief and the information imparted is limited, sharp disagreements emerge about a healthcare decision. The friction often arises because the decisions take the form of conclusions that have been reached without extensive conversations. If there is a true dialogue in the informed consent relationship, reasons for decisions will arise. Then physicians will not feel compelled to argue with patients about the decisions they have reached. Instead, there is a good chance that they will see the reasons behind the decisions and will be able to channel their therapeutic energy and expertise toward helping patients within the patients' value contexts, rather than argue with them because of conflicts in their tacit value agendas.

The last major advantage of informed consent can also be directed toward physicians and other caregivers as well as patients. Informed consent reduces the liability exposure of physicians by maintaining avenues of communication between caregivers and patients. Many malpractice claims occur because patients and caregivers have not communicated fully enough, and such claims can be avoided if effective communication occurs.[121] Consent should never be a perfunctory exercise and should be given only when the patient has received adequate information. A thorough conversation about the issues the patient faces can give the patient the information she needs to make a decision reflective of her values and goals. Often courts are called into a case when such a conversation has not occurred. When there is sound communication between the physician and the patient, contentious issues can be resolved without the need of judicial intervention and resolution. It is interesting that a number of courts, including the New Jersey Supreme Court in *Quinlan*,[122] have indicated the reluctance of judges to become involved in cases that could have been resolved through a more extensive interchange between the caregiver and the patient.

Just as informed consent in the therapeutic relationship can be carried out in a perfunctory manner that simply goes through the motions or in an enriched manner that works with the patient's value system and reflective abilities, so also the Patient Self-Determination Act can be mechanical or enriched in its implementation. In both cases the latter approach takes patient dignity seriously and refuses to yield to the temptation of considering the convenience of caregivers as the highest priority. The Patient Self-Determination Act Reinforces informed consent in the clinical setting and is positioned to guarantee its fulfillment if it is taken seriously. But this can be accomplished only if the spirit as well as the letter of the law is followed.

Decisional Capacity

One of the central issues that arises in the clinical applications of informed consent is the ability of the patient to make decisions.[123] For information can be received and consent given only if the patient has the mental and emotional capacity to make the necessary decisions. If the patient lacks this capacity, then the burden for decision making shifts to the patient's authorized surrogate, who possesses decisional capacity.[124] The matter of decisional capacity is important for the implementation of the Patient Self-Determination Act insofar as the rights accorded by the law apply directly to the patient with decisional capacity and indirectly to the patient's surrogate. Knowing how to deal ethically with the possession (or lack thereof) of decisional capacity is an essential component of the ethical foundations of the Patient Self-Determination Act.

The conditions for decisional capacity have received considerable attention in the past generation in proportion to the increasing emphasis on patient autonomy and informed consent.[125] When the autonomy of patients was not an important matter for consideration and could be readily ignored, then determining decisional capacity was of no consequence. But once respecting autonomy became a cornerstone of healthcare, the conditions for exercising one's autonomy through making healthcare decisions became increasingly significant.[126]

Two authors, Paul Appelbaum and Thomas Grisso, have developed a concise conceptual map of the components of decisional capacity by identifying the following four features.[127] The first component of capacity is the ability of an individual to communicate the choice he wishes to make. Those without this ability cannot meaningfully participate in decisions about their care unless they have done so in advance of their inability to communicate. Thus, the comatose, the catatonic, and those whose communications are incoherent would be considered lacking in decisional capacity.[128]

The second component of capacity is the ability to understand relevant information. This feature does not require that patients have the ability to understand information in every category of knowledge but only in the categories that are relevant for the healthcare decision at hand.[129] Thus, an individual may very well be able to make financial decisions but may be unable to grasp the information necessary to make a sound healthcare decision (or vice versa). It is important for caregivers to give some attention to this characteristic because some tests for orientation may have little to do with deciding decisional capacity. And yet great weight is given to them in the clinical setting.

The third component is extremely difficult to judge in some cases. This constituent is identified as the ability to manipulate information rationally. Caregivers could easily set the standards too high for this test. To satisfy this component, caregivers might be tempted to demand that patients follow the same rules of logic to which they themselves subscribe. However, everyone need not follow the same rules of logic in order to manipulate information rationally. What is basically required is that individuals see the connections between bits of information and that they can establish further connections between the information they have, or are given, and the decisions they make. Thus, it is not illogical for members of the Jehovah's Witness community to refuse blood products. Their decision is logically related to the information they have about God's law.[130] The premises of their decision may simply be different from those of other patients. If the logic is consistent, then the conclusion must be upheld regardless of the content of the decision. Though this may be a difficult standard to apply, its application must include a great deal of latitude for the individual differences among patients and their cultures.[131]

The last feature of capacity that Appelbaum and Grisso identify may very well be one of the most significant. This trait is the ability of a patient to appreciate the situation in which she finds herself and the *consequences* of the situation.[132] If the patient does not possess this ability, then one can confidently say that the patient lacks capacity.[133] For example, an elderly patient with already compromised system function may be facing a possible DNR decision. Thus, to be considered as having the capacity to make such a decision, the patient would have to understand the nature of her condition and the extent to which it is compromised. Additionally, she would have to know the likelihood of a "successful" CPR attempt and the outcomes of such an attempt for someone her age and in her condition.[134] Finally, she would have to know the outcomes of a DNR order, as well as the positive benefits for her care and comfort that a DNR order might provide or foreclose. This is an important feature of capacity because it combines both the canons of informed consent and the trust a caregiver must have in the patient, who may make a decision that may not please the caregiver or the patient's family.

An additional feature to be considered has been identified by Jonson et al. in their manual *Clinical Ethics*.[135] The authors point to the patient's having goals and values as an important component to decisional capacity. This implies that the patient can articulate to some extent the goals and values she possesses and can make decisions consistent with them. Taking into account the values of the patient individualizes the assessment of capacity. As in assessing the ability to manipulate information rationally, here caregivers must guard against the imposition of their own conceptual and value frameworks, as well as their priorities, on the patient. Patients' values may be significantly different from those of the caregivers or family members, but such differences do not point to decisional incapacity in the patient.

The caution has been repeatedly sounded that, in assessing decisional capacity, one must avoid any standard suggesting that agreement with the caregiver would be a primary indicator of capacity.[136] When patients make healthcare decisions that are in agreement with those of their caregivers, the caregivers often simply accept the decision without challenge either to the decision or to the patient's decisional capacity. However, when the decision is in disagreement with the caregivers' agenda, the decision is often challenged, and if it is not changed, the patient's capacity to make the decision often comes into question. Such an approach places the patient in a particularly vulnerable position and virtually strips her of all decisional autonomy unless she can vigorously defend her capacity to make the decision.

The preferable approach to the relationship between the patient's agreement with the caregivers' preferences and the assessment of decisional capacity would be to view agreement as indicating nothing about the patient's capacity.[137] With this approach, the canons of informed consent would be followed for each decision and the tests for capacity would be applied on their own merits and only when concerns arose independently of agreements or disagreements. Every decision would be treated equally and would require the same kind of test for capacity when questions arose.

In the fairly recent past, clinical practice often presumed that the patient, who was rendered vulnerable by disease or injury, did not have the capacity to make healthcare decisions, particularly when there was a history of mental illness.[138] The patient was considered to have been made so vulnerable by the disease that she was out of control both of her lifestyle and the ability to return to it. This was based upon the belief that the information required to make the decision was simply out of reach of the patient. Thus the patient could neither access the information nor manipulate it rationally. Furthermore, the patient's personal stake in the outcomes of the syndrome or therapies was thought to cloud her judgmental abilities. With these beliefs as a background, others, especially the physician, were placed in the primary decision-making role.

In recent times the President's Commission has redirected that attitude.[139] The commission identifies the proper approach as presuming the capacity rather than the incapacity of the patient. This strategy allows for respect for the patient's dignity and autonomy from the outset. The patient is vulnerable only in some aspects in the clinical relationship. There is no justification for presuming that the patient's vulnerability is extended to the ability to make decisions. It may be true that some patients may find their decisional ability compromised by fear or uncertainty. In such cases the proper approach is not to declare them lacking in decisional capacity. Instead they may only need special assistance in making the decisions they face.[140]

The Patient Self-Determination Act has a direct bearing on the issue of decisional capacity. If one takes the approach to the law that it is important to *assist* patients, as the President's Commission suggests, in the decisions that have to be made relative to the law, then decisional capacity can be significantly strengthened in the clinical setting. Taking a mechanical approach to the implementation of the law would result in further compromising the patient's decisional capacity and underlying dignity by failing to promote decisional capacity in those who might be on its functional margins. The superficial approach to informing patients about the stipulations of the law could compromise decisional capacity in the areas of making choices, understanding relevant information, and appreciating their situations and the consequences of their decisions. Finally, the lack of information would compromise their ability to manipulate the information they do have in a rational manner in light of their values and goals. For example, many patients do not realize that they have the right to refuse treatment. Even if they are informed of this right in their initial interview at a healthcare facility, they may not understand its full significance. This might also apply to the matter of drafting an advance directive.

Assisting patients in processing the various concerns of the Patient Self-Determination Act will enhance their decisional capacity by helping them form appropriate choices about their healthcare. Caregivers will be able to identify the information patients need and give them the confidence to demand further explanations when those that have been given to them are insufficient. This assistance will give them a better perspective on their healthcare situations and the results of various treatment alternatives, including no treatment at all. Finally, this approach will make it possible for patients to order the information within the context of their values and goals, which the assistance will help them identify and rank according to their personal priorities. All of these efforts will substantially bolster the patient's dignity.

We can see once again how a perfunctory approach to the Patient Self-Determination Act can diminish the patient in ways that are substantially harmful. This happens when the law is treated as an administrative nuisance to be discharged as conveniently as possible. On the other hand, we can see how careful adherence to the spirit of the law and attempts to make it work fully for the benefit of the patient can enrich the patient's relationship with the caregivers and the institution caring for the patient. The patient's dignity is enhanced, which is one of the primary goals of healthcare.

The Right to Refuse Treatment

The Patient Self-Determination Act explicitly recognizes the right of competent adults to refuse treatment. The law promotes this right not only by acknowledging it but also by ensuring that patients know about it. Until recent years it has generally been assumed by caregivers that patients knew about their right in this regard. However, because of the kind of language used in talking with patients—for example, only offering different *treatments*—and the limited scope of conversations with them, patients often presumed that they had to select some sort of treatment. All too often they did not infer that a legitimate therapeutic approach for a particular condition might be no treatment at all. With the Patient Self-Determination Act this erroneous presumption on the part of patients should no longer occur.

The right to refuse treatment is based on the right of thoroughgoing self-determination that lies at the heart of democratic institutions.[141]

It is a political right that has been accepted in healthcare as the right of individuals to be free from any kind of touching to which they do not give consent.[142] It has also been interpreted by some courts as grounded in a fundamental right to privacy guaranteed by the U.S. Constitution in its First, Fourth, Fifth, Ninth, and Fourteenth Amendments. In chapter 2 we saw how this right was applied in *Quinlan*,[143] *Bartling*,[144] and *Brophy*.[145] In *Cruzan* we saw how the right to refuse treatment has been interpreted as a less rigid constitutional right —namely, as a liberty right, based only on the Fourteenth Amendment.[146] The U.S. Supreme Court has also reaffirmed this right in its decision on physician-assisted suicide: "*Everyone,* regardless of physical condition, is entitled, if competent, to refuse unwanted lifesaving treatment."[147]

If someone has a right, then another individual or organization has a duty to perform some action to help that individual obtain what the right guarantees or to refrain from actions that prevent the person from enjoying the right.[148] The former is called a positive right and the latter is called a negative right.[149] For example, if an individual has a right to Medicare reimbursement for a healthcare service, then the government has the duty to pay for the service. This is called a positive right because it requires an action on the part of the one holding the duty.[150] On the other hand, if an individual has a right to the integrity of her body in such a way that she cannot be touched without consenting to it, then caregivers have the obligation to refrain from touching her without her consent. This is called a negative right because it imposes on others the duty *not* to perform an action.[151]

Though for the most part the Patient Self-Determination Act confers no new substantive rights on patients, it does confer one significant new positive right. It asserts that patients have the *right to know* that they can consent to or refuse treatment, what the hospital policies are regarding limiting treatments, and the stipulations of local state laws regarding advance directives. Therefore, it imposes on healthcare institutions the obligation to engage in an action—namely, to inform patients about their right to refuse treatment, etc. The Patient Self-Determination Act itself does not confer upon patients the right to refuse treatment or the right to sign or draft an advance directive. They already have those rights (conferred by states in the case of advance directives).

Having a right sets a minimal standard for behavior in our society. However, we often do much more for individuals simply because we desire to promote their welfare. And so it is with the Patient Self-Determination Act. In chapter 5 it was noted that healthcare institutions need not go beyond merely *notifying* patients of their rights. However, the mission dimension of the institution may call it to further actions such as *assisting* patients in understanding their rights and helping while they go through the decision-making process as they exercise their rights. If institutions decide not to assist patients in making decisions relative to the rights granted by the Patient Self-Determination Act, they are still fulfilling their basic obligations under the law. There is still a question, however, of how seriously the institution wishes to promote patient dignity because mere no-tification may do little to achieve this goal.

It could surely seem paradoxical to many patients that when they come to a healthcare facility seeking treatment for a disease or injury, one of the first things they hear is that they have the right to refuse treatment. The notification may very well cause wonderment, dismay, or anxiety. Perhaps the first question the interviewer will encounter will be something like: "Why would I want to refuse treatment when I came here to get well?" This would be an opportune moment to educate both patients and their family members not only for the immediate hospital stay but for future stays as well. The limits of healthcare interventions are not an inappropriate topic for patients to consider. Though the Patient Self-Determination Act does not *require* such a discussion, nonetheless it would certainly aid in accomplishing the intent of the law—namely, to help patients become more reflective consumers of healthcare.[152]

One of the reasons for refusing treatment might be that a patient is terminally ill and a particular treatment will not succeed in its attempt to cure. A terminal illness or condition, resulting from disease or injury, is one that is irreversible and causes progressive deterioration. The result is that the patient will die from the condition, and even the use of life-sustaining treatments will only postpone the moment of death.

Life-sustaining treatments, then, are those that, within the context of a terminal illness or condition, only prolong the dying process. They frequently provide little, if any, comfort for the patients or improvement in their quality of life. Thus, some patients, wishing to practice the virtues of acceptance and detachment, may refuse life-sustaining treatments because prolonging the dying process does not fit into their goals for living and dying. On the other hand, some patients may wish life-sustaining treatment because it fits into their values and goals to delay the process of dying. Obviously, this is an intensely personal choice.[153] But it can be a choice only if the patients know that they have the right to refuse treatment.

One of the key questions, then, that patients must ask themselves when approaching the matter of exercising their right to refuse treatment is: "What benefit will the treatment have for me?" Benefits come in a variety of forms. Complete recovery from a disease is one form of benefit, as are the remission of a disease process or the improvement of one's quality of life. Returning an already impaired patient to a previous level of functioning or to a minimally decent quality of life are other benefits. Helping a patient to regain consciousness so that she will be able to interact with her environment and those who care for her is a particular benefit to be considered. Some may consider it beneficial to maintain a permanently unconscious patient in a minimal biological state so that she remains a merely metabolizing body, but others find such a benefit highly questionable.[154]

Each patient must look at his particular condition and decide whether the treatments being considered have a decent probability of achieving a particular benefit. If they do not, then refusing treatment may be the appropriate option. Once again, the patient's value context becomes important in making this decision. For a patient may very well decide that a particular quality of life is not minimally decent for him or that the continuance of a merely biological existence does not fit into his assessment of his finitude and the practice of his virtues within that context.[155]

There is a variation to refusing treatment on the basis of its yielding no benefit. This involves refusing treatment based upon the weighing of the benefits of the treatment against the burdens the treatment imposes upon the patient. In this approach, treatment can be refused even if it provides benefits. The deciding factor is whether the treatment also imposes burdens upon the patient that the patient finds too difficult to bear, in which case the refusal of the treatment is considered morally appropriate. For example it might be perfectly appropriate to refuse CPR even though it might restore the heartbeat if the resulting prospect is languishing for two weeks in an intensive care unit with death at the end of that period. In this context it must always be remembered that patients can refuse treatments for any reason.[156] They can do so even on a whim. They do not need a "good" reason for doing so.[157] Therefore, caregivers and families cannot impose their own criteria on the patient. The patient's preference stands on its own merit. This weighing of benefits and burdens is supported by considerations of both autonomy and beneficence.

The weighing of benefits against burdens involves a whole cluster of considerations, including the patient's value context. Again, the third level of informed consent is shown to be central to good decision making.[158] Patients will have to consider not only whether the proposed treatment will achieve its therapeutic goal—that is, not be futile—but also whether the goal is worth accomplishing and how the goals of the treatment will fit into the patient's lifestyle goals.

A decent estimation of the burdens of an intervention, as compared with the benefits, will also have to be made. For example, patients may select surgery because in spite of the severe discomfort and disability that often accompany it, the long-term benefit makes the short-term difficulties worth enduring. In some cases, however, the burdens may be considered so heavy as to minimize any benefit that might accompany the intervention.

The patient with decisional capacity will be the morally appropriate person to do the weighing because it is the patient who will, in the last analysis, bear the full impact of the burden. When the patient is suffering from incapacity, then the patient's authorized surrogate is charged with the task. Weighing benefits against burdens is a very delicate process and one that requires as much clarity as possible regarding the values and best interests of the patient.

In summary, the process of communicating with individuals so that they can share in the responsibility for healthcare decisions, particularly those that will result in treatment refusals, requires fidelity to the canons of informed consent. Patients must be given accurate information that includes an understanding of their rights, a realistic assessment of their conditions, and what they can expect from treatment interventions. The information must be given in language they can understand. Before they come to a decision, they should be given the opportunity to incorporate the information into their values. It is essential that individuals have a chance to explore their feelings as they are considering a decision and be supported in the decisions they make.[159] Conversations about these important healthcare decisions should occur frequently so that individuals can monitor their situations and reconsider previous decisions in light of changes in their conditions or their additional experiences.

The Patient Self-Determination Act uses the right to refuse treatment as its pivotal point. Information about all the other stipulations of the law revolve around this fundamental right. For this reason, if for no other, special attention must be paid to conversations held with patients on this topic. The quality and extent of the conversations must be a matter of serious concern. Unfortunately, the emphasis in healthcare practice has focused on the more dramatic and tangible issue of advance directives. Effective programs need to be grounded in the underlying right to refuse treatment. Patients who receive this aid will benefit greatly from the implementation of the law while others, left to their own devices, may be left to flounder in this most difficult of healthcare decisions.

Demands for Treatment

If the right to self-determination establishes the right to refuse medical treatment, symmetry would seem to require that patients have a right to demand treatment as well. This would mean that individuals have a right to healthcare. At current writing, this situation is not the case in the United States.[160] Nor is it the case in other countries where there is a right to healthcare that patients have the right to every possible form of healthcare. For even in those countries where universal access to healthcare is guaranteed by the tax dollars collected, there is a rationing at the point of utilization.[161] In countries where universal access is available, rationing is the price individuals have to pay.[162]

A return to the examination of the concept of rights will reveal the reason for the asymmetry in the right to self-determination. It will be recalled from the previous section that a right entails a duty imposed upon someone or some organization to act in certain ways or refrain from acting in certain ways so that the values identified by the right can be realized. Without a duty on another there is no right, only a wish or desire that certain things might happen.[163]

A duty, then, is a burden that someone has to bear in order for others to achieve a certain good that they, or society in general, have deemed worthy of protection. If duties are viewed as burdens, then the asymmetry between the right to refuse treatment and the right to demand treatment begins to make sense. In exercising the right to refuse treatment the patient is only placing upon another the duty to *refrain* from acting. Thus, the burden on the person or institution possessing the duty is a light, or indirect, one requiring no positive actions on the bearer of the duty to promote the welfare of the one refusing treatment. The bearer of the duty does not have to engage in any direct action or bear any special economic burden. At most the individual may have to watch a patient pursue an approach to a healthcare condition with which he does not agree. It may be that such a duty might place a strain on the integrity of the caregiver. But such is the burden caregivers assume (in light of their pledge of beneficence) as a part of the responsibilities of their profession: setting aside their own preferences to promote the good of those whom they have dedicated themselves to serving. In this case the major burden falls on the individual refusing treatment. This individual is the one who may be placing herself in harm's way by her decision and she must bear the consequences.

On the other hand, a right to demand treatment would impose upon another a serious burden in the form of a duty. The individual or institution bearing the duty would be required to engage in positive actions or bear financial burdens that might be considered too heavy to bear. In addition, the bearer of the duty might have to transgress some important professional obligations if he is engaging in some actions that might very well harm the patient demanding the treatment.[164] For example, a patient who asks for healthcare in the form of aid in dying may be imposing an unwarranted burden on the physician if the physician understands that his professional obligations prohibit such assistance.

The principles of bioethics provide another vantage point from which to view demands for treatment. If the patient suffers harm in refusing treatment, the harm is the patient's, under considerations of autonomy. In the case of treatment refusals, autonomy overrides a desire on the part of caregivers to be beneficent by imposing treatment. If the patient enjoys a benefit from refusing treatment, then the benefit is the result of both the autonomy of the patient and the beneficence of the caregiver who has honored the patient's autonomy. If a patient suffers harm in demanding inappropriate treatment, the requirement to produce the harm in the form of treatment imposes a heavy duty on the bearer of the duty—that is, the caregiver, who may be honoring the patient's wishes but who also violates the principle of nonmaleficence, the first step of beneficence.[165] If a patient should benefit from that inappropriate treatment, then the caregiver may have honored the patient's autonomy but only accidentally fulfilled the requirements of beneficence.

In addition, there is often limited financial liability if a patient refuses treatment. However, if a patient can demand treatment and cannot pay for it, someone else must bear the burden of the cost—members of the taxpaying community or members of the insurance pool or both. In exceptional cases, patients could refuse a certain form of healthcare that, if utilized, could improve their situation, but without which they could continue with ongoing healthcare problems. There could be significant costs in such cases, but one would hope that such cases would be rare. Perhaps these sorts of cases indicate that there are hidden costs to the exercise of autonomy.

In summary, then, refusals of treatment ordinarily impose only light, or indirect, burdens on another by way of duties, whereas demands for treatment could impose heavy burdens. As a society we have a tacit commitment to keep burdens at a minimum when possible. This may be one of the reasons why American society, up to this time, has recognized the right to refuse treatment while not granting the right to demand treatment.

Though there is no universal right to healthcare in the United States, there are some limited legal rights to it. Medicare and Medicaid are two forms of these entitlements, and for those who qualify for the programs it can be said that they have a right to some healthcare. Dialysis is a right for every citizen since it is funded by Medicare but is extended to all citizens and is not restricted only to those over sixty-five. Even with Medicare and Medicaid programs, however, there is a form of rationing. For example, transplant surgery is available to members of the programs only on a very limited basis.

In a free market economy one gets what one can pay for either in direct payment or indirect payment through an insurance contract.[166] Any care is available if one can pay the price. In this case the right to healthcare follows from the ability to pay. In healthcare programs, on the other hand, the right to healthcare extends only as far as the providers' willingness to pay for procedures.[167] If the provider is unwilling to pay, then the only way the individual can get the procedures is to pay for it out of pocket or have it provided as an act of charity.

Limits on healthcare provided by taxpayer-supported or insurance programs are ordinarily determined by examining what the programs are willing to provide. Some procedures are considered too costly for the program for the benefits they provide. Sometimes these procedures are called "not costworthy."[168] Sometimes procedures are considered experimental and not clinical.[169] All programs, therefore, stipulate the limits of treatment that they will make available to their subscribers. No program can provide everything. Thus, demands for treatment can never be universally satisfied unless one pays for the treatment out of pocket.

Because of this disparity between refusals of and demands for treatment, conversations about the Patient Self-Determination Act must be very clear about the parameters of self-determination. Though patients must clearly understand that they have the right to refuse treatment, they must also understand that requests or demands for treatments must be considered as their conditions warrant and as treatment options present themselves in their fiscal situations.[170] Any specific limitations on treatments must be discussed with the patient's caregivers. However, at the time of admission, a summary of the healthcare institution's general policies on limiting treatments must be made available to patients or potential patients.[171] This will be a delicate matter to communicate at the time of admission, but it is essential so that patients will be able to decide if they want to continue the admission procedure.[172] It would certainly be unfair to disclose to the patient the information about the institution's policies after the patient is admitted or is made a member of a health maintenance organization.

In examining the matter of a right to demand treatment or a right to healthcare, we have looked at the issue from the standpoint of *legal* rights. Strong positions have been taken in the healthcare reform debate that though we may not have an entitlement to healthcare presently, we still have a *moral* right to healthcare.[173] The difference between the two forms of rights can be briefly outlined in the following manner.[174] Legal rights are those that are codified and specify the individual, group, or institution upon which the duty to act or refrain falls. This identification sets the stage for a judicial process that can be invoked if there is a failure to perform the duty. To put it another way, a legal right guarantees the right to sue. Moral rights, on the other hand, are not codified. They appeal only to the enlightened conscience. Although they may identify the individual, group, or institution upon which the duty should fall, they cannot do so with the force of judicial intervention if the "duty" were to be transgressed.[175] For this reason, moral rights take on the complexion of wishes or desires held by individuals without the power of legal sanctions.[176]

In spite of their limitations, moral rights are not totally anemic. They can be a strong force in society for social change. Legal rights do not emerge from a vacuum. They are developed and codified as the result of prior beliefs and desires in society, which often take the form of expressions of moral rights. As the moral rights that are articulated become more convincing and more pressing, they may be translated into legal rights. This is precisely what is happening in the healthcare debate. The moral right to healthcare has been articulated for a number of years but has only now reached a point where there is widespread agreement that it embodies values worthy of being encased in legal rights.[177] However, even the legal right to demand treatment will have some limitations because of the nature of the conditions of patients, the therapeutic possibilities, and the limitations on the economic resources that can be made available for healthcare.

The Patient Self-Determination Act may be another case of a moral right being translated into a legal right. Since the problem of patients' knowing about the right to refuse treatment emerged in the last generation and new strategies for patients were opened by advance directive legislation in the states, there was a demand that somehow patients ought to know about their rights in these areas. The moral pressure became so great that the law was enacted.

Clinical Futility

One difficult, challenging, and perplexing problem facing contemporary healthcare in a climate of self-determination has come to be known as futile treatment. The difficulty arises from the specific technological and social milieu of contemporary medical practice. Today death does not "automatically" or immediately follow from a critical illness or injury. Many interventions can be interposed between the illness or injury and death. In some cases, the course of the malady can be significantly altered or entirely turned around. But this is not the issue that futility raises.

The significant concern with futility arises when the inevitability of death cannot be faced and the desire to postpone death in vain attempts to "cure" takes over the direction of treatment.[178] The attitude in society of keeping death at arm's length rather than embracing it as an essential component of the human reality fuels the pursuit of futile treatment. Since so many life-extending interventions are currently available, with many more being developed for the future, the boundaries of futile treatment are becoming more and more indeterminate. A clear conceptual map around the issue of futile treatment is badly needed because of the difficulty of defining "futility," but it seems to become more elusive as time goes on.[179] At best it may be possible to identify the values involved and points to be addressed in making such decisions.

Addressing this issue is essential for implementing the Patient Self-Determination Act. Before examining the issues involved in making determinations of futility, its relation to the Patient Self-Determination Act requires some explanation. The law requires that patients be informed that they have the right to refuse treatment. As we have seen, this means that they have the right to refuse any and all treatments regardless of the reason for their refusal. We have also seen that patients may wonder about the clinical reasons for refusing treatments. In response to this very important level of curiosity, patients should be informed that refusals of futile treatment would be very appropriate.[180] In order to give this information to patients there would have to be some explanation about the parameters of futility and what they should look for in their care related to these parameters. A case can be made that only the patient's physician can identify the notion of futility in the case of any given patient.[181] To begin thinking about the matter of futility somewhere early in the treatment process may make it easier to address the issue if it ultimately emerges in the course of treatment.

As we have seen in the previous section, demanding treatments as an expression of self-determination has some significant limits. One of those limits is futile treatments. It has never been a part of the Hippocratic tradition to administer futile treatments.[182] On the contrary, to do so would violate the principle of beneficence. Physicians are required to *benefit* patients and, by definition, futile treatments do not accomplish this end. As a matter of fact, futile treatment may not only not benefit patients but actually do harm to them,[183] by, for example, creating illusions about the possibilities of the treatment or even inflicting additional pain. It may also result in treating patients in ways that are contrary to their conditions, a violation of the principle of justice, itself a form of harm.[184] Thus, it is appropriate to include futility in the discussion of the refusal of treatment.[185]

Since the Patient Self-Determination Act requires that patients be informed of the policies of a healthcare facility or organization regarding the withholding or withdrawing of life-sustaining treatments, the issue of futility may be relevant here as well. Some healthcare institutions and communities are boldly addressing the issue of futile care by developing policies outlining their stance on the issue.[186] These policies are an attempt to address issues of patient welfare, which futile treatments do not promote; caregiver morale, which futile treatments often compromise; and resource allocation, which futile treatments squander.[187] When such policies are developed, patients must know upon admission the general character of the policies and the general manner in which they may be applied in the clinical setting. Patients, or potential patients, must understand that just as self-determination does not extend to demanding treatments that are contrary to acceptable medical practice,[188] so also it does not extend to demanding treatments that are prohibited by institutional policy.

At this point it would be helpful to examine directly the issue of futility to gain a better perspective of the issues involved in making such determinations and to explore any flexibility that might be present in setting its parameters within the context of the Patient Self-Determination Act. In the most general terms, any kind of action is considered futile if it cannot achieve the goal toward which it is directed.[189] Thus, any discussion of futility must begin with a clear definition of the goal to be accomplished. To overcome death as the outcome of treatments directed toward certain types of aggressive cancer is futile. However, introducing remission into the disease process may not be futile. As the goals of interventions change, the determination of the futility of interventions will also change.

If the identification of goals is essential to defining futility, then several significant questions arise. One must first be clear about what kinds of goals are being formulated and who determines them.[190] The clinician would be the likely person to determine appropriate medical goals (e.g., cure, restoration of heartbeat, return of kidney function, etc.) because she possesses medical expertise. The patient, as the primary decision maker, would be the candidate for identifying the appropriate goals insofar as they are consonant with the patient's values. Finally, the patient's authorized surrogate, as the secondary decision maker when the patient is unable to participate in the decisional process, may be considered the appropriate individual to identify the proper goal of an intervention in conjunction with the patient's known values.

The final and perhaps most troublesome question of all may be whether the desired goal itself is suitable. With the issue of identifying the decision maker we have some procedures and criteria to which we have generally agreed as a society. But the propriety of therapeutic goals is often subject to the same variety and lack of agreement as the goals for human life in general in a pluralistic society. This does not mean that it is impossible for clinicians, patients, and institutions to negotiate differences with each other about the goals that are appropriate in the clinical setting. Nor does it mean that parameters for the negotiation cannot be established.[191] It merely means that negotiation and its parameters are essential to addressing the issue of determining futility.

Having seen the general problem of determining futility, we can now examine three different forms of futility. The first form is the one that has received the greatest attention in the current debates. This can be identified as *medical* futility. There is no standard definition for this form of futility. However, a very useful definition might be "any effort to achieve a result [medical] that is possible but that reasoning or experience suggests is highly improbable and that cannot be systematically produced."[192] Another dimension has often been added to the definition by describing a futile intervention as one that does not produce its intended physiological effect or has a statistically very low probability of doing so.[193]

Several issues need to be noted in this dimension of futility. In the first place, since it is a definition of *medical* futility, the determination is made by the physician, with no contribution from the patients. The decision is based purely upon the disposition of the organism and its reaction to therapeutic interventions. The discoveries of scientific investigators provide significant information for the clinician's determination of medical futility. For the determination is made on the basis not of an individual's experience alone or anecdotal evidence from a few colleagues but upon the statistical probability of an intervention's producing a medical outcome. However, any statistical probability that is determined by research efforts must be applied to the particular circumstances of a patient's condition as the patient's physician exercises his clinical judgment.[194]

One of the more difficult issues to address in determining medical futility is certainly the matter of statistical probability. Determining the exact boundaries of futility is impossible. Few medical matters admit of 0 percent probability, although some could be identified if the diagnosis is accurate.[195] There remains, then, the need to determine whether a 10 percent probability of an outcome's being produced by an intervention should determine that the intervention is futile. If not 10 percent, then perhaps 5 percent, or 3 percent, or 1 percent, or 0.5 percent. Relating statistical probability to futility is therefore a matter of judgment. If it is a matter of judgment, then the issue becomes one of identifying whose judgment is most accurate, whose should be the overriding judgment, and what counts as a reasonable judgment. At this point there is little agreement on these questions. If a treatment has a low probability of benefit, it may be inappropriate but not necessarily futile.[196]

Another dimension of the determination of futility can be identified as *personally determined* futility.[197] Personally determined futility describes an effort to achieve a result that may be possible but does not fall within the personally defined goals of the patient (or surrogates who can legitimately speak for patients). As we have seen, each patient approaches the clinical setting with a value history that has helped to define her as a person and some particular goals about her life and what she hopes to accomplish through the therapeutic interventions being considered. In some cases medical interventions may be able to achieve some particular goals that the patient does not consider worthy of attainment. For example, CPR may restore heartbeat to a patient only to leave the patient to languish for an indefinite period of time in an intensive care unit or an extended care facility with ongoing deteriorating function from some disease process. To live in such a way may not fit within the goals of such a patient. Therefore, whereas the CPR may not be futile in the *medical* sense—because restoring heartbeat is the goal of CPR and this can be accomplished—it may be futile in a *personally determined* sense since it cannot achieve the goals of the patient. From the perspective of statistical probability, a physician may think that any result greater than 5 percent is not futile while a patient may think that a 10 percent chance of a favorable outcome is necessary to cross over the line of futility. In many cases, then, the boundaries of personally determined futility may be more limited than the actual possibilities of medicine. In such cases, the Patient Self-Determination Act, with its right to refuse treatment, accommodates the personally determined sense of futility quite nicely.

From the opposite perspective it may be the case that an individual might consider his *personally determined* sense of futility to be broader than the judgment of *medical* futility. In such a case, using the CPR example, a physician may judge that a patient may survive a CPR attempt but would be severely compromised and would never survive to leave the hospital. But for some particular reason the patient may be willing to continue living in spite of the seriously compromised condition. Or the physician may consider a 1 percent chance of a favorable outcome equivalent to futility, but the patient might be willing to pursue treatment on the basis of a less than 1 percent chance no matter how minuscule. In these situations, where there are differences in values rather than facts, the treatment may be inappropriate or inadvisable in the physician's judgment but not futile.[198]

One might well wonder why patients or surrogates would be willing to entertain such broad *personal* determinations of futility. The answer may lie in the fact that many patients and their surrogates cling to even the slimmest of hopes. In fact, they are often encouraged by caregivers to do so instead of being shown that acceptance and detachment are virtues equal in stature to hope. It is often easier to authorize the use of technological interventions than it is to talk to patients about the difficult subject of futility or inadvisable treatments. With its emphasis on treatment refusals and knowledge of hospital (or extended care facility) policies on withholding or withdrawing treatments, the Patient Self-Determination Act may teach patients something of the limitations of life and medicine and they may become less eager to pursue inappropriate aggressive therapies.

However, there are other matters involved in making decisions about futile treatments that must be considered. Often futile treatments are selected and not refused because patients and their families are in a state of denial or grief about the nature of the illness or injury they are facing. Futile treatment is often selected by families for incompetent members as a result of guilt. Guilt is a powerful motive for human actions, especially when it is coupled with years of neglect. Finally, fear on the part of caregivers can be a motive for engaging in futile treatment or limiting discussions about futile treatment with patients and their families in spite of medical indications of futility. Fear of liability is often a reason given for overtreatment. Developing case law demonstrates that the fear of liability in situations where treatments are futile is greatly overstated.[199]

Because of the wide disparity that can occur between the two senses of futility outlined above, a third sense might be considered that may more correctly reflect the nature of the clinical setting and lead to a reconciliation of any differences. This third sense could be called a judgment of *clinical* futility.

Chapter 3 defined the clinical setting as the situation in which both physician and patient are interested parties in the therapeutic outcomes and collaborators in the process of making decisions. The clinical relationship is not a one-sided interaction, with the pathways of the decisions always going in one direction. Instead it is a relationship of mutuality where trust on both sides confers credibility on each partner and where differences are negotiated in such a way that the integrity of both parties is preserved while retaining the well-being of the patient as the primary goal of the clinical encounter.

Because of these dynamics, *clinical* futility can be described as a judgment that integrates considerations of medical futility and personally determined futility into a unified whole and reflects the interests of the total patient and the other individuals who are legitimate participants in the decisional process. Thus, clinical futility considers both the objective research findings coupled with the clinical judgment of the physician and the values and goals of the patient, which have been expressed by the patient herself or her authorized surrogate. This approach to futility opens the path to negotiation when differences occur between patients and caregivers. It allows caregivers to set the parameters for honoring the patient's wishes—when not all wishes can be honored. It also allows patients to push the boundaries of medical futility to allow them to pursue some *reasonable* values and goals, like witnessing a particular event of extraordinary significance to the patient that will occur in the very near future.

There is no easy formula for resolving the negotiations involved in the issue of clinical futility. Ideally, a compromise will be reached by, for example, allowing a patient to pursue a course of treatment for a limited time so she might be able to achieve a personal, but reasonable, goal. Or a patient might be given a time-limited trial, such as an extra week on the ventilator to develop greater certainty in the family about the medical futility of the intervention. However, there may come a time when compromises will not be possible. In such cases, personally determined futility in the form of refusing treatment always overrides a physician's unwillingness to declare an intervention futile.[200] When patients demand an intervention that is clearly medically futile, then judgments of medical futility override the wishes expressed in judgments of personally determined futility.[201] When this situation arises, the interests of effective communication between patient/surrogate and physician require the physician to explain to the patient why the intervention is futile.[202]

When a patient or surrogate requests or demands medically futile treatment, the following alternative approach can be used. Instead of simply responding with the implementation of the treatment, caregivers can address the issues of denial or grief. This should not be done in a way that the patient or family is harmed by the destruction of their defenses. Rather, it can be approached with an attitude of acceptance but with an openness to explore all the relevant issues regarding the patient's condition. This might move the participants in the decision from denial to acceptance and the most appropriate decision that is in the best interests of the patient.

In a similar manner the issue of guilt can be addressed. Guilt is not resolved by recourse to inappropriate technological interventions. Rather, guilt is an internal attempt to cope with the inadequacies of one's behavior. Thus, the only way to address it is to meet it in its own arena. Technology does not confront the matter of guilt; at best, it only delays the engagement. Caregivers must always remember that their covenant is primarily with the patient and only secondarily with the family. Therefore, they cannot, within the context of their traditions and commitments, harm the patient in order to assuage the guilt of family members. It would be ethically inappropriate and contrary to the Patient Self-Determination Act to override a patient's refusal of futile treatment merely to meet the needs of family members.

Thus, when requests or demands for futile treatment are made, an automatic authorization of the technological intervention is often inappropriate.[203] It is more helpful to examine the feelings of the patient or the patient's family or authorized surrogate. With this approach there is a better chance of serving the total good of the patient rather than satisfying some fragment of the patient's clinical presentation such as restoring heartbeat in the presence of multisystem failure. Treating only a fragment of the patient's presentation while all the rest is fatally compromised frequently harms, rather than helps the patient.

Finally, since the issue of legal liability is often identified by caregivers as an additional reason for pursuing medically futile treatment, some perspective is necessary to avoid this pitfall.[204] Liability issues are certainly a major problem in our society, and the importance of being cautious about them should not be minimized. However, they can be overemphasized as well. The obligation of caregivers is to provide medical treatment appropriate to a patient's condition and not to harm the patient. Futile treatment can arguably be said to harm the patient. The best protection against liability problems in the matter of futile treatments may not be the implementation of the treatments but rather full disclosure to patients and their families of the nature of the condition they face and a realistic assessment of the possibilities for a successful outcome.[205] Such an open discussion can have many salutary benefits for patients, families, surrogates, and caregivers alike. Among them will often be the refusal of futile treatments by patients or their authorized surrogates in the context of the Patient Self-Determination Act.

A very practical issue underlies the emerging concern with the utilization of futile treatments. Treatments under these conditions are generally technology-intensive and consequently very costly. In a society that is becoming increasingly concerned about its allocation of resources in all economic areas including healthcare, the lack of cost-effectiveness of futile care cannot be ignored.[206] Though the Patient Self-Determination Act is not intended to address the issue of resource allocation, it can nonetheless have a favorable impact on it because a wise decision maker will not select treatments that are not beneficial in some way, thereby saving the cost of futile treatments.[207]

A final consideration is that of stretching the boundaries of medical futility to accommodate the approach to personally determined futility that represents the values and goals of the patient. Certain interventions may, in the calculated range of probabilities, provide only a very small chance of meeting a medical goal. However, that chance may be sufficient to allow a particular patient to meet an important goal. For example, CPR for an elderly chronically ill patient has a very poor probability of success.[208] However, this patient may wish to witness her grandson's bar mitzvah, which will occur within a short period of time. This may be sufficient reason to attempt CPR even with the extremely limited probability that the patient will survive the attempt with enough mentation to witness the event. This example reveals the other side of the Patient Self-Determination Act, which requires that patients be informed of their right to *consent* to treatment.

Thus, patients who have clearly defined and time-limited goals may best be served by allowing them the latitude to pursue reasonable goals in the face of ultimate medical futility. It is true that some negotiation will have to be conducted about what counts as a "reasonable" goal. But negotiation about matters of this kind is common in the clinical setting.

In summary, then, there are two major difficulties in addressing the issue of futility. The first is the matter of defining futility with the appropriate categories. The Patient Self-Determination Act provides the opportunity to discuss futility with patients in light of their right to refuse treatments and, in some cases, their right to consent to treatment. But, in order for the discussions to be effective, caregivers must have a clear sense of what they are talking about so that the proper parameters of their discussions can be established.

The second difficulty is equally problematic because its definition is often value-laden.[209] It involves the right of competent patients to *demand* futile treatment. Whereas the right to refuse treatment has been well established in both ethics and the law, the right to demand treatment has not been so established except in the case of public healthcare facilities and entitlement programs. Demanding futile treatment is a particular problem because the Hippocratic tradition requires that physicians not harm their patients and, by extension, benefit them when possible. It does not require that they use futile treatment in the care of their patients. Of course, this issue did not emerge with any significant importance until the advent of modern medical technology.

The traditional criteria and principles of bioethics still seem to work. This does not mean that the physician should simply refuse to provide such treatment to her patients. Nor does it mean that she should automatically, and without reflection, authorize futile interventions. Rather, an appropriate strategy might very well be to explore the feelings of patients and their family members that underlie the demand for such treatment. It could be that they mistakenly think they are obligated to accept all possible treatment. In this case, the Patient Self-Determination Act, with its emphasis on the right to refuse treatment, will be very helpful. Or they may not completely understand the issues they face, and then the dynamics of informed consent can be utilized, particularly the third level, which allows them to identify and examine their personal values and goals in order to assess the usefulness of a treatment option.[210]

Ultimately, the matter of futility comes down to the objective findings of research, the clinical judgment of the physician, and the clear identification of the reasonable goals of the patient. Negotiating about these factors in the spirit of the Patient Self-Determination Act will provide the greatest chance of maintaining the integrity of medical practice and the well-being of patients when they are faced with the challenges of determining the futility of proposed treatments.

An Integration of Ethical Issues

The ethical issues outlined in this chapter—the ethical principles, the role of virtues in the clinical setting, informed consent, decisional capacity, the right to refuse and the right to demand treatment, and clinical futility—are all issues that the Patient Self-Determination Act can illuminate and integrate. They have been matters of ongoing concern in bioethics. The Patient Self-Determination Act can provide a new way to approach those issues and can encourage healthcare professionals and providers to develop new ways of thinking about the issues and strategies for resolving problems that arise in patient care. Identifying the power of patients and the limits of that power through a thorough understanding of the Patient Self-Determination Act can create a healthcare environment in which both patients and caregivers will be able to flourish.

NOTES

1. Pellegrino ED, Thomasma DC. For the patient's good: The restoration of beneficence in health care. New York: Oxford University Press, 1988, pages 137–142.

2. Beauchamp TL, Childress JE. Principles of biomedical ethics. 4th edition. New York: Oxford University Press, 1994. This text offers perhaps the most comprehensive and thorough analysis of the principles of bioethics to date.

3. Engelhardt HT. The foundations of bioethics. 2d edition. New York: Oxford University Press, 1996, pages 78–81.

4. Kelly G. Medico-moral problems. St. Louis: The Catholic Health Association, 1961, pages 2–5. See also Arras JD, Steinbock B. (eds). Ethical issues in modern medicine. 4th edition. Mountain View, CA: Mayfield Publishing Co., 1995, pages 20–22.

5. Beauchamp TL, Walters L. Contemporary issues in bioethics. 4th edition. Belmont, CA: Wadsworth Publishing Co., 1994, pages 14–17.

6. Mappes TA, DeGrazia D. Biomedical ethics. 4th edition. New York: McGraw-Hill, Inc., 1996, pages 7–16.

7. For example, when a terminal patient elects a DNR order and the physician agrees to enter the order on the patient's chart, the three principles of autonomy, beneficence, and justice are mutually supportive: autonomy because the patient is exercising her self-determination, beneficence because

the physician is both respecting the patient's autonomy (doing good) and acting with restraint in treating the patient with CPR when it will do no good (avoiding harm), and justice because the patient is terminal and is being treated according to her condition (fairly).

8. Mill JS. On liberty. Buffalo, NY: Prometheus Books, 1986, page 16. "[T]he only purpose for which power can be rightfully exercised over any member of a civilized community against his will, is to prevent harm to others. His own good, either physical or moral, is not a sufficient warrant. He cannot rightfully be compelled to do or forbear because it will be better for him to do so, because it will make him happier, because in the opinions of others, to do so would be wise, or even right. These are good reasons for remonstrating with him, or reasoning with him, or persuading him, or entreating him, but not for compelling him, or visiting him with evil, in case he do otherwise."

9. Application of President and Directors of Georgetown College, 331 F.2d 1010. D.C. Cir. (1964).

10. This stipulation supports the general reluctance of the medical profession to provide assistance in the suicide of terminal patients. See Council on Ethical and Judicial Affairs, AMA. Decisions near the end of life. JAMA 1992; 327:1384–1388. The medical profession views its professional obligation as preserving and promoting life by attempting to heal within the boundaries of the natural processes of life and death rather than taking life. See American College of Physicians. Ethics manual. 3rd edition. Philadelphia: American College of Physicians, 1993, page 4. See also Gaylen W et al. Doctors must not kill. JAMA 1988; 259:2139–2140.

11. Haworth L. Autonomy: An essay in philosophical psychology and ethics. New Haven: Yale University Press, 1986, pages 67–74.

12. Annas GJ. Problems in informed consent and confidentiality in genetic counseling. In Milunsky A, Annas GJ (eds). Genetics and the law. New York: Plenum Press, 1976, pages 111–122.

13. Ingelfinger FJ. Informed (but uneducated) consent. N Engl J Med 1972; 287:465–466.

14. Veatch RM. Medical ethics. 2d edition. Boston: Jones and Bartlett, 1997, pages 6–15.

15. Bok S. Lying: Moral choice in public and private life. New York: Random House, Pantheon Books, 1978, pages 239–246.

16. Balint J. Regaining the initiative: Forging a new model of the patient-physician relationship. JAMA 1996; 275:887–891.

17. The patient may, and frequently does, exercise his autonomy simply by agreeing with the caregiver's recommendation. But this is still an important exercise of autonomy if the dialogue leaves open the possibility of the

patient's refusing the recommendation of the caregiver. See Katz J. The silent world of the doctor and the patient. New York: Free Press, 1984, pages 85–87.

18. President's Commission for the Study of Ethical Problems in Medicine and Biomedical and Behavioral Research. Making healthcare decisions: The ethical and legal implications of informed consent in the patient-practitioner relationship. Washington, D.C.: U.S. Government Printing Office, 1982, page 3.

19. Ibid.

20. This is modified in the matter of advance directives. Advance directives are governed by the principle of autonomy even though the patient lacks decisional capacity when the advance directive is being followed. Thus, the principle of autonomy may cover both present and future decisions of patients when advance directives have been utilized.

21. Drane J. The many faces of competency. Hast Cent Rep 1985; 15:17–21.

22. Brett AS, McCullough LB. When patients request specific interventions: Defining the limits of the physician's obligation. N Engl J Med 1986; 315:1347–1351. The issue of medical futility will be examined later in this chapter. This issue presents very special problems for understanding and implementing the Patient Self-Determination Act.

23. Council on Ethical and Judicial Affairs, AMA. Guidelines for appropriate use of do-not-resuscitate orders. JAMA 1991; 265:1868–1871.

24. On the other hand, clinicians must be cautious about cavalierly identifying a great many personal beliefs as "deeply held," thereby creating an excuse to avoid adjusting their practice patterns to accommodate the autonomy of their patients when such accommodation may be entirely appropriate. This could apply in situations where a patient might elect DNR status—which the physician must respect despite his knowing the patient has a reasonably good (in the physician's eyes) chance of surviving a CPR effort.

25. Wikler D. Ethics and rationing: "Whether," "how," or "how much"? J Am Geriatric Soc 1992; 40:398–403.

26. White BC. Competence to consent. Washington, D.C.: Georgetown University Press, 1994, pages 14–18.

27. Pellegrino ED, Thomasma DC. For the patient's good: The restoration of beneficence in health care. New York: Oxford University Press, 1988, pages 26–27.

28. Lloyd GER (ed). Hippocratic writings. New York: Penguin Books, 1983, page 67. In the Hippocratic oath, "harm" would apply to physical harm, particularly in the matters of abortion and euthanasia. "Injustice" would apply to matters of breaking confidentiality and sexual contact with

patients. For an analysis of the complexities of the notion of "harm" in the Hippocratic Corpus see Jonsen AR. Do no harm. Ann Intern Med 1978; 88:827–832.

29. Goodfield J. Reflections on the Hippocratic oath. Hast Cent Stud 1973; 1:79–92.

30. Pellegrino ED, Thomasma DC. For the patient's good: The restoration of beneficence in health care. New York: Oxford University Press, 1988, page 26.

31. Beauchamp TL, McCullough LB. Medical ethics: The moral responsibilities of physicians. Englewood Cliffs, NJ: Prentice-Hall, Inc., 1984, pages 14–19.

32. For example, consider the breast cancer patient who is presented with the options of surgery or radiation treatment. Her physician determines that surgery will be the most beneficial intervention, but her value agenda and sense of embodiment prompt her to elect radiation. In this situation her autonomy overrides the physician's attempt to be beneficent according to his own agenda.

33. Pursuing futile treatments is a good example of medical practice that is deficient in beneficence. Treatments that are medically futile cannot be construed as beneficial, and thus their use is not an act of beneficence. See Halevy A et al. A multi-institutional collaborative policy on medical futility. JAMA 1996; 276:571–574.

34. A good example of this is not doing CPR on elderly patients in light of the current research indicating the high improbability of success with this population. See Murphy D et al. Outcomes of cardiopulmonary resuscitation in the elderly. Ann Intern Med 1989; 111:199–205. See also Taffet et al. In-hospital cardiopulmonary resuscitation. JAMA 1988; 260:2069–2072. See also Schneider AP et al. In-hospital cardiopulmonary resuscitation: A 30-year review. J Am Board Fam Pract 1993; 6:91–101. The same could be said of the population served in the intensive care setting. See Landry FJ et al. Outcome of cardiopulmonary resuscitation in the intensive care setting. Arch Intern Med 1992; 152:2305–2308.

35. Rescher NP. The allocation of exotic medical lifesaving therapy. Ethics 1969; 79:173–186.

36. Pellegrino ED. Humanism and the physician. Knoxville TN: University of Tennessee Press, 1979, 119–129.

37. Brody BA. Medical futility: A useful concept? In Zucker MB, Zucker HD (eds). Medical futility and the evaluation of life-sustaining interventions. New York: Cambridge University Press, 1997, pages 1–14.

38. Pellegrino ED, Thomasma DC. A philosophical basis of medical practice. New York: Oxford University Press, 1981, pages 183–186.

39. President's Commission for the Study of Ethical Problems in Medicine and Biomedical and Behavioral Research. Making health care decisions: The ethical and legal implications of informed consent in the patient-practitioner relationship. Washington, D.C.: U.S. Government Printing Office, 1982, pages 153–154.

40. Ibid., pages 23–29.

41. Basing the application of the principle of justice on the "nature" of the person implies a particular ontological view holding that all individuals share in a common essence. Such an essentialist view has, at least, three major problems. (1) The very assertion of a common essence, à la Platonic metaphysics, may well be merely an assumption (or at best, a questionable inference) since it has no empirical basis. (2) If there were a common essence, it would be very difficult, if not impossible, to know with any reasonable degree of certainty what the characteristics of the essence were, and disputes about a catalog of those characteristics could never be adequately settled. (3) If there were a common essence, there would still remain the difficulty of applying its requirements in particular situations; whether a specific response would be appropriate could not be decided with any degree of confidence. For the above reasons, and many more, basing justice on the concept of "human nature" may be a perplexing exercise at best.

42. Such a requirement may derive from a value that is placed on an individual's needs (e.g., nutritional assistance when the family breadwinner has unexpectedly lost her employment), a value that flows from the commitment of a professional (e.g., to be available to a client after hours when the client is in a particularly distressful situation), or some socially accepted value (e.g., providing relief to individuals who have suffered in a natural disaster).

43. The role of terminal illness and appropriate responses to it will be elaborated upon later in this section.

44. President's Commission for the Study of Ethical Problems in Medicine and Biomedical and Behavioral Research. Making health care decisions: The ethical and legal implications of informed consent in the patient-practitioner relationship. Washington, D.C.: U.S. Government Printing Office, 1982, pages 155–166.

45. Rawls J. A theory of justice. Cambridge MA: Harvard University Press, 1971, pages 60–62.

46. Engelhardt HT. The foundations of bioethics. 1st edition. New York: Oxford University Press, 1986, pages 356–357.

47. Buchanan AE. The right to a decent minimum of health care. Philosophy and Public Affairs 1984; 13:55–78.

48. It is a common belief among clinicians that the individual physician, who is caring for a particular patient, is not the appropriate person to make deci-

sions about distributive justice. Concern about this matter arises from the nature of the fiduciary relationship between the physician and the patient. The relationship requires that the physician treat the patient for the presenting condition. It is the *condition* that makes the patient *deserving* of the treatment. This is the extent of the justice requirement on the treating physician. Economic matters and the accompanying issues of distributive justice are concerns for others at a distance from the patient's bedside. See Pellegrino ED. The virtuous physician and the ethics of medicine. In Mappes TA, DeGrazia D. Biomedical ethics. 4th edition. New York: McGraw-Hill, 1996, pages 61–64. However, the emergence of managed care, particularly with the gatekeeper role of primary care physicians, is challenging and altering the more traditional view of medical practice represented above. See Emanuel EJ, Brett AS. Managed competition and the patient-physician relationship. N Engl J Med 1993; 329:879–882. See also Auerbach ML. Will managed care alter the art and soul of medicine? West J Med 1994; 160:269–272.

49. Kassirer JP. Managed care and the morality of the marketplace. N Engl J Med 1995; 333:50–52.

50. Engelhardt HT, Rie MA. Intensive care units, scarce resources, and conflicting principles of justice. JAMA 1986; 255:1159–1164.

51. Rawls J. A theory of justice. Cambridge MA: Harvard University Press, 1971, page 73.

52. This basic notion of equality is articulated in no place more succinctly and eloquently than in the equal protection clause of the Fourteenth Amendment to the U.S. Constitution: "All persons born or naturalized in the United States, and subject to the jurisdiction thereof, are citizens of the United States and of the State wherein they reside. No State shall make or enforce any law which shall abridge the privileges or immunities of citizens of the United States; nor shall any State deprive any person of life, liberty, or property, without due process of law; nor *deny to any person within its jurisdiction the equal protection of the laws.*" [Emphasis added]. This equal protection clause requires that those who are similarly situated are to be treated similarly. See Quill v. Vacco. 80 F3d 716 (2d Cir. 1996).

The formal principle of justice has as its complement a material principle that designates what factors or principles should be taken into account when deciding on the similarity or dissimilarity of situations. See Facione PA et al. Ethics and society. 2d edition. Englewood Cliffs, NJ: Prentice-Hall, 1991, page 194. Throughout this discussion of justice these factors are referred to as morally relevant (or possibly morally relevant) differences. A number of candidates for this consideration are identified—for example, (1) whether the patient is functionally self-determining, (2) whether the patient possesses decisional capacity, (3) whether the patient's condition is terminal, (4) whether the patient has decided to refuse treatment, (5) whether the patient has an advance directive, and (6) whether the treatment being considered is futile, etc. Whether the answer to these questions (or material conditions) is yes or no will determine how the formal principle of justice will be applied and whether the patient's situation will be similar or dissimilar to the situation of others who are to be treated in certain ways. For example, if the treatment being considered is indeed futile, then the patient should be treated in the same way as other patients whose treatment falls under the determination of futility. Conversely, if the treatment being considered is not futile because of the patient's condition, then the treatment can be appropriately applied because it is dissimilar to those treatments that are determined to be futile.

53. Several points need to be made when incorporating the notion of "morally relevant differences" in the principle of justice. (1) Morally relevant differences help moral agents to decide when individuals should be treated in similar ways and when they should be treated in different ways. The equal protection clause of the Fourteenth Amendment of the U.S. Constitution is the prime example of the importance of identifying morally relevant differences. See Quill v. Vacco. 80 F.3d 716 (2d Cir. 1996).

(2) Morally relevant differences are not directly derived from a state of affairs. Rather, they flow from some value assessment attached to a state of affairs that in some way is considered warranted by the state of affairs. For example, regarding decisional capacity as a morally relevant difference in considering the just treatment of a patient derives not from the fact of a patient's being able to make a decision but from the importance placed upon a patient's participation in decisions that affect his well-being.

(3) What is determined to be a morally relevant difference is often the result of intense philosophical and political scrutiny that may be conditioned by historical consciousness and circumstances. For example, race and gender were once considered morally relevant differences for many (most?) jobs. Philosophical and political analysis has revealed the fallacy of this judgment. In healthcare, age is currently under careful analysis as to whether and under what circumstances it ought to be considered a morally relevant difference for certain kinds of treatments (e.g., CPR).

(4) There will often be disagreement with the general opinion that a particular feature is morally relevant. For example, parentalists will frequently override the decisions of the elderly even though elderly patients are often quite capable of making healthcare decisions for themselves. In the final analysis, there is no clear formula for deciding what counts as morally relevant differences. They are determined as the result of an ongoing dialogue in society, which has a central role in determining how individuals are to be treated within the context of the principle of justice.

54. Task Force on Ethics of the Society of Critical Care Medicine. Consensus report of the ethics of foregoing life-sustaining treatments in the critically ill. Crit Care Med 1990; 18:1435–1439.

55. Macklin R. The geriatric patient: Ethical issues in care and treatment. In Mappes TA, Zembaty JS (eds). Biomedical ethics. 3d edition. New York: McGraw-Hill, 1991, pages 192–197.

56. Jonsen AR et al. Clinical ethics. 4th edition. New York: McGraw-Hill, Inc., 1998, page 58.

57. Yarmolinsky, A. Supporting the patient. N Engl J Med 1995; 332:602–603.

58. All advance directive legislation places patients in a special situation if they have drafted or signed an advance directive; namely, their physicians are protected from criminal or civil liability if they follow the stipulations in the advance directive. King NMP. Making sense of advance directives. Revised edition. Washington, D.C.: Georgetown University Press, 1996, pages 118–121. As a comparison with the "conscience clause" see also chapter 7, note 29.

59. This is not to say that those under the legal age for consent are excluded from discussions about their healthcare. They can and should be participants in healthcare decisions that affect them because they might very well understand the consequences of their decisions and thus be ethically competent to make them. However, any decisions they might wish to make are not legally determinative. Binding consents to and refusals of treatment can be made only through their proxies. Cf. Garrett TM et al. Health care ethics: Principles and problems. 2d edition. Englewood Cliffs, NJ: Prentice Hall, 1993, pages 31–32.

60. It is a violation of justice because it violates some rights of the patient that healthcare providers have a duty to respect. See Brody BA, Engelhardt HT. Bioethics: Readings and cases. Englewood Cliffs, NJ: Prentice-Hall, Inc. 1987, pages 11–22. These are not just amorphous moral rights that may be open to discussion and argument; they are clearly defined and codified legal rights.

61. Baron CH. Why withdrawal of life-support for PVS patients is not a family decision. Law Med Health Care 1991; 19:73–75.

62. This facet of justice was recognized in the *Quinlan* decision, where the court wrote that "physicians distinguish between curing the ill and comforting and easing the dying; that they refuse to treat the curable as if they were dying or ought to die, and that they have sometimes refused to treat the hopeless and dying as if they were curable." In re Quinlan. 70 N.J. 10, 355 A.2d 647 (1976), page 667.

63. Wanzer SH et al. The physician's responsibility toward hopelessly ill

patients. N Engl J Med 1984; 310:955–959. A more detailed analysis of the issue of futility will be found at the end of this chapter.

64. Cranford RE. The persistent vegetative state: The medical reality (getting the facts straight). Hast Cent Rep 1988; 18:27–32.

65. Council on Ethical and Judicial Affairs, AMA. Guidelines for the appropriate use of do-not-resuscitate orders. JAMA 1991; 265:1868–1871.

66. Tomlinson T, Brody H. Futility and the ethics of resuscitation. JAMA 1990; 264:1276–1280.

67. Cher DJ. Method of Medicare reimbursement and the rate of potentially ineffective care of critically ill patients. JAMA 1997; 278:1001–1007.

68. Murphy DJ et al. Outcomes of cardiopulmonary resuscitation in the elderly. Ann Intern Med 1989; 111:199–205.

69. Schneider AP et al. In-hospital cardiopulmonary resuscitation: A 30-year review. J Am Board Fam Pract 1993; 6:91–101. This study indicates that age alone may not be as decisive a negative indicator of CPR as was once thought. Survival (to leave the hospital) for those 70 to 79 years old was 12.2 percent, and for those aged 80 to 89 it was 10.2 percent. Only for those 89 and over was the survival rate 0 percent.

70. Pearlman RA et al. Insights pertaining to patient assessments of states worse than death. J Clin Ethics 1993; 4:33–41.

71. Murphy DJ et al. The influence of the probability of survival on patients' preferences regarding cardiopulmonary resuscitation. N Engl J Med 1994; 330:545–549.

72. Byock IR. When suffering persists. . . . J Pal Care 1994; 10:8–13. For a discussion of the possibility of advance directives' saving healthcare resources see chapter 7, note 107. Indications are that hospice patients who utilize the Medicare hospice benefit save about 25 percent of cost over those who utilize ordinary treatment modes. See Lewin-VHI, Inc. An analysis of the cost savings of the Medicare hospice benefit. Arlington, VA: National Hospice Organization, 1995. However, the longer the patient is in the program, the less the savings.

73. National Conference of Catholic Bishops. Ethical and religious directives for Catholic health care services. Washington, D.C.: United States Catholic Conference, 1995, part 1.

74. The issue of parentalism was introduced in chapter 3 in the context of the fiduciary relationship. In that discussion parentalism was examined as an attitude that often colors the relationship between one in authority and one who may be her subject through either family ties or social roles. In the current discussion the principle that guides parentalistic actions is the focus of attention.

75. Pellegrino ED, Thomasma DC. For the patient's good: The restoration

of beneficence in health care. New York: Oxford University Press, 1988, pages 3–10.

76. Beauchamp, T. Paternalism. In Reich, WT (ed). Encyclopedia of bioethics. New York: Free Press, 1978, pages 1194–1200.

77. Greenberg DF. Interference with a suicide attempt. New York Univ L Rev 1974; 49:227–269.

78. Zembaty JS. A limited defense of paternalism in medicine. In Mappes, TA, Zembaty JS (eds). 2d edition. Biomedical ethics. New York: McGraw-Hill Book Co., 1986, pages 60–66.

79. American College of Physicians. Ethics manual. 3d edition. Philadelphia, PA: American College of Physicians, 1993, page 2. The position taken in this document is typical.

80. Council on Ethical and Judicial Affairs, AMA. Code of medical ethics: Current opinions with annotations. Chicago: American Medical Association, 1996, page xxxix.

81. Tomlinson T, Brody H. Ethics and communication in do-not-resuscitate orders. N Engl J Med 1988; 318:43–46.

82. American Hospital Association. Values in conflict: Resolving ethical issues in hospital care. Chicago IL: American Hospital Association, 1985, pages 14–15.

83. Pellegrino ED, Thomasma DC. The virtues in medical practice. New York: Oxford University Press, 1993, pages 4–8.

84. MacIntyre A. After virtue. Notre Dame, IN: University of Notre Dame Press, 1981, pages 202–204.

85. Engelhardt HT. The foundations of bioethics. 2d edition. New York: Oxford University Press, 1996, page 289.

86. This would be the position of, for example, the orthodox Christian. See Engelhardt HT. Physician-assisted suicide: Facing death as a Christian in a post-Christian age. Lecture delivered at the University of Dayton, April 9, 1997.

87. Aristotle. Nichomachean ethics. Irwin T (trans). Indianapolis, IN: Hackett Publishing Co., Inc., 1985, pages 49–53.

88. In point of fact they may both be complementary and indispensable to each other. See Pellegrino ED, Thomasma DC. The virtues in medical practice. New York: Oxford University Press, 1993, page 19.

89. This feature of patient life will be explored more fully in chapter 9.

90. Lloyd GER (ed). Hippocratic writings. London: Penguin Books, 1983, page 67. See also Lidz CW et al. Informed consent: a study of decision-making in psychiatry. New York: Guilford Press, 1984, pages 3–5.

91. Katz J. Informed consent in therapeutic relationships: Law and ethics.

In Reich, WT (ed). Encyclopedia of bioethics. New York: Free Press, 1978, pages 770–778.

92. Canterbury v. Spence. 464 F. 2d 772, 150 U.S. App. D.C. 263 (1972).

93. Meisel A, Kuczewski M. Legal and ethical myths about informed consent. Arch Intern Med 1996; 156:2521–2526.

94. Appelbaum PS et al. Informed consent: Legal theory and clinical practice. New York: Oxford University Press, 1987, pages 35–36.

95. President's Commission for the Study of Ethical Problems in Medicine and Biomedical and Behavioral Research. Making health care decisions: The ethical and legal implications of informed consent in the patient-practitioner relationship. Washington, D.C.: U.S. Government Printing Office, 1982, page 41.

96. American College of Physicians. Ethics manual. 1st edition. Philadelphia, PA: American College of Physicians, 1984, page 25.

97. President's Commission for the Study of Ethical Problems in Medicine and Biomedical and Behavioral Research. Deciding to forego life-sustaining treatment: A report on the ethical, medical, and legal issues in treatment decisions. Washington, D.C.: U.S. Government Printing Office, 1983, pages 43–44.

98. Bok S. Personal directions for care at the end of life. N Engl J Med 1976; 295:367–369.

99. Hotchkiss WS. Doctor as patient advocate. JAMA 1987; 258:947–948.

100. Schloendorff v. Society of New York Hospital. 211 N.Y. 125, 105 N.E. 92 (1914).

101. Katz J. Informed consent in the therapeutic relationship. In Reich WT (ed). Encyclopedia of bioethics. 2d edition. New York: Macmillan Library Reference USA—Simon and Schuster Macmillan, 1995, pages 1256–1265.

102. Meisel A, Kuczewski M. Legal and ethical myths about informed consent. Arch Intern Med 1996; 156:2521–2526.

103. Oken D. What to tell cancer patients. JAMA 1961; 175:1120–1128. Patient response to information was often quite the opposite of what physicians feared. Patients object if they are not given appropriate information and often respond very positively to physicians who are honest and open with them. See Alfidi R. Informed consent: A study of patient reaction. JAMA 1971; 216:1325–1329.

104. Katz J. Disclosure and consent in search of their roots. In Milunsky GJ (ed). Genetics and the law. Vol. 2. New York: Plenum Press, 1980, pages 121–129.

105. Jonsen AR et al. Clinical ethics: A practical approach to ethical

decisions in clinical medicine. 4th edition. New York: McGraw-Hill, Inc. 1998, page 55.

106. There is much discussion about how far physicians should go in giving information about risks to patients. Clearly every risk cannot be communicated. The clinical judgment of the physician is central to determining how much information in the area of risks should be communicated. Certainly clinicians should be sensitive to the clues sent by the patient regarding the amount of information he wishes. In general, one might think in terms of mortality and morbidity. When the risk is mortality, then even low probabilities should be communicated. However, when the risk is morbidity, then, depending on the seriousness of the morbidity, there may be a higher tolerance for not disclosing extensive information. See Beauchamp TL, McCullough LB. Medical ethics: The moral responsibility of physicians. Englewood Cliffs, NJ: Prentice-Hall, Inc., 1984, pages 74–75. See also Gorovitz S. Doctors' dilemmas: Moral conflict and medical care. New York: Macmillan Publishing Co., Inc., 1982, pages 35–54.

107. Kassirer JP. Our stubborn quest for diagnostic certainty. N Engl J Med 1989; 320:1489–1491.

108. American Hospital Association. A patient's bill of rights. In American Hospital Association. Values in conflict: resolving ethical issues in hospital care. Chicago IL: American Hospital Association, 1985, pages 77–79.

109. Cousins N. A layman looks at truth-telling in medicine. JAMA 1980; 244:1929–1930.

110. Though the following three levels may often overlap in practice to some extent, they are distinguishable with regard to the focus of the information transfer, the response of patients to the information given, and the participation of patients in appropriating and integrating the information.

111. When informed consent occurs at all, this is often what is likely to happen.

112. Meisel A. Kuczewski M. Legal and ethical myths about informed consent. Arch Intern Med 1996; 156:2521–2526. "A shared process approach does not restrict the physician to providing facts and insists that the patient supply all the values. The physician and patient each have access to interrelated facts and values" (page 2522).

113. Lidz CW, Appelbaum PS, Meisel A. Two models of implementing informed consent. Arch Intern Med 1988; 148:1385–1389.

114. It is an error to think that a signed consent form is informed consent. See Meisel A, Kuczewski M. Legal and ethical myths about informed consent. Arch Intern Med 1996; 156:2521–2526.

115. Here the term "process" functions in much the same way as it did previously in identifying the three distinct levels of informed consent. In both

usages patients' beliefs, values, and wishes are intimately connected to the facts of the medical situation.

116. The ease with which Lidz, Appelbaum, and Meisel draw the distinction between the event and the process model may neglect some of the positive aspects of the event model. Stephen Wear, in Wear S. Informed consent: Patient autonomy and physician beneficence within clinical medicine. Dordrecht: Kluwer Academic Publishers, 1993, calls them to account for this deficiency. Wear contends that the event model is quite sufficient in the majority of cases provided the groundwork in the physician-patient relationship has been adequately laid. "An overall atmosphere of trust, candor, information provision, assessment and feedback is surely essential to the effectiveness and success of any physician-patient encounter" (page 82). His contention is that the atmosphere of the relationship will take care of the issues that Lidz, Appelbaum, and Meisel identify without having to return time and again to assess the therapeutic intervention after it has been initiated (pages 81–82). Wear may be right in many cases. However, one must always remain open to the possibility that the process model may have to be employed as therapy continues. See White BC. Competence to consent. Washington, D.C.: Georgetown University Press, 1994, pages 27–28. Moreover, with regard to the Patient Self-Determination Act, the issues may frequently have to be addressed on an ongoing basis because of their complexity and the changing life situations patients experience.

117. Callahan S. In good conscience: Reason and emotion in moral decision-making. New York: HarperSanFrancisco, 1991, pages 95–113.

118. Zaner RM. Ethics and the clinical encounter. Englewood Cliffs, NJ: Prentice Hall, 1988, page 54.

119. Childress JF. Who should decide? Paternalism in health care. New York: Oxford University Press, 1982, pages 77–80.

120. Strull WM et al. Do patients want to participate in medical decision making? JAMA 1984; 252:2990–2994.

121. Levinson W. et al. Physician-patient communication: The relationship with malpractice claims among primary care physicians and surgeons. JAMA 1997; 277:553–559.

122. *In re Quinlan,* 70 N.J. 10, 355 A.2d 647 (1976).

123. The distinction must be made between "decisional capacity" and "competence." "Competence," the more traditional term, is determined by a judge as the result of a legal proceeding. "Decisional capacity" is a functional assessment made by an attending physician or a psychiatrist that has ethical connotations without a strict legal determination. See The Hastings Center. Guidelines on the termination of life-sustaining treatment and the care of the dying. Bloomington, IN: Indiana University Press, 1987, page 131.

124. President's Commission for the Study of Ethical Problems in Medicine and Biomedical and Behavioral Research. Deciding to forego life-sustaining treatment: A report on the ethical, medical, and legal issues in treatment decisions. Washington, D.C.: U.S. Government Printing Office, 1983, pages 126–136.

125. Buchanan AE, Brock DW. Deciding for others: The ethics of surrogate decision making. Cambridge: Cambridge University Press, 1989. This text focuses upon the issues surrounding proxy decision making and the way patient autonomy and well-being may be extended and enhanced through the proper exercise of the decisional authority of surrogates.

126. One of the most detailed analyses of decisional capacity can be found in White BC. Competence to consent. Washington, D.C.: Georgetown University Press, 1994.

127. Appelbaum PS, Grisso T. Assessing patients' capacities to consent to treatment. N Engl J Med. 1988; 319:1635–1638.

128. This component does not offer a serious problem. However, the issue of making a choice can become a matter of concern if one requires detailed supporting reasons for the choices made. Thus, a competent choice may be a choice expressed by yes or no responses with no reasons attached. See Roth LH et al. Tests of competency to consent to treatment. Am J Psychiatry 1977; 134:279–284.

129. President's Commission for the Study of Ethical Problems in Medicine and Biomedical and Behavioral Research. Making health care decisions: The ethical and legal implications of informed consent in the patient-practitioner relationship. Washington, D.C.: U.S. Government Printing Office, 1982, page 55.

130. Macklin R. Consent, coercion, and conflicts of rights. Perspectives in Biology and Medicine 1977; 20:360–371.

131. This component offers some difficulty for situations of mental impairment. Though the logic of the patient in a psychotic episode may seem flawless, the problem rests with the premises of the logical construction. Religious or cultural beliefs, while not always "rational" according to many schemas of "rationality," are not flawed in the same sense as the premises of the schizophrenic. See Roth LH et al. Tests of competency to consent to treatment. Am J Psychiatry 1977; 134:279–284. A helpful exploration of the importance of being sensitive to beliefs about medical goals and practice in cultures may be found in Pellegrino ED. Intersections of western biomedical ethics and world culture: Problematic and possibility. Cambridge Quarterly of Healthcare Ethics 1992; 3:191–196.

132. This component differs from the third component (manipulating information rationally) insofar as it addresses only the likelihood of results from the

various interventions, given the patient's condition. The third component will very likely involve patient's values, from which a logical conclusion may follow, whereas the fourth component may not have a value dimension at all. Thus, a patient may make a seemingly competent decision for an intervention that will extend life while not genuinely understanding that the limitations of the intervention are such that it may not achieve the goal she has in mind.

133. Jonson AR et al. Clinical ethics: A practical approach to ethical decisions in clinical medicine. 4th edition. New York: McGraw-Hill, 1998, page 58–59.

134. A "successful" CPR attempt can be measured in a variety of ways: (1) restoration of heartbeat, (2) survival to leave the hospital, (3) return to a previous level of functioning, (4) achievement of a minimally decent quality of life. See Landry FJ. Outcome of cardiopulmonary resuscitation in the intensive care setting. Arch Intern Med 1992; 152:2305–2308.

135. Jonson AR et al. Clinical ethics: A practical approach to ethical decisions in clinical medicine. 4th edition. New York: McGraw-Hill, 1998, page 58. See also The Hastings Center. Guidelines on the termination of life-sustaining treatment and the care of the dying. Bloomington, IN: Indiana University Press, 1987, page 131.

136. Roth LH et al. Tests of competency to consent to treatment. Am J Psychiatry 1977; 1344:279–284.

137. The Hastings Center. Guidelines on the termination of life-sustaining treatment and the care of the dying. Bloomington, IN: Indiana University Press, 1987, page 132.

138. Wear S. Informed consent: Patient autonomy and physician beneficence within clinical medicine. Dordrecht: Kluwer Academic Publishers, 1993, pages 10–11. It can be as erroneously easy to presume that patients lack decisional capacity because of their vulnerability as it is to make the presumption simply because patients do not agree with their caregivers. (Roth LH et al. Tests of competency to consent to treatment. Am J Psychiatry 1977; 134:279–284.) Both presumptions seriously violate the dignity of patients. See White BC. Competence to consent. Washington, D.C.: Georgetown University Press, 1994, pages 3–5.

139. President's Commission for the Study of Ethical Problems in Medicine and Biomedical and Behavioral Research. Making health care decisions: The ethical and legal implications of informed consent in the patient-practitioner relationship. Washington, D.C.: U.S. Government Printing Office, 1982, page 62.

140. Ibid., page 60.

141. President's Commission for the Study of Ethical Problems in Medicine and Biomedical and Behavioral Research. Making health care decisions:

The ethical and legal implications of informed consent in the patient-practitioner relationship. Washington, D.C.: US Government Printing Office, 1982, pages 44–47.

142. Schloendorff v. Society of New York Hospital. 211 N.Y. 125, 105 N.E. 92 (1914).

143. In re Quinlan, 70 N.J. 10, 355 A.2d 647 (1976).

144. Bartling v. Superior Court. 163 Cal. App. 3d 186; 209 Cal. Rptr. 220 (1984).

145. Brophy v. New England Sinai Hospital, Inc. 398 Mass. 417, 497 N.E. 2d 626 (1986).

146. Cruzan v. Director, Missouri Department of Health. 110 S. Ct. 2841 (1990).

147. Vacco v. Quill. 117 S. Ct. 2293 (1997).

148. Hart HLA. Are there any natural rights? In Melden AI (ed). Human rights. Belmont CA: Wadsworth Publishing Co., 1970, pages 64–67.

149. Feinberg J. Social philosophy. Englewood Cliffs, NJ: Prentice-Hall, Inc., 1973, pages 59–60.

150. Minogue B. Bioethics: A committee approach. Boston, MA: Jones and Bartlett Publishers, 1996, page 112.

151. Ibid.

152. The interviewer will have to be well trained in discussing the issues raised by the Patient Self-Determination Act. It would not be sufficient to simply assign the task to someone who has only clerical duties. Some healthcare training would be essential for productive conversations on these matters. See Oleson KJ et al. A quality improvement focus for patient rights: Advance directives. J Nurs Care Qual 1994; 8:52–67.

153. This point has been underscored by the Ninth Circuit Court of Appeals in the context of physician-assisted suicide. Compassion in Dying v. Washington. 79 F.3d 790 (9th Cir. 1996). See also Ethics Committee of the Society of Critical Care Medicine. Consensus statement of the society of critical care medicine's ethics committee regarding futile and other possibly inadvisable treatments. Crit Care Med 1997; 25:887–891.

154. Council on Scientific Affairs and Council on Ethical and Judicial Affairs, AMA. Persistent vegetative state and the decision to withdraw or withhold life support. JAMA 1990; 263:426–430. Most of the courts that have addressed the issue of life-sustaining treatments for patients in a persistent vegetative state have considered the continuance of life in such a state to be nonbeneficial. The only court to consider life in a persistent vegetative state to be a benefit to the patient has been the Supreme Court of Missouri in the case of Nancy Cruzan. See Cruzan, by Cruzan v. Harmon, 760 S.W. 2d 408 (Mo. en banc 1988).

155. In spite of attempts to "objectively" assess the quality of a patient's life, it still remains largely a subjective factor and one about which patients must continue to make personal decisions. See Konopad E et al. Quality of life measures before and one year after admission to an intensive care unit. Crit Care Med 1995; 23:1653–1659.

156. Davis NA. The right to refuse treatment. In Beuchamp TL. (ed). Intending death: The ethics of assisted suicide and euthanasia. Upper Saddle River, NJ: Prentice Hall, 1996, pages 109–130.

157. Note again the U.S. Supreme Court's statement: "Everyone, *regardless of physical condition,* is entitled, if competent, to refuse unwanted lifesaving medical treatment." Vacco v. Quill. 117 S. Ct. 2293 ad 5 (1997) [emphasis added].

158. See the previous section in this chapter on informed consent.

159. Ivey AE, Authier J. Microcounseling: Innovations in interviewing, counseling, psychotherapy, and psychoeducation. 2d edition. Springfield IL: Charles C. Thomas, 1978, pages 80–83.

160. Engelhardt HT. The foundations of bioethics. 2d edition. New York: Oxford University Press, 1996, pages 376–379.

161. President's Commission for the Study of Ethical Problems in Medicine and Biomedical and Behavioral Research. Securing access to health care. Washington, D.C.: U.S. Government Printing Office, 1983, pages 115–119.

162. Rodwin MA. Medicine, money, and morals: Physicians' conflicts of interest. New York: Oxford University Press, 1993, pages 158–160.

163. Macklin R. Moral concerns and appeals to rights and duties. Hast Cent Rep 1976; 6:31–38.

164. Pellegrino ED. The place of intention in the moral assessment of assisted suicide and active euthanasia. In Beauchamp TL (ed). Intending death: The ethics of assisted suicide and euthanasia. Upper Saddle River, NJ: Prentice Hall, 1996, pages 163–183.

165. Pellegrino ED, Thomasma DC. For the patient's good: the restoration of beneficence in health care. New York: Oxford University Press, 1988, pages 26–27.

166. Engelhardt HT. The foundations of bioethics. 2d edition. New York: Oxford University Press, 1996, pages 387–390.

167. Managed care contracts have underscored this feature, which has always been a part of healthcare insurance contracts. The provider decides what level of healthcare will be provided. The insured, by agreeing to the contract, also agrees to the reimbursement limitations for healthcare costs. The rights of the insured (patient) and the duties of the provider are limited to the terms of the contract. Zibelman AM. The practice standard of care and liability of managed care plans. J Health Hosp Law 1994; 27:204–217.

168. The Hastings Center. Guidelines on the termination of life-sustaining treatment and the care of the dying. Bloomington, IN: Indiana University Press, 1987, pages 120–126.

169. In vitro fertilization was not covered (and, in some situations, is still not covered) in its early implementation because insurers considered it experimental rather than clinical in spite of the fact that its success rates in fertility centers was well established.

170. Some of the conditions for unwarranted demands for treatment will be considered in the next section, which examines the issue of futile treatments. The parameters of decisional authority in cases of demands for futile treatments will be explored in that discussion.

171. An example of such a statement is provided to patients by Grandview Hospital and Medical Center, Dayton, Ohio with regard to its "Medical Staff Guidelines on Determining Futile and Inadvisable Treatments" (1998).

172. This becomes a particularly important issue when seniors are seeking admission to extended care facilities. If they have particular beliefs about the extent of healthcare they wish to receive, they should be sure at the time of admission that the policies of the extended care facility complement their wishes.

173. Buchanan AE. The right to a decent minimum of health care. In Beauchamp TL, Walters L. (eds). Contemporary issues in bioethics. 4th edition. Belmont CA: Wadsworth Publishing Co., 1994, pages 695–700.

174. Feinberg J. Social philosophy. Englewood Cliffs, NJ: Prentice-Hall, Inc., 1973, pages 55–68 and 84–88.

175. While moral rights may be compelling and may ultimately be codified in the law, they do not confer upon the bearer the power to sue, which is present only with legal rights.

176. Macklin R. Moral concerns and appeals to rights and duties. Hast Cent Rep 1976; 6:31–38.

177. McCullough LB. The right to health care. Ethics in Science and Medicine 1979; 6:1–9.

178. Of course, the notion of futility does not arise only in end-of-life decisions. Any treatment can be futile if it cannot achieve its goal, as we shall see shortly. End-of-life decisions provide a dramatic example of the issue of futility because the stakes are so high.

179. Brody BA, Halevy A. Is futility a futile concept? J Med Philos 1995; 20:123–144. The authors point out four conceptual types of futility definitions: (1) physiologic futility, (2) imminent demise futility, (3) lethal condition futility, and (4) quality-of-life futility. In their view, the different conceptual approaches serve to complicate the development of a workable definition of futility.

180. On one level, the "refusal" of futile treatment is only possible when the futile treatment is offered. There is much (but certainly not universal) agreement that treatment determined to be futile should not even be offered to patients and/or surrogates. See Jecker NS, Schneiderman LJ. Medical futility: The duty not to treat. Camb Q Healthc Ethics 1993; 2:151–159. On another level, the refusal of futile treatment can take the form of agreement with a healthcare professional that a particular intervention is futile and, thus, the treatment will be declined.

181. The patient's physician finds herself in this position because she can integrate the objectives research findings regarding a particular syndrome and its natural course with the way in which the patient manifests the disease and the particular patient's health history. This is the clinical judgment of the physician and, though there is an inevitable component of subjectivity in such a judgment, this is a professional clinical standard for making a prognosis. See Bioethics Advisory Committee. Medical staff guidelines on determining futile and inadvisable treatments. Dayton, OH: Grandview Hospital and Medical Center, 1998, and Committee on Ethical Responsibility. Clinical decisions and the determination of futile treatments. Kokomo, IN: Saint Joseph Hospital and Health Center, 1995. See also Ethics Advisory Committee. Clinical futility: Position, policy, and guidelines. Anderson, IN: Saint John's Health System, 1995, and Santa Monica-UCLA Medical Center. Futile care guidelines. Santa Monica, CA: Santa Monica Hospital Medical Center, 1991.

182. Blackhall LJ. Must we always use CPR? N Engl J Med 1987; 317:1281–1285. As foundation to this tradition is the statement in the Hippocratic Corpus, The Science of Medicine: "First of all I would define medicine as the complete removal of the distress of the sick, the alleviation of the more violent diseases and the *refusal to undertake to cure cases in which the disease has already won the mastery,* knowing that everything is not possible to medicine." Lloyd GER (ed). Hippocratic writings. New York: Penguin Books, 1983, page 140 [emphasis added].

183. This action would, then, violate the nonmaleficence form of beneficence.

184. Engelhardt HT. Ethical issues in aiding the death of young children. In Kohl M (ed). Beneficent euthanasia. New York: Prometheus Books, 1975, pages 180–192. The author here sees harm as sometimes taking the form of "the injury of continued existence" (pages 185–188).

185. Miles SH. Informed demand for 'non-beneficial' treatment. N Engl J Med 1991; 325:511–515.

186. Whether developing such policies is a wise move on the part of healthcare institutions is a matter of considerable debate. See Hudson T. Are

futile-care policies the answer? Hospitals and Health Networks 1994; 68:26–32. On the negative side of this question see Spielman B. Community futility policies: The illusion of consensus? In Zucker MB, Zucker HD (eds). Medical futility and the evaluation of life-sustaining interventions. New York: Cambridge University Press, 1997, pages 168–178. On the other hand, the lack of a futile care policy can lead to situations such as the Gilgunn case in Massachusetts, which is currently under appeal. Gilgunn v. Massachusetts General Hospital. No. 92-4820 (Super. Ct. Mass. April 21, 1995). Wagg D, Reardon F. Treatment decisions in Massachusetts: The legal landscape. Forum 1995; 16:5–7. In this case Joan Gilgunn sued Massachusetts General Hospital and two physicians for the emotional distress she suffered when her mother's physicians entered a DNR order on her mother contrary to Gilgunn's wishes and those of her comatose mother, whom she represented. The physicians and the hospital contended that CPR would have been futile in this case. The jury was instructed that it would first have to determine whether the CPR was indeed futile before it could award damages to Gilgunn. On April 25, 1995 the jury determined that the care was futile, and Gilgunn was unable to recover damages. Gilgunn, her mother, her mother's physicians, and the hospital might all have benefited from a clear policy for determining futility. Minimally, a procedural policy for determining futile interventions might have helped. See Halevy A, Brody BA. A multi-institution collaborative policy on medical futility. JAMA 1996; 276:571–574. For additional futility policies and guidelines cf. note 181 above.

187. Murphy DJ. The economics of futile interventions. In Zucker MB, Zucker HD (eds). Medical futility and the evaluation of life-sustaining interventions. New York: Cambridge University Press, 1997, pages 123–135.

188. President's Commission for the Study of Ethical Problems in Medicine and Biomedical and Behavioral Research. Making health care decisions: The ethical and legal implications of informed consent in the patient-practitioner relationship. Washington, D.C.: U.S. Government Printing Office, 1982, page 3.

189. Jonsen AR et al. Clinical ethics: A practical approach to ethical decisions in clinical medicine. 4th edition. New York: McGraw-Hill, 1998, pages 22–32.

190. Younger SJ. Who defines futility? JAMA 1988; 260:2094–2095.

191. Engelhardt HT. The foundations of bioethics. 2d edition. New York: Oxford University Press, 1996, page 308.

192. Schneiderman LJ et al. Medical futility: Its meaning and ethical implications. Ann Intern Med 1990; 112:949–954, page 950.

193. Younger S. Futility in context. JAMA 1990; 264:1295–1296. Ethics Committee of the Society of Critical Care Medicine. Consensus statement of

the society of critical care medicine's ethics committee regarding futile and other possibly inadvisable treatments. Crit Care Med 1997; 25:887–891.

194. Schneiderman LJ et al. Medical futility: Response to critiques. Ann Intern Med 1996; 125:669–674.

195. PVS patients will not return to consciousness. See Cranford RE. The persistent vegetative state: The medical reality (getting the facts straight). Hast Cent Rep 1988; 18:27–32. Patients admitted to a hospital with a dissecting aneurysm will not survive CPR to leave the hospital. Patients with a cerebral vascular accident with accompanying hemorrhage have a CPR success rate of only 1.4 percent (about as close to 0 percent as one can find). Patients over ninety years of age have a 0 percent success rate for CPR. See Schneider AP. In-hospital cardiopulmonary resuscitation: A 30-year review. J Am Board Fam Pract 1993; 6:91–101.

196. Callahan D. Controlling the costs of health care for the elderly—fair means and foul. N Engl J Med 1996; 335:744–746.

197. Wicclair MR. Ethics and the elderly. New York: Oxford University Press, 1993, pages 22–29.

198. Ethics Committee of the Society of Critical Care Medicine. Consensus statement of the Society of Critical Care Medicine's ethics committee regarding futile and other possibly inadvisable treatments. Crit Care Med 1997; 25:887–891. An inadvisable treatment in this situation might be described as a clinical intervention that a physician, relying on the medical literature and his clinical judgment, determines is highly unlikely to produce a beneficial outcome for the patient, will be detrimental to the patient's quality of life, or will not meet a patient's or authorized surrogate's reasonable goals.

199. Kapp MB. Futile medical treatment: A review of ethical arguments and legal holdings. J Gen Intern Med 1994; 9:170–177.

200. Wanzer SH et al. The physician's responsibility toward hopelessly ill patients. N Engl J Med 1984; 310:955–959.

201. Council on Ethical and Judicial Affairs, AMA. Guidelines for the appropriate use of do-not-resuscitate orders. JAMA 1991; 265:1868–1871.

202. Halevy A, Brody BA. A multi-institution collaborative policy on medical futility. JAMA 1996; 276:571–574.

203. Ruark JE et al. Initiating and withdrawing life support: Principles and practices in adult medicine. N Engl J Med 1988; 318:25–30

204. Meisel A. Legal myths about terminating life support. Arch Intern Med 1991; 151:1497–1502.

205. Kapp MB. Futile medical treatment: A review of ethical arguments and legal holdings. J Gen Intern Med 1994; 9:170–177. See also Kapp MB. Treating medical charts near the end of life: How legal anxieties inhibit good patient deaths. University of Toledo L Rev 1997; 28:521–546.

206. Cher DJ, Lenert LA. Method of Medicare reimbursement and the rate of potentially ineffective care of critically ill patients. JAMA 1997; 278:1001–1007. The authors here take the position that more careful attention to clinical judgments when the possibility of futility ("potentially ineffective care") arises in the course of caring for the critically ill elderly could save a considerable amount of money. They estimate an annual savings of $48 million in the Medicare population of California alone.

207. Lewin-VHI, Inc. An analysis of cost savings of the Medicare hospice benefit. Arlington, VA: National Hospice Organization, 1995. See also Murphy DJ. The economics of futile interventions. In Zucker MB, Zucker HD (eds). Medical futility and the evaluation of life-sustaining interventions. New York: Cambridge University Press, 1997, pages 123–135.

208. Murphy DJ et al. Outcomes of cardiopulmonary resuscitation in the elderly. Ann Intern Med 1989; 111:199–205. See also Taffet GE et al. In-hospital cardiopulmonary resuscitation. JAMA 1988; 260:2069–2072.

209. Gewirtz P. On 'I know it when I see it.' Yale Law J 1996; 105:1023–1047. See also Ethics Committee of the Society of Critical Care Medicine. Consensus statement of the Society of Critical Care Medicine's ethics committee regarding futile and other possibly inadvisable treatments. Crit Care Med 1997; 25:887–891.

210. See the earlier section on informed consent in this chapter.

7

Advance Directives

The Patient Self-Determination Act requires that patients be informed upon admission to a healthcare facility or healthcare program of their rights under their state's laws regarding advance directives. It does not require states to have such laws, nor does it set forth a requirement for the form such laws should take. Patients merely have the right to know their local laws. We have seen, in chapter 2, how the *Cruzan* court looked favorably upon advance directives as constituting clear and convincing evidence of the wishes of a patient lacking decisional capacity when healthcare decisions had to be made.[1]

The stipulation in the Patient Self-Determination Act about advance directives has received the most attention from those who are attempting to implement the law.[2] However, as we have seen in chapter 6, the right to consent to or *refuse* treatment, as an expression of self-determination, is actually the foundation of the law. Since the role of advance directives has become a matter of increasing consequence in healthcare practice and since they are a highly significant concrete expression of the law, special attention must be paid to them if they are to become effective tools for healthcare decision making.[3]

The Nature of Advance Directives

The history of advance directives has been a troubled one in the United States. The social reasons for this will be explored in the next section. For now it is important to define advance directives and examine their various forms.

The purpose of advance directives is to allow patients to have some influence on the healthcare choices made for them after they have lost decisional capacity. Advance directives are intended to extend the autonomy of patients beyond the point of this loss.[4] They allow patients to set their own healthcare agenda in the process of dying so that decisions can reflect the patient's own beliefs, values, and goals rather than those of others. Advance directives, then, are primarily an expression of the wishes of patients, regardless of the forms they take. The correlation between the patient's wishes and the forms in which those wishes are expressed can create some problems, which we will examine later in this chapter.

Advance directives are intended to be instruments of communication.[5] That is, they are not merely private expressions of patients' wishes that are made public only when the advance directives are to be invoked. They are optimally used as methods of communication between patients and their families and patients and their physicians.[6] If they are not seen as opportunities for communication, their effectiveness may be considerably reduced. We shall return to this important function of advance directives after surveying the forms they may take.

There are three basic forms for advance directives: (1) oral directions for the course of care, (2) living wills, and (3) durable powers of attorney for healthcare, or, more generally, healthcare proxies.[7] We shall explore each of these in turn.

Oral directions, given by individuals to others who might be involved in decisions about their healthcare, are probably the most common form of advance directive.[8] These are often communicated in conversations that arise spontaneously and are often triggered by some news event or experience of a friend or relative in the healthcare setting. For example, a visit to a friend or relative in a hospital or extended care facility might prompt a comment such as "I don't ever want to be in a situation like Charlie's" or "Don't ever let that happen to me." Such informal comments are often just as accurate in expressing an individual's wishes as any written advance directive that might be framed. Oral expressions can indicate the individual's wishes about the parameters of healthcare that she would find tolerable or intolerable. These expressions are not to be discounted in the clinical set-ting.[9] They often are followed in the form of family members telling physicians that "Charlie would not want this kind of intervention," meaning that if Charlie could speak he would definitely refuse this kind of treatment. Physicians then write the appropriate orders.

Oral expressions of a patient's wishes may be effective advance directives up to a point. Since they may be assumed to express the patient's wishes, they are to be considered seriously. Even though they may not possess all the reflective background that one might expect from a formal exercise with written documentation, they may still express legitimate consents to or refusals of treatment.[10] It must be remembered that patients can refuse treatments for any reason.[11] They do not have to have "good" reasons,[12] nor do their refusals have to result from extensive reflection. If this is true of patients with decisional capacity, and if advance directives are intended to extend patient autonomy beyond the loss of decisional capacity, then a strong argument can be made that oral advance refusals should carry serious weight in determining the direction of healthcare for patients who have lost decisional capacity. The loss of decisional capacity does not eliminate the interest patients have in their welfare and the moral harms they may have to suffer if their wishes are not followed.[13]

If everyone—family member or surrogate—who has a legitimate interest in the healthcare decisions for the patient with an oral advance directive agrees that the report of the wishes of the patient expressed orally is accurate, and if the physician trusts the individuals who report the wishes, then there is no good moral reason for the oral advance directive not to be honored.[14] The major problem with informal oral advance directives occurs when there is a disagreement among those who have an interest in the decisions being made for the patient about what the patient actually said, or would have wanted, or if the physician has a particular problem with the decision being suggested.[15] Without an independent written statement that provides documentation of the patient's wishes, there is no way to solve disputes satisfactorily about what the patient truly wanted. In the case of disputes, other mechanisms must be utilized that may or may not yield the kind of decision the patient is reported to have wanted.[16] Patients who limit themselves to oral advance directives are taking a great risk about whether their wishes will be honored. We have already seen how Nancy Cruzan's case became such a problem precisely because she had only an oral advance directive. This did not count as clear and convincing evidence in Missouri, which required such a standard for removing life-sustaining treatments from an incompetent. Had she executed a written advance directive, her case would never have gone beyond the initial court hearing and, very likely, would not have had to go to a hearing at all.

Another form of oral advance directive is an expression of one's wishes to one's physician. This conversation will frequently be considered more formal than the casual exchange that might occur between one's relatives or friends, especially if the physician documents the conversation in the patient's chart. Because of the covenant relationship between the physician and the patient, oral exchanges between them are considered to carry more weight than oral exchanges between others.[17] Such expressions of wishes are considered more reflective than others because of the nature of the conversations between the parties involved and the pledges of fidelity and trust that are exchanged. The documentation in the chart functions as a written expression of the patient's wishes and can generally function in the same way as other legislated forms of advance directives.

Frequently patients will pursue conversations with their physicians rather than with family members because they do not want to trouble their family members with conversations that are often considered unpleasant. Another reason for taking this approach might be that patients find written advance directives intimidating and refuse to draft or sign them, but they are quite willing to talk over the matters with their physicians.[18] The important thing is that patients express their wishes. If the most they can tolerate is a documented conversation with their physicians, then this approach is far better than nothing, if nothing is the only alternative.

The second form of advance directive is the written living will. It is called a "living" will because, unlike an "estate" will, which goes into effect to distribute the estate after an individual has died, the living will goes into effect while the individual is still alive. Both documents are drafted or signed while an individual possesses decisional capacity. Ordinarily the living will takes the form of refusing medical treatments that the author does not consider beneficial under certain circumstances.[19] However, living wills may also direct that certain approaches to care be continued or instituted after decisional capacity has been lost.[20] In certain rare instances, the living will may stipulate that all possible care be continued up to the moment of the patient's death.[21]

Early in the development of living wills two qualifications were generally considered prerequisites for the implementation of such a document. The patient had to be terminally ill and to have irreversibly lost decisional capacity.[22] Once these two conditions were present, the directions in the living will were supposed to be honored. Many states include permanent loss of consciousness—that is, persistent vegetative state—on a par with terminal conditions even though there is strong professional opinion that PVS is not, strictly speaking, terminal.[23] As living will legislation has progressed, the stipulation that patients be "terminally ill" for the directive to be honored has sometimes been eliminated, although it is still a common feature.[24] When this diagnosis of terminal illness occurs, "no hope of recovery" seems to be sufficient to implement a living will.

The stipulation requiring an irreversible loss of decisional capacity is included so that patients who have only temporarily lost decisional capacity can once again directly participate in decisions about their healthcare after they have recovered that capacity. The moral issue here is the need to allow the patient to become functionally autonomous once again. However, it is conceivable that a patient may foresee that the chances of regaining decisional capacity are so remote and the harms to be endured while waiting for that possibility to materialize so great that the language of "irreversibility" might very well be changed to the language of "probability." Thus, they may want their living will to go into effect even though there might be a slight chance that they could recover decisional capacity.[25]

The terminal illness prerequisite has often been considered a central part of living will documents because of the deteriorating condition of the patient and the possibility that continued interventions might do no more than prolong the dying process. However, we saw in chapter 6 that there can be considerable disagreement or latitude in the definition of a terminal illness. This problem generally revolves around whether the definition is formulated in terms of temporality—how soon the patient will die—or according to functional considerations—the nature of the deterioration being experienced by the individual.[26] State laws generally indicate some preference for considerations of temporality, however vaguely they might be worded.[27] However, there may be compelling moral reasons, based on respect for the patient's dignity, to prefer the functional interpretation over the temporal one. Thus, conditions that some consider chronic, such as advanced Alzheimer's disease or persistent vegetative state, may be defined by the patient as terminal "enough" to warrant the enforcement of an advance directive.[28] We shall see more of this later when we discuss the exercise of writing a living will.

A living will can state a patient's wishes either in broad strokes or in specific detail. It lets those who have some involvement in the patient's care know the limitations the patient desires for her care. It is intended by the authors of such documents that the expressed wishes impose an obligation on family members and caregivers alike to follow the wishes contained in the document.[29] Its moral force is powerful even though its legal force may be somewhat weaker, given some state laws formulated about these documents.[30]

The second written form of advance directive is the durable power of attorney for healthcare (or some variation known as a healthcare proxy).[31] The durable power of attorney is an appointment by the author of the document (known as the "principal") designating someone whom she trusts (known as the "attorney-in-fact") to act in a decision-making capacity for the principal when healthcare decisions are to be made and the principal is unable to make those decisions. This document, or another attached to it, may carry specific instructions to the attorney-in-fact outlining the parameters of the decisions, or specific decisions, that the principal wishes to be followed in determining the course of her healthcare.

Unlike a regular power of attorney, which ceases when the principal loses decisional capacity, the durable power of attorney continues after the loss of decisional capacity; hence the term "durable." A durable power of attorney may cover a variety of functions but does not necessarily include healthcare decisions. The durable power of attorney *for healthcare* is specific for healthcare decisions and goes into effect only when the principal has lost decisional capacity.[32] Other durable powers of attorney, such as for financial transactions, may function both before and after the loss of decisional capacity.

The texture of the authority of the attorney-in-fact in a durable power of attorney for healthcare is designated by the laws of the individual states.[33] In addition to variation from state to state, these laws, like living will legislation, are frequently revised and refined.[34] In general, the attorney-in-fact can make healthcare decisions for the principal whether the principal has *irreversibly* lost decisional capacity or not. In some states, if the loss of decisional capacity is temporary, the attorney-in-fact may not refuse life-saving or life-sustaining treatments.[35] In these states the attorney-in-fact can refuse life-sustaining treatments on behalf of the principal only if the loss of decisional capacity is permanent.

Whereas some states (e.g., Ohio)[36] require that the patient be terminally ill, or in a permanently unconscious state (PVS), for the attorney-in-fact to be permitted to withhold or withdraw life-sustaining treatments, other states give the attorney-in-fact comprehensive authority to make all healthcare decisions for patients lacking decisional capacity.[37] The same moral concerns arise in defining the notion of terminal illness and the irreversible loss of decisional capacity in a durable power of attorney for healthcare as were outlined earlier in the discussion of living wills.

The appointment of an attorney-in-fact is no small matter for an individual. The gravity of the decision may be indicated by the notion that the attorney-in-fact is someone who is trusted deeply enough by the principal to be empowered to make life-and-death decisions for the principal.[38] Special reflective care must be taken to ensure that the principal knows whom he can trust to make such decisions. This appointment can be a member of the family or a friend outside the family. Whether or not the attorney-in-fact is a member of the family, her authority takes precedence over that of other family members in making healthcare decisions for the principal.

When an attorney-in-fact is designated, the fiduciary relationship that the physician previously had with the patient is enlarged to include the attorney-in-fact. Thus, all the principles and procedures that govern the dynamics of informed consent must be directed to the attorney-in-fact. The mutual trust that animates the physician-patient relationship must incorporate the physician-attorney-in-fact relationship on behalf of the patient. The physician has no more right to second-guess the decisions of the attorney-in-fact than she does to second-guess the decisions of the patient. For the attorney-in-fact has been designated as a trustworthy spokesperson for the patient/principal. The authority of the attorney-in-fact is indeed awesome and no less than that of the patient who has decisional capacity.

When the attorney-in-fact makes decisions on behalf of the patient, the principle of substituted judgment is the preferred principle to be followed.[39] This holds that the individual making the decision should substitute for his own judgment the judgment that the person for whom he is making the judgment would make if she could do so.[40] This means that the decision of the attorney-in-fact may not be the one he would have made if he had been able to follow his own preferences. The attorney-in-fact, then, makes the healthcare decision through the "value eyes" of the principal/patient rather than through his own "value eyes." He is doing what the patient would have wanted.

It is not always easy to determine what the principal's decision would have been. Three ways of identifying the bases for substituted judgment can be considered. (1) The principal may have left specific instructions with the attorney-in-fact—for example, an accompanying living will document or a similar set of specific instructions—and the latter simply carries out the instructions because they clearly represent what the principal would have wanted. (2) The principal may have left some incomplete verbal clues from which the attorney-in-fact can draw inferences about what the principal would have wanted in a set of circumstances the principal may not have envisioned—for example, "I don't think I would like to live like. . . . " (3) The principal may have engaged in certain behaviors in analogous circumstances or made lifestyle choices from which inferences may be drawn about what she might like to have happen in the current situation—for example, a formally physically- and intellectually-active person may be assumed not to wish to be confined to a persistent vegetative state.[41]

The best approach might be for the principal to leave specific instructions for the attorney-in-fact. However, this is no guarantee that the patient's wishes will be followed.[42] Providing specific instructions is not always possible in healthcare decisions, but some guidelines may be possible and indeed quite helpful.[43] Minimally, the patient should include a statement of trust in the ability of the attorney-in-fact to make a good decision for the patient, given the realities of the clinical situation, which, admittedly, the patient cannot foresee in exquisite detail. To do less is to place the attorney-in-fact in a difficult decision-making position. Incorrect inferences may be drawn and erroneous decisions could follow. But the whole point of trusting an individual whom one appoints as an attorney-in-fact is the belief that he will make the best judgment of which he is capable, knowing full well that he may be the victim of human error, but also trusting that the attorney-in-fact will never act out of self-interest.

Many times individuals simply cannot bring themselves to anticipate healthcare crises for themselves and leave few clues as a foundation for substituted judgments. But they may still wish to appoint an attorney-in-fact. An attorney-in-fact who is appointed under these circumstances and who cannot really make a decision based upon the principle of substituted judgment can only resort to the principle of best interest.[44] This principle requires a decision maker to make the decision that a reasonable person would make given all the known facts and that seems to promote what is best for the patient. For example, if a form of care is not going to provide a decent benefit for a patient, then that intervention can be refused. In this way the best interest of the patient is preserved even though the patient has not herself identified that interest.

Here again the matter of trust enters the decisional arena. Even though a principal may have no tolerance for making or anticipating difficult healthcare decisions, she may trust another to make those decisions for her when the time comes. Thus, the attorney-in-fact is appointed with the understanding that he will act in the best interest of the principal when the time comes to make end-of-life decisions. This should not stop the attorney-in-fact from periodically reviewing the appointment and attempting to solicit some instructions from the principal.[45]

There is probably no one right way for individuals to make their wishes known in advance directives. The best way is the strategy that makes patients feel most comfortable. Each way has its own assets and liabilities, as will be examined below. We have already seen that the written documents have the advantage over oral advance directives in providing a means to settle disputes. Living wills allow patients to speak for themselves, and durable powers of attorney place someone in a decisional position who can assess the particular circumstances firsthand. Many individuals who opt for written forms choose both a living will and a durable power of attorney for healthcare. In this case the living will may function as a set of instructions for the attorney-in-fact. If there is a substantive conflict between what is stated in the living will and a decision made by the attorney-in-fact, then the living will, in most cases, is the document to be honored (based on the principle of autonomy) because it is the patient speaking directly for herself.[46]

Regardless of the approach used, advance directives allow patients to retain some measure of control in the decisions made in their healthcare. They are no longer consigned to the role of victims of someone else's value agenda. They can still exercise their autonomy, and in that way advance directives can play a major role in preserving the personal dignity of patients.

The Social Justification for Advance Directives

The interest in advance directives came about as a result of two major influences in modern medicine. The first was the technological advancements of contemporary medical practice. Medicine reached a point of being able to maintain patients in critical conditions far longer than ever before. It became possible to prolong dying as well as living. This skill was often exercised without the patient's being aware of it. Along with the ability to prolong dying came the skill of doing so long after patients had lost contact with their surroundings and their inner states. Many were quick to perceive that such an extension of the dying process not only provided no benefit to them but was positively harmful.[47] It was perceived by many that the aggressiveness of medical practice had to be curtailed in some way.

The second major influence was the developing concern about patient autonomy over the last two generations.[48] The era of parentalistic medical practice began to wane seriously in the 1950s and the movement toward patient control over, or at least participation in, the decisions about their healthcare began to grow.[49] Many patients no longer wanted to trust themselves solely to the value agendas of others, whether they were physicians or family members, in making intensely personal decisions about the manner of their dying.[50] They wanted not only to exercise their autonomy as decisions were being made during their periods of awareness but to extend their autonomy to those clinical situations where their awareness was dimmed or totally eliminated. Some vehicle for expressing the wishes of patients was necessary if that interest in autonomy was to be preserved and promoted. Patients needed some way to prevent situations from arising or continuing that they perceived to be harmful.

Early forms of advance directives met with little respect from the medical profession. All too often the language contained in them was vague to the point of being useless.[51] Additionally, the documents were often not utilized as open pathways of communication but were presented in the clinical setting in such a way that physicians found it difficult to verify their meaning or the intent of those who had signed them. In 1983 the President's Commission took the bold step of endorsing the durable power of attorney for healthcare as an effective form of advance directive.[52] As late as 1984, when the American College of Physicians produced the first edition of its *Ethics Manual,* only a brief reference was made to advance directives,[53] alluding to the fact that some patients complete such documents but that physicians need not take them too seriously.[54]

During the 1980s a number of cases came before the courts related to issues of withholding or withdrawing treatments.[55] In these cases the courts used the wishes of the patients involved as the first benchmark for making decisions about the level of care to be given to the patients. At the same time there was a flurry of activity as state legislatures debated advance directive laws. In view of this judicial and legislative emphasis on the importance of considering the wishes of incompetent patients, advance directives became so significant that, in the second edition of its *Ethics Manual* in 1989, the American College of Physicians revised its opinion about advance directives and not only endorsed their importance for medical practice but also laid out a strategy to make them more effective for patients and physicians.[56] By 1989, the American Medical Association supported advance directives as an appropriate component of healthcare decision making.[57] At the same time physicians and medical societies across the country began cooperating with state legislators to draft legislation on advance directives that would accomplish the dual purpose of protecting both physicians and patients.[58]

The final turning point came with the *Cruzan* decision in the U.S. Supreme Court in 1990.[59] The court endorsed advance directives as a desirable approach to dealing with healthcare decisions for those who have lost decisional capacity. Such documents were considered by the court to constitute clear and convincing evidence of a patient's wishes for withholding or withdrawing life-sustaining treatments. Advance directives, then, were given the highest court's approval as a way for patients to govern the course of their treatments after the onset of decisional incapacity.

The Patient Self-Determination Act, with its clear identification of the right of patients to refuse treatments, has added further support to the advance directive movement. Every state now has some form of advance directive written into its legislation.[60] The power and the authority of advance directives have reached a new high in the United States, and the directives have profoundly affected the delivery of healthcare in those institutions that take the Patient Self-Determination Act seriously. But even with the added emphasis on advance directives, estimates are that only 15 percent of the population have them.[61]

Advance directive legislation has significantly enlarged the range of individuals who can serve as authorized surrogates for individuals who have lost decisional capacity. Prior to advance directives physicians frequently made decisions about the termination of treatment. When the physician determined that the treatment was no longer accomplishing its goal, the intervention would end. If anyone participated in the decision to end treatment, it was a family member. Common law designated that the next of kin was the one with the final decisional authority. (In recent years this common-law designation has been codified by a number of state legislatures.)[62] If there were no family members or the family members were unable to fulfill their decisional function, then a guardian was appointed by the court to make the decisions.

Among the surrogates who had decisional authority prior to advance directive legislation, no one was explicitly appointed by the patient. Physicians came the closest insofar as they were chosen by the patient to treat them. (Family members are not *chosen* because patients are born into that network, and guardians are appointed by the court with little or no input from the patient.) The development of the durable power of attorney for healthcare as a form of advance directives allowed patients, for the first time, to appoint a decision maker in case they were suspicious of the physician's agenda, distrustful of family members, or fearful of whom the court might appoint as their guardians. There is a qualitative difference between the attorney-in-fact and all the others because the attorney-in-fact is the patient speaking indirectly as a result of the explicit trust the patient has shown in her. This is the reason the attorney-in-fact has a preeminent position as decision maker. The social role of the attorney-in-fact may prove to be one of the most significant innovations in the current climate of healthcare.

One of the social issues that often emerges as a reason for the development of advance directives is the litigious nature of contemporary society. In healthcare, physicians are often held responsible for negative outcomes even when the action of the physician did not cause them. The tendency of many patients to place inappropriate responsibility on physicians has cast a pall over medical practice. In order to protect themselves in this climate physicians tend to test patients excessively and often overtreat them to the point of violating the principle of nonmaleficence.[63] Physicians have become fearful of what survivors and their lawyers will do if they do not press on in their treatment of patients to the bitterest of ends.[64]

Advance directives were developed to address some of these issues as well as the concern for maintaining the dignity of patients. They address the litigation issue by holding physicians blameless if they follow the wishes of patients that are expressed in their advance directives. This includes following the decisions of the attorney-in-fact who has been appointed by the patient. Survivors of patients cannot sue physicians if, as a result of following the advance directive, the patient dies earlier than she would have if treatment had continued.[65]

There is a kind of asymmetry in this protection for the physician, however. All advance directive laws protect the physician in the manner described above. However, they do not *require* the physician to follow the wishes of patients that are expressed in their advance directives. This is consistent with the practice in medicine of allowing a physician to remove herself from a case if the patient is requesting the physician to engage in unethical or unsound medical practice.[66] The "conscience" clause, therefore, applies equally to patients possessing decisional capacity and those who must speak through their advance directives.[67] Physicians need to be honest about whether an unwillingness to treat a patient stems from a genuine disagreement about the morality of an action (e.g., abortion) or a violation of a professional standard (e.g., assisted suicide) or simply from an unwillingness to stretch their practice standards to encompass the reasonable wishes of the patient. In the last case, the conscience clause does not properly excuse the physician from caring for the patient, although the physician may recommend that the patient seek another physician whose practice patterns are more in line with the patient's wishes.

Physicians are directly protected by advance directive legislation that makes them immune from prosecution, but patients are not protected to the same extent. Patient dignity may seem to suffer because of a societal preference for protecting physicians more strongly. This is not necessarily the case. Protecting the physician also protects the patient because the physician is not forced by fear of survivors or other court actions to provide treatment for patients if they have expressed their wishes about forgoing treatment. There is thus a much greater likelihood that the physician will follow the wishes of the patient.

The possible misuse of a conscience clause adds greater urgency to the communication that should occur between physicians and patients in drafting an advance directive.[68] Patients need to let their physicians know about their intention to draft or sign an advance directive, and they should go over the content of the document together.[69] This should reduce the likelihood of a physician's questioning the legitimacy of such a document if it should ever have to be invoked. If the physician has any qualms about honoring an advance directive, that should become apparent in such a conversation. At that time, the patient can decide whether to take a chance with the current physician or seek out another physician who has a more positive attitude toward advance directives in general or the patient's particular instructions.

As a result of the *Cruzan* decision, one might be tempted to assume that treatment cannot be withheld or withdrawn from a patient who has lost decisional capacity unless the patient has completed an advance directive. This is not the case.[70] The principle of best interest has not been totally supplanted by the principle of substituted judgment embodied in an advance directive; substituted judgment has only been given greater emphasis. For example, futile care is always inappropriate whether or not it is refused through an advance directive.[71] Imposing undue burdens on a patient who will enjoy only minimal (or no) benefit is inappropriate. Finally, violating the best interests of a patient to satisfy the self-interest of another, whether it be a family member or a caregiver, is improper.[72] Without an advance directive it may be more difficult to end or withhold a particular intervention, but it is not impossible to do so. Conversely, withholding or withdrawing treatments is much easier if patients have taken the time to anticipate the situation and give directions about the course of their care through advance directives.

In summary, society has become more complex in its interactions in the healthcare setting through advances in technology. And because of a growing respect for the autonomy of patients and the permeating force of litigation, the time for advance directives has surely arrived. Though advance directives do not guarantee a totally smooth administration of healthcare when end-of-life decisions have to be made,[73] they can provide a mechanism for making many of those decisions easier on behalf of patients who have lost decisional capacity if communication is included as an adjunct. Patients can remain in control and take comfort in the fact that their agenda will continue to carry weight even in their last days.

General Problems with Advance Directives

From the earliest days of the passage and implementation of the Patient Self-Determination Act concerns have been raised about its usefulness.[74] These reservations cover a broad spectrum. A brief survey of these problems might be helpful before launching into a detailed examination of advance directives. The analysis in the following four sections may give some clues to the composition of advance directives and strategies for developing and implementing them. Perhaps these suggestions will also reduce some of the misgivings about the effectiveness of advance directives and the Patient Self-Determination Act.

(1) There have been suspicions that patients do not want to talk about end-of-life decisions, and there has been evidence that even

when they express a desire to speak with their physicians about these matters, they do not have the actual conversations or do not actually sign a living will.[75] Concerns were expressed that conversations about advance directives are too time-consuming and require too much training. Forms came under attack. General forms were considered too vague, and specific forms with specific directions about interventions were considered the gateway to inappropriate care.[76] Concerns were also raised about whether proxies can make appropriate decisions for patients when they are appointed in a durable power of attorney for healthcare.[77]

Few, if any, of these early concerns have been resolved. There is evidence to support both sides of the controversies. Thus, the indications are that more evidence needs to be gathered on virtually every issue related to the Patient Self-Determination Act.[78] But in spite of its problems and some early evidence to the contrary,[79] the Patient Self-Determination Act does seem to work in some cases.[80] Some recent research indicates that even with specific instructions given in advance directives, care is inconsistent at best in half the cases studied.[81] Additionally, one study has found that advance directives enhance neither physician-patient communication nor decision making about resuscitation.[82] Much work still needs to be done, not just in answering the question of whether it is working, but also in developing strategies that will make the law truly effective.[83]

(2) Perhaps the central problem has to do with the difficulty of talking about specifics with physicians. One study has shown that advance directives have not actually enhanced communication between patients and physicians.[84] There seems to be a significant reluctance on the part of physicians to talk about advance directives.[85] Reasons may range from lack of time for discussions to discomfort with talking about dying to difficulty in predicting what patients' medical needs will be in end-of-life situations.[86] On the other hand, some physicians actively solicit patients' advance preferences and spend considerable time discussing them.[87]

(3) Questions have been raised about whether patients will change their minds subsequent to signing an advance directive or whether their choices will remain stable. In spite of concerns in this area there does seem to be some evidence that once one has decided to forgo treatment in an advance directive, he remains consistent in that deci-

sion.[88] Thus, one may approach advance directives with some confidence in their reliability.

(4) There will always be borderline cases regarding the implementation of advance directives, and these cases present particularly difficult problems in surgery.[89] How one is to interpret patients' wishes expressed in an advance directive when unanticipated conditions arise has been, and will probably always remain, troublesome, particularly if physicians do not have somewhat detailed conversations with their patients.[90]

(5) The patient's understanding of the purpose of advance directives can be a matter of some concern. But of greater concern are the methods to be used by patients in formulating them. Some very detailed methods have been suggested, and they have considerable merit for those patients who have a tolerance for exquisite detail.[91] A question still remains, however, as to the appropriate approach for those who are not enamored of such specificity. A further question remains about the correct way to interpret advance directives if they are couched only in general terms.

(6) The lack of general use of advance directives is troublesome. If only 15 percent of the population signs or drafts advance directives, is their limited use worth the effort?[92] Granted that with time and further familiarity there may be an increase in the use of advance directives, the question still remains as to whether the increase will justify the effort needed to promote them. On the other hand, the low numbers may not be as big a concern as whether advance directives can improve the quality of care of the patients who have them.[93]

(7) Educational programs are essential for the implementation of the Patient Self-Determination Act. The questions that need to be addressed are what sort of programs are needed and whether educational programs can really help increase patients' comprehension of advance directives, their moral usefulness, and the legal requirements that govern them.[94] The failure of some programs may only mean that there are still challenges that can be met if creative educators turn their attention to them.[95]

(8) Empirical evidence indicates that there is a great willingness to discuss end-of-life decisions and advance directives.[96] This interest is present on the side of both patients and physicians, a fact suggesting that conversations about advance directives can be effective. How-

ever, less optimistic are the results of the SUPPORT study, which indicate that, in spite of extensive efforts at communication, these efforts may not substantially change physician practices and the way patients are treated in end-of-life situations.[97] Perhaps, as the SUPPORT study suggests, greater and more creative efforts must be made at communication.

(9) Even if advance directives are developed, there is still a concern about whether they will be accessible when they are needed.[98] If advance directives are not produced when they need to be implemented, or if they are not followed by their caregivers, the effort to generate them may have no value. The transmission of the advance directive remains a matter of serious concern.

(10) Finally, a matter of ongoing debate is whether the use of advance directives is economically advantageous in managing the resources of healthcare. Some studies indicate that advance directives have a positive influence on resource management,[99] while other studies argue that any result is negligible.[100] Further studies will be needed in this area together with closer observance of the stipulations of the advance directives themselves. A related matter is whether advance directives really function as a promotion of patient autonomy or are actually used to limit care, primarily for the purpose of reducing healthcare costs.[101]

The problems raised by the use of advance directives and their role in the Patient Self-Determination Act cannot be minimized. However, they must also be seen in perspective. Advance directives have only recently appeared upon the healthcare scene and have only more recently been taken seriously by caregivers and healthcare institutions. An instrument with such complex implications cannot be expected to be perfect so early in its use. What may be needed at this point is not to allow the problems of advance directives to overwhelm healthcare delivery, but to bend every effort to making them work and fulfill the promise that they hold for improving the quality of patient care at the end of life. If nothing else, the societal discussion of advance directives has sparked some changes in the communication patterns between patients and physicians, a variety of educational programs, and some actual changes in the practice patterns of some physicians. Even if advance directives fail in the long run, these changes can have a salutary effect on the practice of medicine and the welfare of patients.[102]

Advantages and Disadvantages of Advance Directives

From the observations in the previous three sections we can begin to see emerging some of the advantages and disadvantages of advance directives. In the first section this matter was directly addressed with oral advance directives. Now is the time to attempt to identify clearly the advantages and disadvantages of written advance directives. This effort should assist caregivers who are talking to patients about advance directives in their facilities. For, as was said earlier, advance directives are not for everyone, and a particular form of advance directive is not necessarily appropriate for all patients.

There are many advantages to drafting an advance directive. An advance directive, particularly a detailed living will or special instructions to a physician or an attorney-in-fact, can provide a documented portrait of the author by delineating her wishes and values. One cannot compose such a document without seriously reflecting upon the meaning of her life, the values that drive her, the goals she wishes to obtain, and the virtues she wishes to practice. Furthermore, such an exercise places the author within the natural rhythms of life by acknowledging that death is an integral part of the life process.[103]

An important ethical advantage is that an advance directive promotes personal autonomy by extending the making of choices beyond the loss of decisional capacity. This extension promotes continuity of care because it ensures that beliefs and attitudes toward treatment that the author had prior to the loss of capacity will continue to be honored. The advance directive also acknowledges the dignity of the author by allowing her to accept the moral risks that are a necessary part of her decision making as a moral agent.

This last feature—namely, the element of risk taking—causes some to allege that advance directives are unreliable and the risks attendant to attempting to forecast the clinical future constitute their major disadvantage. Many would claim that no one can anticipate all contingencies or even enough contingencies about future healthcare decisions to make meaningful clinical decisions in anticipation of the onset of decisional incapacity.[104] Though not all contingencies can be anticipated, many of them can be.[105] The ability to anticipate future decisions would require the author to monitor her healthcare circumstances and adjust or reinforce the stipulations of her advance directive in light of unfolding clinical conditions.[106] This may mean that an advance directive that an individual wrote while she was in a relatively healthy state should be reviewed when a terminal diagnosis is returned or as a chronic disease progresses.

The anticipation of contingencies raises another important issue. Some individuals are more willing than others to take risks. The taking of moral risks in making decisions was identified in chapter 4 as an important dimension of human dignity. Risk taking is a virtue that is sometimes practiced with considerable ease. Even if one is taking greater risks than a healthcare professional might like, respect for her dignity requires that those wishes, along with the risks they assume, be respected.

Advance directives also provide benefits to others as well as the author herself. A well-drafted advance directive will relieve others of the need to second-guess the wishes of the author. Feelings of guilt can also be relieved because others (e.g., surrogates) will know that they are making decisions as the author would want them and are respecting her dignity by honoring her wishes. The fear of lawsuits against caregivers who honor the author's wishes can be muted because state laws that recognize advance directives ordinarily grant immunity from prosecution or civil procedures to those who honor the wishes of patients when they comply with the stipulations of the advance directives and the law.

Once again resource allocation issues become an element for consideration. Currently, a good deal of our healthcare resources are being allocated to the care of those lacking decisional capacity who have not expressed their wishes about the extent of their care. If individuals are encouraged to express their wishes, some of those resources in individual cases may be saved or allocated for other important societal purposes.[107]

The legal freedom of a physician to refuse to honor an advance directive was discussed in the previous section. Suffice it to say that advance directives have the advantage of acting as a compelling moral force on the way caregivers participate in healthcare decisions about their patients. The disadvantage is that advance directives do not bind caregivers absolutely. The dynamics of informed consent enter into this situation, for both patients and caregivers need to know each other's attitudes so they can negotiate with each other in light of those attitudes while the patient still has decisional capacity.[108] In this way the advantage/disadvantage facet of advance directives can preserve both the dignity of the patient and the integrity of the caregiver.

There are some special advantages and disadvantages that can be identified for the two forms of advance directives. Living wills have the advantage of allowing patients to speak for themselves. They are particularly advantageous if patients have taken the time to achieve some degree of specificity about treatments.[109] The disadvantage of living wills is that patients must anticipate situations they *might* face;[110] they are not actually face to face with the situation. This exercise is always accompanied by some degree of uncertainty. Thus, patients are not able to make decisions based upon their immediate experience of the clinical situation. Nor can they weigh the contingencies that accompany their circumstances.

The disadvantage of living wills in terms of foreseeing the future is countered by the advantage of the durable power of attorney. For the attorney-in-fact is able to make a decision based upon the immediate experience of the principal's clinical situation and can weigh the variables of the exact situation carefully before making a decision.[111] On the other hand, the attorney-in-fact can speak for the patient only in light of the patient's trust for him. The attorney-in-fact is not the patient and so the nuances of the attorney-in-fact's decision may not be a mirror image of the patient's. The principal can minimize the differences by giving directives to the attorney-in-fact about the course she wishes her healthcare to take and by articulating her trust in the attorney-in-fact. A living will that has some degree of specificity could function as such a directive. Thus, those who want the fullest protection may want to complete both a living will and a durable power of attorney for healthcare.

When all the advantages and disadvantages are taken into account, the former seem to outweigh the latter.[112] However, apprehension, fear, anxiety, or neglect often stands in the way of individuals' completing advance directives.[113] In such cases—and they are the vast majority—periodic reminders about considering advance directives may need to be given to patients as their life experiences and healthcare circumstances change. Though they might not be ready at one time to think seriously about advance directives, they might be ready at another time. For this reason ongoing educational programs conducted by healthcare institutions, such as those discussed in chapter 5, are vital.

Writing an Advance Directive

One of the major problems with advance directives is that many are too general to give sufficient guidance. Language such as "no use of *heroic means*" tends to cloud the issues because there is no universal understanding of what constitutes "heroic means." Frequently, there is virtually no advance discussion between patients and physicians about the proper interpretation of this sort of directive.

If an advance directive is to function effectively, it must be credible and contain some measure of specificity.[114] In *Cruzan*, for example, the Supreme Court indicated that advance directives that are specific with regard to treatment and condition meet the clear and convincing evidence criterion that states are permitted to establish in cases of withdrawing life-sustaining treatments from patients lacking decisional capacity.[115] The Court did not mean that all states should require clear and convincing evidence, preferably taking the form of specificity, but only that states could require it if they wished.

The credibility of the document refers to the intention and motivation of the author.[116] Documents that contain only a signature on a form may have doubtful credibility.[117] The reader may have no way of knowing whether the individual signing the document really knows the significance of the document or has thought seriously about it. The author may not have accurate information about her healthcare condition or the options available to her. A credible document would have some indication about the intent of the author and the significance the author attaches to the document. It would also establish a value profile of the author so that the selection or refusal of treatment can be seen as being consistent with the value context that provides a framework for it.[118] A discussion between the patient and the physician that focused upon the intention, motivation, and values of the patient could go a long way toward guaranteeing that the advance directive would be honored.

The specificity of the document refers to the identification of the treatments the author desires or does not desire.[119] Specificity in an advance directive could also identify those outcomes the author would like to achieve, or at least be able to tolerate, and those he would like to avoid. This level of specificity may be difficult to accomplish in exquisite detail because no one can anticipate the future with accuracy. And it may be beyond the author's level of tolerance or ability to achieve such precision. But some indication about outcomes could communicate an idea of the author's treatment wishes and the conditions where it would be appropriate to implement them.[120] One cannot expect to produce an ideal document, but this should not stop him from producing a good one.

Though credibility and specificity may be the most desirable characteristics of an advance directive, it would seem that many states do not consider them important since they mandate a definite form cast with (general terms, or at least, some precise language.)[121] Forms required by state law with a signature line, though not ideal, are a beginning insofar as they can identify the parameters of a patient's wishes. Caregivers in the state are familiar with them, and signatures on them may bear increasing weight as the Patient Self-Determination Act is implemented. One should use a mandated form because it gives protection in those states where specific language is required by law. In those states a personally designed advance directive cannot provide the same protection. If there is a recommended form that is in wide circulation, this should also be used because healthcare institutions will not have to study the form to determine its validity. However, if the patient wishes to go beyond the forms, there is nothing to stop her. Patients are always free to write what they wish as an addendum when there is a required form, provided the form is properly signed. The supplemental document can indicate that the patient wishes to add to the standard form and then go on to state the author's explicit reflections and wishes.

Communication remains one of the most important functions of an advance directive.[122] To whom the author's wishes are communicated is as important as the wishes themselves. The author's physician and family or friends are the appropriate objects of the communication.[123] Several steps to this communication process can be identified. The first is to be taken when the author is considering signing or drafting an advance directive. At this time, some discussion with her physician can be very helpful. The physician can explain the significance of the document, present the various approaches to treatment, dispel any misunderstanding the patient might have, and emphasize the physician's commitment to honoring the author's wishes. Documents that do not include the physician in the loop of the reflections may not be accepted if they are presented only at the time they must be implemented.

The family members or significant others are the second important objects for communication. Often treatment decisions are delayed or made inappropriately because there is division among family members about the way a patient who lacks decisional capacity should be treated. As the second step in the communication process there could be discussion with family members at the time an advance directive is being considered. Such a discussion can give them the opportunity to listen to the convictions of the author and come to terms with them as well as to work out any differences in interpretation of the directive that might arise. Allowing the family dynamics to play out before a crisis develops will not solve every problem in implementing an advance directive, but such conversations may solve many of them and will surely mitigate some of the need for second-guessing the intentions of the author.

The final step in the communication process occurs once the appropriate documents are signed. The signed copies should be given to the physician and suitable family members or other surrogates. Giving copies to one's attorney and religious leader might also be appropriate. Keeping the copies only in a desk drawer, safe deposit box, or a lawyer's files will likely make them inaccessible at the very time they are needed. The Patient Self-Determination Act requires healthcare facilities to document advance directive information in the patient's records. In many states, and for many institutions, this has meant keeping a copy of the advance directive itself on the patient's chart, at least while the patient is currently in the institution or program.[124] Keeping the advance directive as a part of the permanent record for a patient may create some problems in case a patient changes the directive in any way at a later time.

Once an advance directive is written, it should not be considered unchangeable. This is particularly the case when certain specifications are given to the document or when an attorney-in-fact has been appointed. New technologies could be introduced to the healthcare setting or, over time, the success rate of current technologies could improve or decline. Life experiences and relationships may change an individual's perception of the direction her advance directive should take. For example the attorney-in-fact may die or may no longer be considered trustworthy for the task the principal has designated.

Of particular importance is the periodic review of a document or one's instructions to the attorney-in-fact after the document has been written or signed. Healthcare professionals might have difficulty implementing an advance directive that was twenty years old or more. Reviewing one's advance directive every three to five years would be helpful to communicate that beliefs about end-of-life decisions prompting the directive are relatively current.[125] If all remains the same, the author of the directive can sign the document again and enter the new date. This procedure lets others know that the authors have reflected again on their decisions and that their directives truly represent their current state of mind. If their healthcare condition radically changes, the advance directive should be reconsidered and updated. In light of a specific healthcare future rather than a vague future, the author may wish to incorporate alterations into the document. As patients go through the process of a terminal illness, they may also have new insights into their goals and the values they consider important to pursue. This experience may be a reason for additional changes. Approaching an advance directive as a "work in progress" underscores the narrative character of the author's dignity and helps to preserve that dignity by keeping reflections on end-of-life decisions up to date.

Whenever these changes are made, they should be communicated to those who have a direct interest in the decisions and care of the author. In this way changes will not be countered with the presentation of older documents that might represent different views. Older documents may be destroyed or kept to show the continuity in the author's thinking if that should ever be a problem in making healthcare decisions.

Advance directives are tools to promote patient dignity, but this outcome does not occur automatically. Patients must assume a large measure of responsibility in developing strategies to help them achieve this end. There are limits to what healthcare facilities can do to assist patients in writing their advance directives. Ultimately the responsibility for the clarity of the documents and appropriate communication about them must be borne by the patient. If patients want their personal dignity preserved, they must become active in the process. The Patient Self-Determination Act provides the opportunity; the patient must do a good deal of the work.

Content of Advance Directives

When an individual is thinking about writing an advance directive either as a primary document or as a document that is supplemental to a standard form required or recommended by state law, there are some elements that it would be helpful to include. Recall that the two most important features of the document are its credibility and its specificity. In addressing these issues, authors may wish to be very detailed or they may have a tolerance for only limited details. There is no single way the issues in the documents should be stated.[126] The amount of detail to be contained in any particular document will depend on the disposition of the author and the kind of assistance he receives in writing the document.

Nonetheless, elements that make a document credible could include an explicit statement about the reasons for writing the document, which convey vital information to those who will read the document and have to implement it. Possible reasons might include giving guidance to caregivers and family, preserving the author's dignity, eliminating guessing about the author's wishes by secondary decision makers, avoiding unwanted treatments, avoiding prolonged dying, extending life, or saving costs to the estate. The reasons demonstrate that the author has reflected upon what is important to him; the advance directive is not based on a whim, is not just an automatic response to some social force, and is not the result of coercion.

Another essential way to communicate credibility is to identify clearly one's values and the goals one seeks to achieve with the decisions being made. This approach explicitly identifies what is most important to the author. The value narrative, which was discussed in chapter 4, provides a context for the treatment decisions one will make in the document. Included in this section would be a statement about the minimum quality of life the author would be willing to live. Thus, any condition that irreversibly falls below that minimal level would activate the implementation of the advance directive.[127]

A final way to establish credibility would be for the author to make some statement about his views regarding the way death fits into his life process and acceptance of death.[128] This topic is often avoided by patients and physicians alike.[129] However, inclusion of this issue in an advance directive indicates that the document must be taken seriously by those who are called upon to execute it. Also one might include some statement about the way he sees his role in anticipating contingencies when making these sorts of healthcare decisions. This is particularly important since authors must realize that they cannot anticipate every clinical contingency. Those who implement the document would be helped to know that the author has accepted this fact but wants his wishes to be followed in spite of uncertainties. Comments about the way he views the virtue of risk taking,[130] a very significant facet of human dignity, would also be most helpful.

The author will determine the appropriate level of specificity. We have seen earlier that vague or general language is seldom useful unless there is some documented conversation that interprets the language used. One of the reasons for pressing the point of specificity is that the more comprehensive the detail, the easier it will be to extrapolate and fill gaps that may not have been anticipated. For example, if a patient specifies that she does not want nasogastric tube feedings or a gastrostomy but has neglected to include hyperalimentation, the conclusion can be drawn that she would refuse the hyperalimentation as well. Another advantage is that some specificity will put one in a position to meet any clear and convincing evidence standard the state may have or may institute in the future.

Frequently, advance directives are implemented when two conditions are present—a terminal illness, many times defined in terms of the imminence of death, and the irreversible loss of decisional capacity. Unfortunately, there is enough disagreement in society about what constitutes a terminal illness and decisional incapacity that it might be helpful if the author addressed this matter. If she considers a terminal illness one in which she will die within a relatively brief period of time, as some state laws suggest, then she might want to indicate that understanding. On the other hand, if the time element is not a concern, then she should indicate that perception as well and specify the conditions under which the advance directive should take effect. This would allow for a treatment refusal to be honored earlier than might otherwise happen.

If the author interprets decisional incapacity as the total and permanent loss of consciousness, this could be stated.[131] If, however, she regards it as loss of the ability to respond to her environment in any meaningful or purposeful way, it would be helpful for caregivers to know that as well.[132] If, as was suggested earlier, a patient wants to indicate a refusal of treatment in spite of a low probability of a return to decisional capacity, this provision can also be made.

Even though a state's laws sometimes place certain restrictions on the implementation of advance directives through particular interpretations of matters such as what constitutes a terminal illness or decisional incapacity, authors of such documents may still wish to give their own interpretations of these issues. If the wishes of patients are to be honored in terms of their values and goals, then this information should carry strong moral weight with those who would implement the advance directive.[133] Special precautions may be taken to avoid an entanglement with state laws that do not reflect clinical realities. Or family members may wish to appeal to the courts for a ruling on following a patient's wishes even though they may not conform precisely to the state's laws. A court may look favorably on a document that is very specific because, after all, honoring the wishes of the patient is paramount and may very well take precedence over a law that has been generated as a compromise among various special interest groups in the state legislature.

In relation to the notion of specificity, it would be important for the author of an advance directive to indicate what she knows about her healthcare condition. If the author is terminally ill when the advance directive is drafted, this information is vital, for it allows any misunderstandings about the condition to be corrected or clarified. If the author suffers from some chronic disease or conditions that could result in sudden crisis or death, then her understanding here should be discussed and included. Informed consent becomes an important issue here. For, in spite of even good communication with one's physician, there is always the possibility that the patient may miss or misinterpret some information. If the author is normally healthy, general healthcare conditions, family history of disease, or the possibility of injury might be included in the document.

When it comes to selecting or rejecting the actual treatments themselves, their relative benefits and risks, the futility of their further pursuit, and the accomplishment of particular life goals must all be considered. Not every possible intervention can be mentioned but the major interventions deserve some attention—for example, transplants, dialysis, antibiotics, respirators, transfusions, etc. The utilization of CPR, the scope of resuscitation efforts, and medically administered nutrition and hydration are interventions that should be explicitly mentioned in an advance directive.[134] The reason for specificity in these areas lies in the fact that the interventions cited are often futile and can best be judged only against realistic medical goals and the personally determined goals of the patient.[135]

Moreover, there is much controversy in society currently about CPR and tube feedings.[136] The controversy about DNR orders is related to both terminal conditions and advanced age. CPR is often considered futile in both cases.[137] DNR should be explicitly addressed as a part of the protocol in extended care facilities, particularly because the possibility of eventual loss of decisional capacity looms large. The controversy around medically administered nutrition and hydration focuses on whether they are to be considered medical treatment or simply comfort care.[138] Even though the *Cruzan* decision considered them medical treatment, the matter has not been settled in many minds. A statement in an advance directive expressing the author's wishes regarding this intervention is one of the few ways in which one can be relatively sure that her wishes will be honored.[139]

The recent Supreme Court ruling on physician-assisted suicide gave special attention to the issue of pain medication and pain control.[140] This matter was addressed in both the majority opinion and in particular was singled out in Justice O'Connor's concurring opinion. It was the opinion of the Court that pain medication, even in high doses which might shorten the life of the patient, is an appropriate way to address the needs of patients in end-of-life situations. This approach was justified by the principle of double effect.[141] The issue of terminal sedation was given special attention.[142] When terminal sedation is utilized as a method of pain control a further decision is required regarding the use of tube feedings.[143] Patients may wish to include in their advance directives some consideration of their desired level of pain control, particularly when faced with the possibility of such a radical form of pain control as terminal sedation and its accompanying decisions about nutrition and hydration.

In considering the various treatments, patients can decide which they want and under what circumstances they might wish to consent to them or refuse them. For example, a patient might wish to consent to the administration of antibiotics if they will keep him more comfortable. But the same patient might choose to refuse antibiotics for a lethal infection and go the route of purely palliative care because he views the antibiotics as prolonging his dying.

Most advance directives focus on healthcare conditions and treatments, but a statement about the outcomes of treatment would also be helpful.[144] This would relate to what was said earlier about reflections on what counts as a minimally decent quality of life. The author may identify the outcomes she would want to avoid—for example, living in a persistent vegetative state or in a permanent condition in which she could not meaningfully receive stimuli from, or respond to, her environment. Or she could identify the outcomes she would be willing to tolerate within the context of her disease process. This factor would provide great help to caregivers when a full range of treatments cannot be, or is not, specified. If the author has clearly indicated that she would not want to continue to live with a particular outcome, then the caregivers can withhold or withdraw interventions that might perpetuate that outcome.

In summary, advance directives are important moral and legal protections and should be carefully considered by all individuals while they are still capable of understanding their options and making healthcare decisions, no matter how tentative they may be. The more explicit the documents can be and the more extensive the communication at the time they are being drafted, the greater the chance of their being honored.[145] They should be reviewed periodically as life conditions change so that both patients and caregivers can be confident that the document represents the most recent thinking of its author.

Assistance in Writing Advance Directives

The extensive analysis above indicates that drafting or signing an advance directive is no simple matter. Minimally, it requires a clear understanding of what advance directives are and what they can do. Maximally, it requires a reflective life with a keen sense of what is important to the patient and a discerning ability to develop the strategies to bring it about. Few patients possess the skill to draft an advance directive without some assistance.

Prior to the last two decades the culture of patients has been dominated by almost total reliance on healthcare professionals.[146] Patients have been encouraged to listen to healthcare professionals, accept their opinions, and follow their directions with docility. Trust in the professional has been one of the major characteristics of the patient. The movement toward patient autonomy in the last two generations has gradually shifted the focus for many patients from docility and blind trust to inquisitiveness and responsibility. Many patients no longer wish to relay on others to make decisions for them. They want to be active participants in the decisions that govern their healthcare.

But this is an unfamiliar role for patients, and they need considerable assistance in discharging it. The Patient Self-Determination Act sets the stage for patients to become active participants in the decisions governing their healthcare, but it cannot function without some help in its implementation. For patients who are strangers to this new role in healthcare, considerable assistance may be required. Entering into a role of being a responsible patient is not an automatic transition, nor can it be easily accomplished.[147]

Recall that the Patient Self-Determination Act requires only a *notification* of rights. Giving information does not necessarily guarantee that the rights and the manner in which they can be exercised will be understood. The mere shuffling of paper is a poor substitute for the more human contact necessary for implementing the spirit of the Patient Self-Determination Act. There will be a great need for developing the art of conversation with patients in order to help them become wiser consumers of healthcare.[148] There is no substitute for the interactive context of the conversation that allows for information to be exchanged and immediate reaction to it to be processed. Conversations, if carried out skillfully, make patients active in thinking about the direction of their healthcare. Conversations are particularly important to put patients at ease when dealing with difficult topics such as refusing treatment and formulating advance directives. The informality of the conversation may significantly reduce the level of the intimidation fostered by the clinical setting. Thus, simple as it may seem, the first form of assistance for patients will be simply to talk with them in an unhurried and respectful manner, allowing for the free flow and exchange of information and impressions.

The Patient Self-Determination Act requires that patients be notified about their rights under their state's laws regarding advance directives. This looks like a simple piece of information to provide to patients except that many of these laws are so lengthy and convoluted that even trained attorneys have difficulty interpreting them. In Ohio, for example, the law that went into effect there in 1991 was 75 pages long and required 27,500 words to cover all that the legislature had to say.[149] Even written simplified versions of these laws often do not give patients enough command of their requirements and applications for patients to effectively understand, sign, or develop an advance directive. Thus assistance will have to come in the form of conversations with patients in which they can ask questions and be enlightened about what the law says to them.

Understanding how a durable power of attorney for healthcare works is another area in which patients will have to be assisted. They will need to know how it differs from other powers of attorney and the extent of, and expectations for, an attorney-in-fact who is designated. The notion of substituted judgment will need careful explanation. In appointing an attorney-in-fact, individuals may need assistance in identifying an individual whom they trust to carry out such an appointment with diligence.

Reflecting on their life experiences to identify their beliefs, values, and goals is sometimes a very difficult exercise for those not accustomed to it. This may be particularly difficult when applying them to healthcare decision making at a time when the technological imperative is so strong. Some help may be necessary to facilitate this exercise as a beginning point for drafting an advance directive if one chooses a more personal expression of her wishes.

Without a doubt individuals will need some assistance to work through their fear of confronting their own finitude as death becomes a real possibility for them. They will need to understand the difference between death by natural causes, suicide, and the technological prolonging of dying.[150] These are matters of common confusion in our society. Patients, or potential patients, have no easier time distinguishing them than anyone else. They will need to understand the role of the virtue of acceptance in completing an advance directive and how to interact with others who may not be able to practice this virtue at the same time the patient wishes to practice it.

Assistance will often be necessary in the process of communicating with others about the role of the advance directive in the individual's life. Often others—physicians and family members—will be reluctant to enter into discussions with those who desire to complete an advance directive. Those who would have such documents in these circumstances will need support and strategies to open, and keep open, the lines of communication.

Finally, and perhaps most important, individuals may need assistance in determining whether there is a role for an advance directive in their lives. Many are uncertain about the value of advance directives and, after some reflection, may wish to forgo them at a particular time.[151] Such a decision should not be an automatic decision but one resulting from careful consideration of a directive's function and the consequences of not having one. A mere exchange of paper at the time of admission to a healthcare facility could never accomplish this level of reflection.

Perhaps nothing speaks more eloquently to the contemporary significance of advance directives than the Ohio legislation mentioned earlier. In less complex times when a patient came to die, he simply spoke his farewells to his family and friends and said, "I am ready to die." Then he lapsed into unconsciousness and died. Or, if he was already unconscious, the family members would say, "He is ready to go; he won't suffer any more." And then he died. Or, the physician would say, "There is nothing more we can do but keep him comfortable; he has suffered enough." And then he died. Ohio's advance directive law has taken 27,500 words to allow the same end. And even then there are a variety of interpretations of it. As decisions around the process of dying become more and more perplexing, every avenue must be explored to make them less cumbersome. In many clinical situations advance directives can provide one of those avenues.

NOTES

1. Cruzan v. Director, Missouri Department of Health. 110 S. Ct. 2841 (1990).

2. The reason for this emphasis may lie in the fact that advance directives are more tangible components of the law than most of its other elements. They also seem to hold the promise of more direct influence on treatments. It may also be the case that advance directives, as living wills, simply capture the imagination of patients and caregivers more than other issues raised by the Patient Self-Determination Act. This is not to say that these reasons are *good* reasons, particularly in light of the many problems raised by advance directives in the clinical setting. See Greco PJ et al. The Patient Self-Determination Act and the future of advance directives. Ann Intern Med 1991; 115:639–643.

3. Emanuel LL et al. Advance directives for medical care: A case for greater use. N Engl J Med 1991; 324:889–895.

4. President's Commission for the Study of Ethical Problems in Medicine and Biomedical and Behavioral Research. Deciding to forego life-sustaining treatment: Ethical, medical, and legal issues in treatment decisions. Washington, D.C.: U.S. Government Printing Office, 1983, pages 136–141 and 145–151.

5. Emanuel LL, Emanuel LJ. The medical directive: A new comprehensive advance care document. JAMA 1989; 261:3288–3293.

6. Markson L et al. The doctor's role in discussing advance preferences for end-of-life care: Perceptions of physicians practicing in the VA. JAGS 1997; 45:399–406.

7. Annas GJ. The health care proxy and the living will. N Engl J Med 1991; 324:1210–1213.

8. American College of Physicians. Ethics manual. 3d edition. Philadelphia, PA: American College of Physicians, 1992, page 16.

9. Joint Commission for the Accreditation of Health Care Organizations. 1997 comprehensive accreditation manual for hospitals. Oakbrook Terrace, IL: Joint Commission on Accreditation of Health Care Organizations, 1996. Standard RI.1.2.4.

10. Wishes may be expressed in a multitude of valid ways. A particular structure does not make a wish any more or less representative of the accuracy of the wish. Certain structures may fulfill criteria for particular social conventions such as a signed advance directive. But other structures may very well be just as accurate portrayals of what an individual wishes to happen in particular situations.

11. See chapter 6.

12. Rubenfeld J. The right to privacy. Harvard L Rev 1989; 102: 737–807.

13. In re Colyer. 99 Wash 2d 114, 660 P.2d 738 (1983).

14. This was the centerpiece of the decision about Brother Fox, who had

not written a formal advance directive but let his wishes be known in a formal discussion (more structured than simply a "casual" conversation) about Karen Ann Quinlan and the use of life-sustaining treatments. The court ruled that written documentation was not necessary in such an expression of patient wishes. Oral statements were enough to allow withdrawal of life-sustaining treatments. In re Storar (In re Eichner) 52 N.Y.2d 363, 438 N.Y.S.2d 266, 420 N.E.2d 64, cert. denied, 454 U.S. 858 (1981).

15. Without clear and unambiguous direction about the patient's wishes, the physician often has to fall back on her own judgment, utilizing the principle of beneficence. Such judgments often take the form of continued treatment. Council on Ethical and Judicial Affairs, AMA. Decisions near the end of life. JAMA 1992; 267:2229–2233.

16. Such mechanisms might include patient care committees, ethics committees, probate hearings, etc.

17. The covenant relationship is richer than simply a relationship of agreement and cooperation. It also involves a deep sense of trust and fidelity based upon roles that seek the intrinsic good of the partners to the covenant. Pellegrino ED, Thomasma DC. The Christian virtues in medical practice. Washington, D.C.: Georgetown University Press, 1996, page 80. See also May WF. The physician's covenant: Images of the healer in medical ethics. Philadelphia: Westminster Press, 1983 pages 106–144.

18. Lynn J. Why I don't have a living will. Law, Medicine & Health Care 1991; 19:101–104.

19. Walker RM et al. Living wills and resuscitation preferences in an elderly population. Arch Intern Med 1995; 155:171–175.

20. Emanuel L. The health care directive: Learning how to draft advance care documents. J Am Geriatr Soc 1991; 39:1221–1228.

21. State of Indiana. Healthcare consent law. Indiana Code § 16-8-11 (West Supp. 1988). This is called a "Life-Prolonging Procedures Declaration."

22. Collins ER, Weber D. The Society for the Right to Die. The complete guide to living wills: How to safeguard your treatment choices. New York: Bantam Books, 1991, pages 50–51. Attached to the stipulation "terminal illness" is sometimes found a time qualifier—for example, "we consider terminally ill patients as those whose condition is irreversible whether treated or not and who most likely will die within 3 to 6 months." American College of Physicians. Ethics manual. 3rd edition. Philadelphia: American College of Physicians, 1992, page 19.

23. American Academy of Neurology. Position of the American Academy of Neurology on certain aspects of the care and management of the persistent vegetative state patient. Neurology 1988; 39:125–126.

24. Choice in Dying. Refusal of treatment legislation. New York: Choice in Dying, 1996, Introduction page 2.

25. Such a stipulation might be made in the case of an Alzheimer's patient. See King NMP. Making sense of advance directives. Revised edition. Washington, D.C.: Georgetown University Press, 1996, page 10. A detailed advance directive would be required, however, such as the one suggested by Linda Emanuel in The health care directive: Learning how to draft advance care documents. JAGS 1991; 39:1221–1228. This issue is discussed further in a later section of this chapter.

26. American Academy of Neurology. Position of the American Academy of Neurology on certain aspects of the care and management of the persistent vegetative state patient. Neurology 1988; 39:125–126.

27. Thus we find phrases such as "death will occur in a relatively short period of time," "death is imminent," "death will occur in a short period of time" etc.

28. This attitude is endorsed by a good many physicians who believe that no aggressive therapeutic interventions whatsoever, including artificial nutrition and hydration, should be used for PVS patients. See Payne K et al. Physicians' attitudes about the care of patients in the persistent vegetative state: A national survey. Ann Intern Med 1996; 125:104–110.

29. However, physicians do not always have to honor the wishes expressed in an advance directive. See King NMP. Making sense of advance directives. Revised edition. Washington, D.C.: Georgetown University Press, 1996, pages 153 and 251; see also Choice in Dying. Refusal of treatment legislation. New York: Choice in Dying, 1996, Introduction pages 2–3, just as they do not always have to honor every wish of a competent patient. In Indiana, the physician who feels that he cannot honor a patient's advance directive must attempt to help the patient find another physician who can do so. Indiana Code Ann. § 16-36-1-1 to 16-36-1-14 (Burns 1992). In Ohio, a physician can refuse to honor a patient's advance directive as a matter of "conscience," but the patient may be transferred to another physician. State of Ohio: Senate Bill 1, 1991.

30. In Cruzan v. Director, Missouri Department of Health. 110 S. Ct. 2841 (1990), the Court held that advance directives can act as clear and convincing evidence of the wishes of an incompetent. It *did not* require that the incompetent be in a terminal condition for the advance directive to function in this way. Nor did it *require* that physicians comply with advance directives. Such matters are left to state laws.

31. Peterson L. Advance directives, proxies, and the practice of surgery. Am J Surg 1992; 163:277–281.

32. Collins ER, Weber D, The Society for the Right to Die. The complete

guide to living wills: How to safeguard your treatment choices. New York: Bantam Books, 1991, pages 68–69.

33. Ibid., page 117.

34. Choice in Dying. Refusal of treatment legislation. New York: Choice in Dying, 1996, Introduction page 2.

35. Ohio is an example of a State with such a stipulation. State of Ohio: Senate Bill 1, 1991.

36. Ibid.

37. See Choice in Dying. Refusal of treatment legislation. New York: Choice in Dying, 1996, Introduction pages 3–4.

38. The trust factor is particularly important if the attorney-in-fact is permitted to make decisions about life-sustaining treatments for patients who have only temporarily lost decisional capacity. An example of this feature might be found in Rhode Island. R.I. Gen Laws §§ 23-4.10-1 to 23-4.10-2 (1989).

39. Jonsen AR et al. Clinical ethics: A practical approach to ethical decisions in clinical medicine. 4th edition. New York: McGraw-Hill, Inc., 1998, page 87.

40. The problem here, as with all advance directives, is that the patient cannot foresee all future circumstances. Thus, the attorney-in-fact may not be able to duplicate exactly the judgment the principal might have exercised prior to the onset of decisional incapacity. For this reason the principal might want to be careful not to be unduly restrictive in giving instructions to the attorney-in-fact. The attorney-in-fact may have to massage new information into the "substituted" judgment. This is an added reason for the element of trust in choosing the attorney-in-fact, who may have to consider new information while, at the same time, remaining faithful to the spirit of the beliefs, values, and preferences of the principal.

41. Only number 1 would, without difficulty, satisfy the clear and convincing evidence standard, which was the centerpiece of the holding in Cruzan v. Director, Missouri Department of Health. 110 S. Ct. 2841 (1990). In rare cases number 2 might work if the clues were specific enough and had been communicated to a variety of individuals. Clear and convincing evidence would probably never encompass number 3. The focus on clear and convincing evidence (in those states where it is required) gives added weight to the need to clearly express one's wishes before the onset of decisional incapacity. Making others draw too many inferences is fraught with risk.

42. Teno JM et al. Do advance directives provide instructions that direct care? JAGS 1997; 45:508–512.

43. King NMP. Making sense of advance directives. Revised edition. Washington, D.C.: Georgetown University Press, 1996, pages 126–129.

44. Jonsen AR et al. Clinical ethics: A practical approach to ethical decisions in clinical medicine. 4th edition. New York: McGraw-Hill, Inc., 1998, page 87.

45. At the time of drafting or signing advance directive documents, individuals may be reluctant to get too specific because of anxiety or the perceived weight that such documents carry. After a period of time they may become more willing to talk about the import of their advance directives. Family members and attorneys-in-fact should seize this opportunity to gain a clearer perspective on the author's/principal's wishes. This conversation becomes particularly important since surrogates often have difficulty in determining what a patient would want without the patient's guidance. (See Seckler AB et al. Substituted judgments: How accurate are proxy predictions? Ann Intern Med 1991; 115:92–98.)

46. Collins ER, Weber D, The Society for the Right to Die. The complete guide to living wills: How to safeguard your treatment choices. New York: Bantam Books, 1991, page 69.

47. Here again, "harm" is considered in the moral sense—that is, a transgression against one's sense of dignity—rather than in a physical sense, which would involve physical injury or the inflicting of pain.

48. Veatch RM. A theory of medical ethics. New York: Basic Books, 1981, pages 47–49.

49. Beauchamp TL. Paternalism. In Reich WT (ed). Encyclopedia of bioethics. 2d edition. New York: Macmillan Library Reference USA—Simon and Schuster MacMillan, 1995, pages 1914–1920.

50. The notion of exercising control over the manner of one's dying as an intensely personal decision reached a highly sophisticated articulation in the decision of the Ninth Circuit Court of Appeals on physician-assisted suicide. Compassion in Dying v. Washington. 70 F.3d 790 (9th Cir. 1996).

51. Phrases such as "no heroic measures" or "no extraordinary means" were virtually useless because of the ambiguity of the words "heroic" and "extraordinary." Collins ER, Weber D, The Society for the Right to Die. The complete guide to living wills: How to safeguard your treatment choices. New York: Bantam Books, 1991, page 44.

52. President's Commission for the Study of Ethical Problems in Medicine and Biomedical and Behavioral Research. Deciding to forego life-sustaining treatments: Ethical, medical, and legal issues in treatment decisions. Washington, D.C.: U.S. Government Printing Office, 1983, pages 149–153.

53. American College of Physicians. Ethics manual. 1st edition. Philadelphia: American College of Physicians, 1984, pages 29–30.

54. Ibid.

The so-called "living will" has excited considerable interest that will continue in the future. . . . Physicians who practice in states that have enacted living will statutes are urged to seek local legal counsel as to the exact rights and responsibilities encompassed by that state's statute. . . . In those states that have not enacted living will statutes or that have expressly provided that living wills are not legally enforceable within that state . . . the physician is under no binding legal obligation to follow the instructions or information contained in the document unless the physician has specifically agreed with the patient or guardian to be bound by its content. All physicians would be well advised to be aware of the thoughts and desires of the patient expressed in the document, but need only consider that language to be instructive and *not* determinative of the way in which the physician will treat the patient.

55. See Emanuel EJ. A review of the ethical and legal aspects of terminating medical care. Am J Med 1988; 84:291–301.

56. American College of Physicians. Ethics manual. 2d edition. Philadelphia: American College of Physicians, 1989, pages 32–33:

Importance of Advance Directives. Recognizing the difficulty of assessing preferences when a patient lacks decision-making capacity, physicians should encourage competent patients to make plans about treatment in advance of medical crises. This advance planning should specifically address two key points: the type of treatment the patient would wish to receive in different circumstances and the person whom the patient wishes to have serve as the surrogate decision-maker when he or she becomes unable to participate in decision-making. This process of discussion with the patient informs the physician of the patient's preferences and values, improves communication between physician and patient, and often reduces the patient's anxieties because the patient knows the physician is willing to discuss these highly sensitive issues and will be responsive to the patient's wishes. Discussions about the wishes of patients should be documented in the medical record. Patients should be encouraged to formalize their advance directives, for example by using a living will or through a durable power of attorney.

Living Wills. These documents are valid ethically because they provide insight into a patient's preferences at a time when the patient lacks the capacity to communicate. Physicians must apply clinical judgment to know whether the general language of a living will applies to the specific circumstances of a particular patient. Therefore, when a patient prepares a living will, the patient should be encouraged to provide a copy of it to the physician, so that it can be discussed and understood and entered in the medical record. This will ensure that the patient's wishes are known, even when the patient comes under the care of different physicians in various institutional settings. Because patients can and do change their minds, both oral conversations and written directives should be updated periodically so that choices made by the patient are contemporary with the progress of treatment, and thus carry greater weight.

57. "A competent adult patient may, in advance, formulate and provide a valid consent to the withholding or withdrawal of life-support systems in the event that injury or illness renders that individual incompetent to make such a decision. The preference of the individual should prevail when determining whether extraordinary life-prolonging measures should be undertaken in the event of terminal illness." Council on Ethical and Judicial Affairs, AMA. Code of medical ethics: Current opinions. Chicago IL: American Medical Association, 1992, § 2.21.

58. Physicians are directly protected insofar as they are immune from criminal and civil liability if they follow the wishes of a patient as expressed in an advance directive (provided the wish itself is not contrary to the law, such as assisted suicide in some states). Weir RF, Gostin L. Decisions to abate life-sustaining treatments for nonautonomous patients: Ethical standards and legal liability for physicians after *Cruzan*. JAMA 1990; 264:1846–1853. Physicians are also protected if, as a matter of conscience, they cannot follow the wishes expressed in a living will. This is the same sort of protection physicians have if a competent patient wishes to pursue a form of treatment that a physician, in good conscience, cannot provide because it transgresses a deeply held belief or sound professional practice. President's Commission for the Study of Ethical Problems in Medicine and Biomedical and Behavioral Research. Making health care decisions: The ethical and legal implications of informed consent in the patient-practitioner relationship. Washington, D.C.: U.S. Government Printing Office, 1982, page 3. In cases affected by matters of conscience, patients are encouraged to seek out another physician.

Patients are protected by advance directives indirectly through the protection given to physicians. They can generally rely on physicians to follow their wishes because they know that physicians are immune from prosecution if they do so. It is still an open question whether an advance directive actually (legally) *requires* a physician to follow it. Such cases have not yet been tested in the courts. In the cases that have come to judicial hearings, physicians have been protected if they followed an incompetent patient's wishes, but they have not been *required* to do so. The physician can always step aside. On the other hand, institutions have been *required* to follow a patient's wishes. See In re Jobes. 108 N.J. 394, 529 A.2d 434 (1987). As practice patterns develop after the Patient Self-Determination Act and as ethical guidelines become clearer, one can generally expect physicians to follow advance directives even without an explicit legal requirement.

59. Cruzan v. Director, Missouri Department of Health. 110 S.Ct. 2841 (1990).

60. Every state except Alaska has some form of proxy authority, although not every state authorizes a living will. New York, Michigan, and Massachusetts do not authorize living wills. See Choice in Dying. Maps. New York: Choice in Dying, 1997.

61. Hanson LC, Rodgman E. The use of living wills at the end of life. Arch Intern Med. 1996; 156:1018–1022.

62. Indiana (Indiana Code Ann. § 16-36-1-1 to 16-36-1-14 (Burns 1993)) and Ohio (State of Ohio: Senate Bill 1, 1991) are two examples of this movement.

63. Wanzer SH et al. The physician's responsibility toward hopelessly ill patients. N Engl J Med 1984; 310:955–959.

64. Kapp MB. Treating medical charts near the end of life: How legal anxieties inhibit good patient deaths. University of Toledo L Rev 1997; 28:521–546.

65. Meisel A. Legal myths about terminating life support. Arch Intern Med 1991; 151:1497–1502.

66. American College of Physicians. Ethics manual. 3d edition. Philadelphia: American College of Physicians, 1993, pages 4–5.

67. Pellegrino ED, Thomasma DC. The Christian virtues in medical practice. Washington, D.C.: Georgetown University Press, 1996, page 123. See also Miles SH et al. Conflicts between patients' wishes to forgo treatment and the policies of health care facilities. N Engl J Med 1989; 321:48–50. The "conscience" clause can be explicitly found in the advance directive statutes of a number of states, such as New York (New York Pub. Health Law § 2984 (McKinney Supp. 1991)) and Ohio (State of Ohio: Senate Bill 1, 1991).

68. Singer KL. Talk about death with healthy patients? I always do. Medical Economics 1994; August 22:69–76.

69. Dunn PM et al. A method to communicate patient preferences about medically indicated life-sustaining treatment in the out-of-hospital setting. J Am Geriatr Soc 1996; 44:785–791.

70. Council on Ethical and Judicial Affairs, AMA. Decisions near the end of life. JAMA 1992; 267:2229–2233.

71. Drane JF, Coulehan JL. The concept of futility: Patients do not have a right to demand medically useless treatment. Health Progress 1993; 74:28–32.

72. Beauchamp TL, McCullough LB. Medical ethics: The moral responsibilities of physicians. Englewood Cliffs, NJ: Prentice-Hall, Inc., 1984, pages 31–39.

73. Teno, J et al. Advance directives for seriously ill hospitalized patients: Effectiveness with the Patient Self-Determination Act and the SUPPORT intervention 1995. J Am Geriatr Soc 1997; 45:500–507.

74. Wolf SM et al. Sources of concern about the Patient Self-Determination Act. N Engl J Med 1991; 325:1666–1671.

75. Gamble ER et al. Knowledge, attitudes, and behavior of elderly persons regarding living wills. Arch Intern Med 1991; 151:277–280.

76. Brett AS. Limitations of listing specific medical interventions in advance directives. JAMA 1991; 266:825–828.

77. Seckler AB et al. Substituted judgment: How accurate are proxy predictions? Ann Intern Med 1991; 115:92–98.

78. One of the strongest challenges to the Patient Self-Determination Act has come from the SUPPORT study. (See Connors AF et al. (SUPPORT principal investigators). A controlled trial to improve care for seriously ill hospitalized patients: The study to understand prognoses and preferences for outcomes and risks of treatments (SUPPORT). JAMA 1995; 274: 1591–1598.)

79. Emanuel EJ et al. How well is the Patient Self-Determination Act working? An early assessment. Am J Med 1993; 95:619–628.

80. White ML, Fletcher JC. The Patient Self-Determination Act: on balance, more help than hindrance. JAMA 1991; 266:410–412.

81. Teno JM et al. Do advance directives provide instructions that direct care? J Am Geriatr Soc 1997; 45:508–512.

82. Teno JM. Advance directives for seriously ill hospitalized patients: Effectiveness with the Patient Self-Determination Act and the SUPPORT intervention 1995. J Am Geriatr Soc 1997; 45:500–507.

83. It is toward the achievement of this goal that this text is aimed.

84. Virmani J et al. Relationship of advance directives to physician-patient communication. Arch Intern Med 1994; 154:909–913. See also Teno JM. Advance directives for seriously ill hospitalized patients: Effectiveness with the Patient Self-Determination Act and the SUPPORT intervention 1995. J Am Geriatr Soc 1997; 45:500–507.

85. Morrison RS et al. Physician reluctance to discuss advance directives: An empiric investigation of potential barriers. Arch Intern Med 1994; 154:2311–2318.

86. McCue JD. The naturalness of dying. JAMA 1995; 273:1039–1043.

87. Markson L et al. The doctor's role in discussing advance preferences for end-of-life care: Perceptions of physicians practicing in the VA. J Am Geriatr Soc 1997; 45:399–406.

88. Danis M et al. Stability of choices about life-sustaining treatments. Ann Intern Med 1994; 120:567–573.

89. Peterson LM. Advance directives, proxies, and the practice of surgery. Am J Surg 1992; 163:277–281.

90. Durable powers of attorney for healthcare were developed to deal with precisely this problem.

91. Emanuel LL. The health care directive: Learning how to draft advance care documents. J Am Geriatr Soc 1991; 39:1221–1228.

92. LaPuma J et al. Advance directives on admission: Clinical implications and analysis of the Patient Self-Determination Act. JAMA 1991; 266:402–405. See also Hanson LC, Rodman E. The use of living wills at the end of life. Arch Intern Med 1996; 156:1018–1022.

93. Oleson KJ et al. A quality improvement focus for patient rights: Advance directives. J Nurs Care Qual 1994; 8:52–67. The SUPPORT study raises some genuine issues of concern in this matter. (See Connors AF et al. (SUPPORT principal investigators). A controlled trial to improve care for seriously ill hospitalized patients: The study to understand prognoses and preferences for outcomes and risks of treatments (SUPPORT). JAMA 1995; 274:1591–1598.)

94. Siegert EA et al. Impact of advance directive videotape on patient comprehension and treatment preferences. Arch Fam Med 1996; 5:297–312.

95. DesRosiers M, Navin P. Implementing effective staff education about advance directives. J Nurs Staff Dev 1997; 13:126–130.

96. Reilly BM et al. Can we talk? Inpatient discussion about advance directives in a community hospital: Attending physicians' attitudes, their inpatients' wishes, and reported experience. Arch Intern Med 1994; 154:2299–2308.

97. Connors AF et al. (SUPPORT principal investigators). A controlled trial to improve care for seriously ill hospitalized patients: The study to understand prognoses and preferences for outcomes and risks of treatments (SUPPORT). JAMA 1995; 274:1591–1598.

98. Morrison RS et al. The inaccessibility of advance directives on transfer from ambulatory to acute care settings. JAMA 1995; 274:478–503.

99. Chambers CV et al. Relationship of advance directives to hospital charges in a Medicare population. Arch Intern Med 1994; 154:541–547.

100. Schneiderman LJ et al. Effects of offering advance directives on medical treatments and costs. Ann Intern Med 1992; 117:599–606.

101. Levinsky NG. The purpose of advance medical planning—autonomy for patients or limitation of care? N Engl J Med 1996; 335:741–743.

102. Hanson LC. Can clinical interventions change care at the end of life? Ann Intern Med 1997; 126:381–388.

103. McCue JD. The naturalness of dying. JAMA 1995; 273:1039–1043. We saw the importance of addressing many of these issues in chapter 4, where we examined the issue of human finitude.

104. Brett AS. Limitations of listing specific medical interventions in advance directives. JAMA 1991; 266:825–828.

105. What can never be anticipated is how patients would feel about an intervention once they experienced their malady in the framework of actually implementing an advance directive. It often happens that patients do think differently about an intervention once they experience a disease or injury. Many say they would never undergo chemotherapy, but when the cancer develops they elect it. Many say they could never live as a paraplegic, but after an accident they are grateful for another chance at life, even from a wheelchair. Would an Alzheimer's patient who has elected a DNR order really prefer CPR when the arrest occurs? Or would someone in a PVS really prefer to live life that way? On one level these two questions seem to make no sense because such patients have lost contact with the world and, presumably, their inner states. But one cannot help but wonder. Hence the factor of taking risks.

106. In one study, most patients (85%) who initially decided to forgo life-sustaining treatments did not change their minds. However, this does not mean that it is not helpful for patients to review their wishes from time to time, especially as their clinical situations change. See Danis M et al. Stability of choices about life-sustaining treatments. Ann Intern Med 1994; 120:567–573. Besides helping patients, such a review, particularly if documented, would give caregivers greater confidence in following the wishes of patients because they would have a series of articulations of wishes rather than having to rely on just one.

107. Some studies of the relationship between advance directives and resource allocation have not indicated, in general, that there is a *dramatic* savings of resources by the use of advance directives. See, e.g., Schneiderman LJ et al. Effects of offering advance directives on medical treatments and costs. Ann Intern Med 1992; 117:599–606, where the effect was negligible. See also Teno JM et al. Do formal advance directives affect resuscitation decisions and the use of resources for seriously ill patients? J Clin Ethics 1994; 5:23–30, where similar effects were reported. See also Emanuel EJ, Emanuel LL. The economics of dying: The illusion of cost savings at the end of life. N Engl J Med 1994; 330:540–544, where the savings

represent a meager 3.3 percent. On the other hand, other studies indicate as much as a 68 percent reduction in cost in a Medicare population using advance directives. See Chambers CV et al. Relationship of advance directives to hospital charges in a Medicare population. Arch Intern Med 1994; 154:541–547. Though the studies indicating little to no savings cannot be minimized, it must be noted that in individual cases cost savings could be substantial. See previous computations on Nancy Cruzan in chapter 5, note 40.

108. Molloy DW et al. Treatment preferences, attitudes toward advance directives, and concerns about health care. Humane Med 1991; 7:285–290. See also Walker RM et al. Living wills and resuscitation preferences in an elderly population. Arch Intern Med 1995; 155:171–175.

109. This will be further examined later in this chapter.

110. Edinger W, Smucker DR. Outpatients' attitudes regarding advance directives. J Fam Pract 1992; 35:650–653.

111. Peterson LM. Advance directives, proxies, and the practice of surgery. Am J Surg 1992; 163:277–281.

112. White ML, Fletcher JC. The Patient Self-Determination Act: On balance, more help than hindrance. JAMA 1991; 266:410–412.

113. Markson LJ et al. Implementing advance directives in the primary care setting. Arch Intern Med 1994; 154:2321–2327.

114. Emanuel LL et al. Advance directives for medical care—a case for greater use. N Engl J Med 1991; 324:889–895. See also King NMP. Making sense of advance directives. Revised edition. Washington, D.C.: Georgetown University Press, 1996, pages 126–128. On the other hand, some evidence suggests that specificity in advance directives fulfills the promise of enhancing healthcare decision making in barely 50 percent of cases. See Teno JM et al. Do advance directives provide instructions that direct care? JAGS 1977; 45:508–512. Of course, by some standards, 50 percent success may not be entirely insignificant.

115. Cruzan v. Director, Missouri Department of Health. 110 S. Ct. 2841 (1990).

116. Peterson LM. Advance directives, proxies, and the practice of surgery. Am J Surg 1992; 163:277–281.

117. Ulrich LP. The Patient Self-Determination Act: A training program for healthcare professionals. Kettering, OH: Breckenridge Bioethics, 1991, pages 95–97.

118. Value histories are particularly helpful in developing this dimension of an advance directive. See Monagle JF, Thomasma DC (eds). Medical ethics: Policies, protocols, guidelines & programs. Gaithersburg, MD: Aspen Publishers, Inc., 1995, section 8:1.

119. Emanuel LL. The health care directive: Learning to draft advance care documents. J Am Geriatr Soc 1991; 39:1221–1228.

120. Pinch WJ, Parsons ME. The ethics of treatment decision making: The elderly patient's perspective. Geriatr Nurs 1993; 14:289–293.

121. See State of Ohio: Senate Bill 1. 1991. See also states (such as Indiana in Choice in Dying. Refusal of treatment) legislation. New York: Choice in Dying, 1996.

122. Virmani J. Relationship of advance directives to physician-patient communication. Arch Intern Med 1994; 154:909–913. Although this study demonstrates that little communication actually occurred between patient and physician in the population studied, it nevertheless indicates the need for such communication.

123. The SUPPORT study surmises that greater success might have been achieved if the patients had spoken to their physicians directly rather than through nurse intermediaries. Connors AF et al (SUPPORT principal investigators). A controlled trial to improve care for seriously ill hospitalized patients: The study to understand prognoses and preferences for outcomes and risks of treatments (SUPPORT). JAMA 1995; 274:1591–1598.

124. Monagle JF, Thomasma DC (eds). Medical ethics: Policies, protocols, guidelines & programs. Gaithersburg, MD: Aspen Publishers, Inc., 1995, section 5.

125. Carney MT, Morrison RS. Advance directives: When, why, and how to start talking. Geriatrics 1997; 52:65–73 suggests an annual review and revision. This may be a bit too demanding for the average healthy person. But even more frequent reviews might be appropriate for those suffering from serious or critical illness.

126. Ulrich LP. The Patient Self-Determination Act: A training program for healthcare professionals. Kettering, OH: Breckenridge Bioethics, 1991, pages 161–166.

127. Statements about the patient's perception of his quality of life would be particularly important since there is much agreement that what counts as an acceptable quality of life has a very large subjective component. See Jonsen AR. Clinical ethics: A practical approach to ethical decisions in clinical medicine. 4th edition. New York: McGraw-Hill, Inc., 1998, pages, 107–115, and Gula RM. Quality of life: A focus on the patient's total good. Health Progress 1988; 69:34–39. Determination of one's quality of life can admit of a number of different benchmarks. One could focus upon functional attributes and perceptions of one's well-being such as those Spitzer et al. identified: (1) active involvement in an occupation, (2) activities of daily living, (3) perception of one's health, (4) support of family and friends, and (5) outlook on life. Spitzer WO et al. Measuring the quality of life of cancer

patients: A concise QL-index for use by physicians. J Chron Dis 1981; 34:585–597. In any case an assessment of one's quality of life and the value of its pursuit can best be determined by the individual himself as he evaluates his ability to flourish—to fulfill his potentials and goals.

128. Rinpoche S. The Tibetan book of living and dying. San Francisco: Harper San Francisco, 1992, pages 29–31.

129. Seravalli EP. The dying patient, the physician, and the fear of death. N Engl J Med 1988; 319:1728–1730.

130. See chapter 4.

131. This could cover the persistent vegetative state even though some may not consider this a terminal condition. See The Multi-Societal Task Force on PVS. Medical aspects of the persistent vegetative state. N Engl J Med 1994; 330:1499–1508, and, 1994; 330:1572–1579.

132. This approach could cover conditions such as Alzheimer's, which cause the patient to lose cognitive contact with the world, and which the patient could consider "terminal" even though death may not be imminent.

133. The emphasis in Cruzan v. Director, Missouri Department of Health. 110 S. Ct. 2841 (1990), and Vacco v. Quill. 117 S. Ct. 2293 (1997), on the right of patients to refuse treatment "regardless of physical condition," as stated in the latter case, may give renewed impetus to the movement to honor advance directives even if there is not a "terminal" condition present. The key issues would then be the loss of decisional capacity and the desire of the patient to avoid a prolonged state where recovery is hopeless.

134. Emanuel LL. The health care directive: Learning how to draft advance care documents. J Am Geriatr Soc 1991; 39:1221–1228.

135. Wicclair MR. Ethics and the elderly. New York: Oxford University Press, 1993, pages 22–29.

136. Additionally, CPR and artificial nutrition and hydration are the two major issues (along with ventilator support) that have been addressed by the courts from *Quinlan* to the present day.

137. Council on Ethical and Judicial Affairs, AMA. Guidelines for the appropriate use of do-not-resuscitate orders. JAMA 1991; 265: 1868–1871.

138. Lynn J (ed). By no extraordinary means: The choice to forgo life-sustaining food and water. Bloomington, IN: Indiana University Press, 1986. This entire volume examines this difficult issue.

139. Ten states have various stipulations in their advance directive legislation about the ability to forgo artificially supplied nutrition and hydration. See Choice in Dying. Maps. New York: Choice in Dying, 1997.

140. Vacco v. Quill. 117 S.Ct. 2293 (1997).

141. There is a long history of the use of the principle of double effect in eth-

ics. See Paris JJ. McCormick RA. The Catholic tradition on the use of nutrition and fluids. America May 2, 1987, pages 356–361. The conditions of the principle of double effect require that (1) the act performed be either good or neutral, (2) the good effect must be intended, (3) the bad effect must not be the means to produce the good effect, and (4) there must be a proportionate reason for tolerating the bad effect. See Beauchamp TL. Introduction. In Beauchamp TL (ed). Intending death: The ethics of assisted suicide and euthanasia. Upper Saddle River, NJ: Prentice-Hall, Inc., 1996, pages 11–13.

142. Truog RD et al. Barbiturates in the care of the terminally ill. N Engl J Med 1992; 327:1678–1682. In this procedure pain medication is titrated upwards to the point where the patient's pain is controlled by producing an unconscious state in which the patient will die.

143. Quill TE et al. Palliative options of last resort: A comparison of voluntarily stopping eating and drinking, terminal sedation, physician-assisted suicide, and voluntary active euthanasia. JAMA 1997; 278: 2099–2104.

144. Pinch WJ, Parsons ME. The ethics of treatment decision making: The elderly patient's perspective. Geriatr Nurs 1993; 14:289–293.

145. An example of the kind of document that could be generated as a result of the guidelines outlined above can be found in Cantor NL. My annotated living will. Law, Medicine & Health Care 1990; 18:115–119.

146. Emanuel EJ, Emanuel LL. Four models of the physician-patient relationship. JAMA 1992; 267:2221–2226.

147. This dimension of being a responsible patient will be explored in chapter 9.

148. The SUPPORT study suggests this as a possible inference from its results. (Connors AF et al. (SUPPORT principal investigators). A controlled trial to improve care for seriously ill hospitalized patients: The study to understand prognoses and preferences for outcomes and risks of treatments (SUPPORT). JAMA 1995; 274:1591–1598.) Helpful suggestions for conducting these conversations are found in Jonston SC et al. The discussion about advance directives: Patient and physician opinions regarding when and how it should be conducted. Arch Intern Med 1995; 155:1025–1030, and Carney MT, Morrison RS. Advance directives: When, why, and how to start talking. Geriatrics 1997; 52:65–73.

149. State of Ohio: Senate Bill 1. 1991.

150. Beauchamp TL. Introduction. In Beauchamp TL (ed). Intending death: The ethics of assisted suicide and euthanasia. Upper Saddle River, NJ: Prentice Hall, 1996, pages 2–11.

151. Caregivers should not be discouraged by patients' rejections of the advance directive exercise. Widespread acceptance of advance directives as

clinical instruments for decision making may require a series of conversations taking place over a long period of time, perhaps years. However, the study of Murphy et al. shows that many patients can be influenced by conversations with their caregivers and can make reflective judgments if given appropriate information and time to do so. Murphy DJ et al. The influence of the probability of survival on patients' preferences regarding cardiopulmonary resuscitation. N Engl J Med 1994; 330:545–549.

8

The Roles of Healthcare Professionals

As was noted in chapter 5, the Patient Self-Determination Act places responsibility for its implementation upon institutions. For this reason, the success of the act rests primarily with institutions and their commitment to following, at the very least, the letter of the law. However, it was argued, institutions can go beyond the minimalist conformity to the law and attempt to raise the level of awareness of their patients as they go through the process of making decisions about their healthcare. This broader approach may require allocating some additional resources to implement not only the letter but also the spirit of the law. This argument was placed within the context of the mission commitments of healthcare facilities.

But there is another component to fostering the success of the Patient Self-Determination Act. The other part of this success story will be fashioned by the talents of the healthcare professionals who bring all their skills to bear on developing meaningful conversations with patients about the act, its intent, its implementation, and its implications. For many it will require the development of new knowledge, attitudes, and skills. These discussions with patients, as we have tried to indicate, are about topics that society as a whole tends to disregard or avoid, such as limitations on our human lives, our moral responsibility for decisions about our well-being, and the inevitability of death. The task set by the Patient Self-Determination Act will require self-reflection, proficiency, courage, and a considerable measure of professional dedication.

Institutions have varied widely in the avenues they have established for conveying the information about the Patient Self-Determination Act, including institutional policies regarding the withholding and withdrawing of life-sustaining treatments.[1] Some of the choices they have made have demonstrated whether the conversations required by the act have become enriching opportunities for patients or merely bureaucratic exercises.[2] Some have assigned the task to admissions personnel.[3] others to nursing, and still others to social services. Regardless of who carries out the function initially, it is important to view the Patient Self-Determination Act exercise as an interdisciplinary effort that can utilize a range of clinical professionals in order for the conversations to be effective.

As has been noted, the notification part of the law can be carried out fairly briefly, although the explanation of the rights regarding advance directives may be somewhat complex, depending on the state's laws. It is important that all the information to be communicated be massaged into manageable and nonthreatening packages.[4] The exact sequence in which this communication occurs is largely a matter of the personnel assigned to the task and their degree of creativity and responsiveness to patients' needs.

Because of the variety of healthcare professionals who may be involved in conducting conversations about the Patient Self-Determination Act, it may be helpful to examine the special contributions each profession can bring to these conversations. Each will have a special range of skills and perspectives that can be tapped as important institutional resources for benefiting patients as they attempt to come to grips with these difficult issues highlighted by the Patient Self-Determination Act. No one profession has an exclusive claim on the skills necessary for implementing the act. For this reason the more the various professions work together, the more their patients will benefit.

Preparing the Professional

From the outset caregivers ought to realize how important it is for them to come to grips with the issues the Patient Self-Determination

Act raises if they expect to communicate effectively with patients about them.[5] Patients can quickly sense discomfort in caregivers if the caregivers have not addressed the issues in their personal lives. Much of what has been said in the earlier chapters applies to caregivers and patients equally. If advance directives are important for patients, they must be important for caregivers, who will one day become patients. If it is important for patients to become clear about the personal beliefs, values, and goals that drive them in making decisions about their healthcare, particularly in the area of consenting to and refusing treatments, it is just as important for caregivers to clarify them for themselves. It is contradictory for caregivers to expect more of their patients than they themselves are willing to undergo.[6] In walking meaningfully with someone along the path of acknowledging the frailty of human existence and the difficulty of critical decisions,[7] the companions cannot be very far apart.

There are many approaches to the moral life and many ways to address the issues that arise in healthcare ethics. For those who would approach the task of integrating ethical considerations and medical practice, careful reflection is necessary and moral commitments are required. But from beginning to end, self-awareness and the openness to negotiation are essential in maintaining both the integrity of caregivers and the dignity of patients.[8]

Patients, families, surrogates, and caregivers do not always share the same moral perspectives, values, and goals. The challenge of healthcare ethics in general, and the Patient Self-Determination Act in particular, is to recognize that no one occupies an absolutely privileged position in determining the goods of the moral life.[9] For those who would serve individuals as they struggle with the difficult issues of personal health, deterioration, and death, compassion and tolerance are key ingredients for a successful professional life. The challenge and the indispensable key to interacting with patients effectively is to be willing to converse with them and explore with them the various ways of developing sound judgments about those most difficult of all issues, end-of-life decisions.

The Role of the Physician

The Patient Self-Determination Act imposes no requirements on physicians. From the outset this omission has been puzzling, particularly since the topics covered by the law touch on extremely sensitive areas that are intimate components of the fiduciary relationship.[10] It is very likely that those who drafted the law considered the regulation of physicians in this area to be impossible. They probably thought there would be a greater chance of supervision if the requirements were limited to institutions.[11]

However, the exemption of explicit physician responsibility does not mean that they can have no part to play in the implementation of the Patient Self-Determination Act. They can still play a vital role in helping patients address the issues of the law.[12] A case might even be made that they, as the fiduciaries of the patients, are in the best position to help patients understand the issues and incorporate them into their decision making.

Contemporary expectations of the physician-patient relationship are identified in a variety of ethical codes and essays related to physician behavior. A summary characterization would be that the role of the physician is one of patient advocate.[13] The notion of patient advocacy holds the key to the involvement of the physician in the Patient Self-Determination Act. The primary role of the physician is to reduce the vulnerability of the patient caused by disease or injury.[14] This function is discharged in a number of ways. Primarily, the physician counters the ignorance of the patient with expert knowledge in diagnosis, prognosis, and therapy. In the last analysis, this is the reason that patients come to physicians. As patient advocates, physicians ally themselves with their patients as they confront the problem they share—namely, disease or injury.

Informed consent opens the pathways of knowledge and empowerment whereby the physician initially discharges the role of patient advocate.[15] The dynamics of informed consent involve both mutual trust and mutual empowerment.[16] The fiduciary relationship that makes informed consent possible lies at the heart of what it means to be a patient and a vulnerable human being facing the contingencies of our finitude.[17] The expert knowledge of the physician makes a highly significant contribution to dispelling the patient's vulnerability.

In addition to the vulnerability of ignorance that the patient brings to the clinical setting, there is also the vulnerability caused by the difficulty of deciding about approaches to treatment. Patients often do not know which way to turn in the maze of medical information and therapeutic possibilities. Weighing the benefits and burdens of various therapeutic approaches can itself be enormously trying. Because of this problem of making decisions, patients and physicians often lapse into the default therapies prompted by the technological imperative.[18] Few things make a patient more out of control than simply pursuing a therapeutic course because it is too difficult to process and evaluate the necessary information to make a clear decision about consenting to or refusing the treatment. One of the most devastating accompaniments to this phenomenon is that it provides no frame of reference for evaluating the therapy at a latter time in order to consider alternative approaches to the patient's condition. We saw how important this reevaluation was in the process model of informed consent, which offers the greatest promise of preserving patient dignity.[19]

In response to this vulnerability and in addition to providing medical expertise, the physician occupies a special position in the clinical setting for assisting the patient in the decision-making process.[20] The physician can provide not only information but also a vantage point for evaluating it. The physician can show the patient the medical benefits and risks of the procedures under consideration and, in doing so, discharges the role of patient advocacy in the highest form possible. Unfortunately, the skill with which physicians discuss such serious matters with their patients is often limited.[21] Physicians frequently substitute careful attention to effective communication with an unsubstantiated belief that they know what patients want.[22]

In becoming a conscientious patient advocate in the broadest possible sense, the physician is not only responding to the patient's needs but also creating the role for the patient as collaborator.[23] The notion of collaboration in the clinical setting is an important element in the efforts of the physician. To work with an active, rather than passive, patient and to solve the common problems together will forge a solid bond between the patient and the physician from which both can benefit. This benefit takes the form of the promotion of the autonomy of the patient and respect for the integrity of the physician. The dignity of all parties in the clinical relationship is thereby enhanced.

In effectively implementing the Patient Self-Determination Act physicians may have to make some alterations in their professional culture.[24] Leaders among physicians may need to move other physicians into new practice patterns.[25] Hospital cultures themselves may have to change to incorporate a physician's more "conversational" role with her patients.[26] Finally the "reimbursement obstacle" will have to be overcome. Physicians complain that they are not reimbursed for talking with patients or counseling them.[27] They are reimbursed only for "treating" patients. Managed care will have to address this issue creatively so that patients, physicians, and providers can mutually benefit.[28]

Nothing can replace the fiduciary relationship that exists between physicians and their patients. As we shall see in the next two sections, social services, chaplaincy, and nursing professionals can begin the conversations around the Patient Self-Determination Act and generate reflection on the issues by patients or their authorized surrogates.[29] But those conversations are never complete until physicians have had a chance to explore the results of their reflections with their patients. For only the physician has the authority to write treatment orders for patients.[30] It is in this area of physician-patient communication that the bonds of mutual trust are forged and where the patients' confidence in the quality of their care is firmly established.[31]

But the physician does not have to wait until others initiate the conversations about treatment refusals or advance directives.[32] Ideally these conversations should begin in the physician's office, where they can be conducted in the atmosphere of trust that should permeate the fiduciary relationship.[33] If physicians take the initiative and begin the conversations with patients, their patients will be well prepared when they have to be admitted to a healthcare facility. The institutional conversations may no longer frighten them because they have already had them with the person whom they trust most with their healthcare.[34]

Other caregivers can talk about treatments and outcomes in general terms, but physicians have a special authority when talking about these matters with their patients.[35] Physicians are in an ideal position to help patients through the agony of choice either about treatment consents, treatment refusals, or advance directive decisions relative to their own peculiar circumstances. By entering into this dialogue, physicians can help individuals become more careful decision makers.

In human affairs the best decisions are achieved by applying general knowledge to specific situations. And this is what is needed by the patient in making healthcare decisions.

By openly communicating her beliefs, values, goals, and wishes to the physician, the patient makes it possible for the physician to be a "good" physician. For a "good" physician attempts to integrate his medical expertise into the value life of each patient. Medical efforts can then be concentrated on achieving this integration as closely as possible within the boundaries of sound medical practice, rather than forcing an artificial set of priorities upon the patient.

Documentation of conversations with patients and the decisions they make during these conversations will be vital tools upon which to rely in case patients never commit their beliefs and desires to paper themselves.[36] For many patients will never write down their wishes. This does not mean they do not have them; it may only mean that they could not bring themselves to express them in writing. Oral communications between a physician and a patient that have been documented by the physician constitute persuasive evidence of the patient's wishes.

Just as the Patient Self-Determination Act poses a strong challenge to the mission of a healthcare institution, it poses an equally strong challenge to the professionalism of the physician.[37] Physicians may have to redesign their practices to make time to conduct the conversations with patients that the spirit of the Patient Self-Determination Act can stimulate,[38] particularly in an era where managed care may introduce artificial restrictions on the time physicians can devote to conversations with their patients.[39] They will need to establish the communication patterns that will be necessary to make those conversations effective.[40] They will need to promote and participate in educational programs that will give patients the chance to begin thinking about the stipulations and rights expressed in the Patient Self-Determination Act. Finally, they will have to develop restraint in pursuing only their own therapeutic agenda with their patients.[41] Patients' refusals of treatment and their advance directives will sometimes move in a direction counter to what the physician might like. Setting aside one's own value agenda in order to defer to that of the one she serves is often the calling of the true professional and requires much discipline.[42] To the extent that physicians respond to these challenges, society and patients will see a renewed respect for the noble calling of medicine.

The Role of Social Services and Chaplaincy

In implementing the Patient Self-Determination Act social services and chaplaincy can play a very significant role. The term "social services" designates those healthcare professionals who are specially trained in communication skills and who work with patients at the level of values exploration, goal setting, and developing coping skills to meet problems that arise in the course of their healthcare.[43] Included in this group are social workers, healthcare counselors, and psychotherapists. Chaplains and those working in the many areas of pastoral care are parallel professionals. They discharge many tasks that are similar to those of social services with the added spiritual dimension that flows from both their training and their convictions.

These professionals, with their special clinical roles, move healthcare beyond merely addressing the symptoms of a particular disease or the failure of an organ system. They enlarge the scope of healthcare by making it holistic—that is, including all the patients' beliefs and behaviors in addition to the disease or injury that afflicts them. They address the social, emotional, and spiritual needs of patients as they move through the healthcare system.[44] They can add to the quality of care for patients and thus enlarge the capability of the physician.[45]

It is vitally important for this group of highly skilled professionals to have a role at the early stages of the admissions process when the requirements of the Patient Self-Determination Act are first addressed. One of the first tasks might be to determine whether there is someone who has decision-making authority for the patient if a need to consult him arises. At this time the basis for that authority can be determined—that is, whether that person holds a durable power of attorney with healthcare decision-making authority, is a family member, or has some other relationship with the patient. Establishing the nature of the authority early on can save much time later if the surrogate's authority has to be invoked. If the patient has not designated someone to make these decisions when the need arises, or if the authority has not been properly conferred, then the discussion can turn to the appointment of an attorney-in-fact or some form of healthcare representative.

If there is question about the decisional capacity of a patient, some initial assessment may need to be made so that the proper medical personnel can be utilized to make the authoritative clinical judgment about that capacity.[46] Since the conversations necessitated by the Patient Self-Determination Act cannot be held with those lacking capacity, it would be necessary to make some determination about the matter of capacity early in the admissions procedure. If capacity to make healthcare decisions is not present or is questionable, then the patient's legitimate surrogate must be included in the conversations.

If the institution is committed to going beyond the minimum required by the law, another important task of social services could be to gather a values history of the incoming patients by identifying the values that have been important in guiding their lives and assessing ways in which they can be promoted while they are living under the institution's care.[47] Chaplaincy may be particularly helpful here, especially if the patient has a strong religious bent.[48] If the patient is not clear about those values, some attempt should be made to help her achieve some clarity about them. These exercises will provide essential information to set the context for the discussion about the right to refuse treatments. In keeping with the intent of the Patient Self-Determination Act, it will be necessary for social service personnel to help those admitted into the institution's care to understand the consequences of treatment refusals for their personal lives and lifestyle choices.

In addressing the matter of advance directives, those in social services and chaplaincy, supplementing any initial efforts by physicians, will be in an excellent position to (1) inquire whether the patient has an advance directive, (2) if there is an advance directive, check to be sure it conforms to the laws in that state, (3) assist patients in reviewing and revising their advance directives if appropriate, (4) assist patients in understanding the purpose and importance of advance directives, and completing one in conformity with the law if desired, and (5) assist patients in writing down any specific wishes to make subsequent decision making easier. In all these activities surrounding the reviewing or drafting of an advance directive, those in social services can provide invaluable assistance to the patient by helping her think through her personal goals and values, which will have a profound impact on the content of her advance directive. In spite of the effort to discuss advance directives,[49] patients must be reassured that if they do not have directives, they will not suffer any discrimination from healthcare professionals.

Special attention will have to be paid to the need for reviewing or revising advance directives. Although it is estimated that only about 15 percent of the population currently have advance directives,[50] a fairly significant proportion of these will have advance directives of long standing. Some may predate current state laws and do not fulfill the legal requirements. These will have to be revised and brought into compliance with the stipulations of the state's laws. Some may have been drawn up a number of years before and no longer represent the current thinking of the patient. These documents should be revised to include patients' current beliefs, values, and expectations for their healthcare, as well as significant advances in healthcare technology that might influence patients' decisions. Finally, in those instances where the documents do comply with the law and reflect the patients' current thinking, it might be well to have the patients update and sign the documents again to demonstrate that the review has occurred and that the patients still hold the same position.

In helping patients develop a statement of their wishes to supplement any advance directive standard form or simply state their wishes, care should be taken to help them consider (1) treatments they would want and would not want, (2) the outcomes of interventions they would not like to bear, (3) the healthcare conditions they would or would not like to continue, and (4) the quality of life they hope to, or are willing to, experience as they live out their lives. Social service or chaplaincy personnel can help the patient develop the value context in terms of beliefs and issues of importance that govern the patient's life in order to give perspective to the preferences she wishes to express. Articulating a value system in light of spiritual beliefs may be a particular strength of those in chaplaincy services. Credibility and specificity in these documents, discussed in chapter 7, should be guiding factors in this activity.

In order to accomplish this task, a variety of forms or grids have been developed that systematically outline possible outcomes and treatments.[51] Patients can select from them the options they desire in each circumstance. Though such grids may be helpful for patients who are highly organized in their lives and disposed to be very systematic, many patients will probably find the approach intimidating and much too impersonal. It may be helpful for those assisting patients in designing an advance directive to have such a schema in mind, but it will generally be most helpful if the decisions flow from the patient through some sort of counseling modality.[52] This approach will allow patients to integrate their goals and values more naturally into the process of selecting treatments and to call an end to the exercise when they can tolerate no more, without artificially forcing them to enter territory into which they are not prepared to venture.

These professionals can also impress upon patients the advantages of designating an attorney-in-fact if one has not been designated. They can explore the issue of trust with the patient and help her think through the selection of someone to fulfill that role.[53] If there is an attorney-in-fact already designated, the professional can help to establish pathways of communication between the patient and the attorney-in-fact so that he will be in the best position to make judgments about the patient's healthcare if called upon to do so.[54] This includes the communication and documentation of the patient's wishes and expectations about the course of her healthcare.

A checklist of matters covered in the conversations with the patient would be helpful for the social service or chaplaincy professional so that all the necessary items will be addressed. This provides a record that can be consulted while the individual is in the care of the institution, or, perhaps, a managed care group, so that issues can be revisited from time to time as the opportunity or need arises. It is an ongoing challenge to develop forms of documentation that both record what has transpired and make that information available for subsequent use.

Not all of the Patient Self-Determination Act conversations will accomplish their purposes, nor can it be expected that they will achieve their ends on the first encounter. The culture of patients will have to change just as the culture of healthcare delivery does.[55] Patients will have to become accustomed to approaching healthcare from a new vantage point. Patients can seldom be expected to enter into these conversations eagerly or completely and come out with a definite plan. Perhaps the best we can hope for is that *with each encounter* the patients' awareness of the importance of becoming more actively involved in the decisions about their healthcare will be increased and that they will make some steps in that direction. Incremental improvement is certainly better than no improvement at all.

The beginning of a hospitalization may not be the best time to draw up a hurried advance directive or even sign a standard one. But it is a time to begin thinking about it and securing help during the hospital stay to start the process that will ultimately end with a reflective advance directive. Any progress will make the next healthcare admission easier. If extended care is involved, the process can occur over a moderately extensive period of time.[56]

Although the Patient Self-Determination Act applies to conversations at the time of admission to a healthcare institution, there is no reason for its concerns to be confined to that period. Pursuing the initial conversations during the patient's stay in an institution can be helpful in deepening her awareness of the issues involved and possibly bringing to closure some of the tasks related to the spirit of the law. Some return to the conversations might also be appropriate at the time of discharge planning, a function generally reserved for social services. Here the unfinished business that the patient might do well to reflect upon can be recalled and reexamined. For example, a patient may want to avoid talking about an advance directive at the time of admission, but in discharge planning, suggestions can be made about considering the matter in the future. The continuity of the conversations will be significant both to help patients move in the direction of fulfilling the opportunities established by the law and to impress upon them the importance of doing so.

There is a definite place for social services and chaplaincy in the ongoing educational programs that institutions are obliged to conduct. Because of their training in communication they may be the premier educators in this area. They can conduct, or significantly participate in, the programs discussed in chapter 5. They can also be the contact person for members of the community who would like to pursue some of the ideas presented in such programs. In this way they serve not only the healthcare institution but the community at large.

Like all healthcare professionals, those in social services and chaplaincy have a unique set of resources to provide to patients. If patients are to become better consumers of healthcare by becoming more reflective decision makers, this group of professionals can be largely responsible. No good decision can be made without situating it in a value context that will point to the option to be chosen. Only the highly reflective individual can identify and articulate her value framework without assistance. All others will need and benefit greatly from those dedicated men and women who have committed themselves professionally to social services and chaplaincy.

The Role of Nursing

Nurses, because they are in many ways independent professionals,[57] will find themselves in a peculiarly delicate situation if an institution has a commitment to moving beyond the basic requirements of the Patient Self-Determination Act and providing assistance to patients in addressing the issues the law raises.[58] The nursing code of ethics requires nurses to "provide services with respect for human dignity and the uniqueness of the client."[59] Here again, the notion of promoting the dignity of patients seems to take priority and the nurse is to some extent an advocate for the patient to ensure the preservation of the patient's dignity.[60] In discharging their duties toward patients, nurses often find themselves in a conflicted situation resulting from changing roles in the clinical setting. Traditionally their role was to be subservient to the physician who made all the significant therapeutic decisions about patient care.[61] In some instances nurses were to take the initiative in patient care but make it look as though it was actually the physician who was making the decisions.[62] In contrast with the traditional role and its variations, the suggestion is sometimes made that the nurse should act as a strong patient advocate who promotes patient self-determination[63] and may often have to confront and even defy physicians to protect patients.[64]

Discussions about the medical dimension of a patient's care should normally fall within the scope of the fiduciary relationship between patient and physician. The omission of physicians from the requirements of the Patient Self-Determination Act means that nurses may often find themselves required to give medical information to patients when they show an interest in it or express a need for it in an attempt to make decisions about consenting to or refusing treatment or drafting an advance directive. In fulfilling this role nurses can quite appropriately give the patient a great deal of general information about certain kinds of treatment—what happens during CPR, what medically administered nutrition and hydration are designed to do, the results of pain control, etc. Depending upon their interpretation of their role, and their understanding of the physician's authority, they may or may not state specifically what the effect of an intervention might be for a particular patient.[65]

Perhaps one of the most significant aspects of the nurse's role relative to the Patient Self-Determination Act is to attempt to bring the patient's physician into the loop of the conversations. Without the physician's having a direct encounter with the patient, the physician may never really understand the patient's decisions or be able to respect them with conviction. In bringing the physician and the patient together, the nurse is making it possible for both to discharge their decisional roles more effectively.

The role of the nurse as generally intermediary between physician and patient, as well as exercising the role of communicator,[66] was the reason for choosing nurses for the position they discharged in the SUPPORT study.[67] The study describes the role of the nurse in the study: "The intervention nurse also undertook time-consuming discussions, arranged meetings, provided information, supplied forms, and did anything else to encourage the patient and family to engage in an informed and collaborative decision-making process with a well-informed physician."[68] In spite of these efforts there was no improvement in discussions or timing of DNR status, days spent in ICU, or hospital resource use. This information, coupled with evidence that advance directives have only minimal impact when patients are hospitalized, indicates that conversations about matters related to the Patient Self-Determination Act have been quite ineffective.[69]

Nurses, who seem to be likely candidates for being effective communicators, do not seem to have made a significant difference in the implementation of the goals of the Patient Self-Determination Act. The SUPPORT study does not fault nurses in this regard. It concludes by noting that it is still a "worthy vision" to have patients more involved in decision making in life-threatening illnesses and that to accomplish this goal there need to be "more proactive and forceful attempts at change."[70]

In spite of recent studies to the contrary and the delicacy of their situations vis-à-vis physicians,[71] it is still possible for nursing professionals to contribute to the process by which patients or their surrogates make healthcare decisions or consider approaches to treatments. Because of their specialized training, they can lead the exploration into the general nature of interventions that might be considered, their purpose, the risks and benefits that may accompany them, and the available alternatives. They can join with the social service and chaplaincy professionals in helping the patient to examine carefully the consequences of treatment refusals and to formulate any necessary questions for the physician.[72]

Nurses can examine the different types of benefits that may be open to patients such as complete recovery, the remission of a disease process, an improved quality of life, continued relief from pain, a return to a previous level of functioning, and the restoration of awareness. They can then recommend that patients explore these various possibilities with their physicians.

On the other hand, they can help patients, their families, and surrogates understand the burdens patients may face as the result of particular interventions, such as decreased functioning capabilities, compromised mentation, discomfort, and treatment that is inconsistent with their status. Finally, they can also make individuals aware that some treatments may be futile insofar as they will not reach their physiological objectives or help patients achieve some of the personal goals for which they had hoped. Such discussions are invaluable for patients who may be drafting advance directives or revising previous advance directives.

As with the conversations with social service or chaplaincy professionals, these conversations should be documented according to the procedures of the institution's policy. Such documentation is helpful not only to provide a record of what was discussed but also to set the stage for subsequent conversations with patients. Nurses can review the Patient Self-Determination Act checklist that the social services, chaplaincy, or admissions personnel began and note where they can be helpful in addressing the requirements of the Patient Self-Determination Act or the institution's commitment to go beyond them.

Social services and nursing professionals have a special obligation to make it clear to patients and others on a continuing basis through both words and behaviors that they will help patients live with hope for the essentials that can be provided as they are living out their lives within the context of their finitude. When patients face decisions like treatment refusals or withdrawing specific treatments in terminal cases through advance directive decisions, they inevitably experience fears of abandonment, isolation, and pain.[73] These professionals can reassure patients that they will not be abandoned or isolated from those they love or their caregivers. Furthermore, they can assure them that every effort will be made to manage their pain if that is their wish,[74] and that they will receive the care and respect they can rightfully expect as a part of their human dignity.[75]

Nursing professionals, like social services and chaplaincy, can play a vital role in the institutional and community educational programs that healthcare institutions are required to conduct according to the stipulations of the Patient Self-Determination Act. Of those professionals employed by healthcare institutions who are not physicians, nurses are the ones with the greatest knowledge in the area of medical interventions and the greatest experiential sensitivity to the issues at stake in making decisions about medical care. They are well equipped by training and experience to explain clinical realities and the range of realistic options. They can also convincingly impress upon public audiences the importance of developing a value context for making such decisions. Interdisciplinary efforts involving nursing, social services, and chaplaincy approaches to public education can enrich the decision making of potential patients by demonstrating the need to integrate healthcare decisions fully into all facets of one's life. Nursing professionals can illustrate convincingly how this can be done.

Perspective

We have seen in this chapter that each healthcare profession, identified above, brings a special set of skills and resources to the conversations that can help realize the goals of the Patient Self-Determination Act. Each profession has a special focus in its healing arts. Each in its own way benefits the patient with its healing power. Working together as teams, the various professionals may be able to develop the creative approaches over time that the SUPPORT study indicates may be essential for more active patient participation in those decisions relative to the Patient Self-Determination Act.

The concept of healing cuts a broader path than alleviating symptoms by reducing pain, eliminating colonies of microbes, mending broken bones or broken hearts, removing diseased organs, and restoring organic functioning. Healing also involves overcoming the fragmentation we all experience in a society that moves too fast and is often too technologically sophisticated for ordinary people to grasp. Healing involves restoring dignity to those who are marginalized by esoteric enterprises that purport to help them while neglecting many of their most fundamental needs.

The Patient Self-Determination Act establishes a context for a more comprehensive form of healing by letting patients know that what they believe and desire really does matter. The context clearly identifies the rights of patients and opens the possibility that those rights will be taken seriously. It invites those who are engaged in other forms of the healing arts to broaden the scope of their endeavors, to converse with patients about very difficult issues, and to help patients develop frameworks for making wise decisions about their healthcare. The law makes it possible for each patient to overcome the feeling of fragmentation that the lack of information and power conveys in the clinical setting. It makes it possible for the lesions in respect for patient dignity to be healed if all healthcare professionals make their best efforts and cooperate in the project.

NOTES

1. Monagle JF, Thomasma DC (eds). Medical ethics: Policies, protocols, guidelines, & programs. Gaithersburg, MD: Aspen Publications, Inc. 1996, sections 5 and 6.

2. A bureaucratic exercise will focus on giving a limited amount of information with brochures, asking patients formula questions that allow only yes or no answers, and providing no follow-up while patients are in the institution. An enriching opportunity will be characterized by conversations with the patient about the meaning of the Patient Self-Determination Act, the way it may impact on the patient's values and decisions, and its role in the patient's care in the future, and by subsequent conversations with patients about matters that may hold some interest for them, such as the drafting or signing of an advance directive in the future.

3. There are special problems with this approach, which were noted in chapter 5. See also Oleson KJ et al. A quality improvement focus for patient rights: Advance directives. J Nurs Care Qual 1994; 8:52–67.

286The Patient Self-Determination Act

4. One need only be reminded of the importance of presenting information to patients in language they can understand. See Lidz CW et al. Barriers to informed consent. Ann Intern Med 1983; 99:539–43. An example of such a package is Ethics Advisory Committee. Building a healthy partnership with your physician and Saint John's. Anderson, IN: Saint John's Health System, 1992.

5. It has been a long-standing criticism of healthcare professionals, particularly physicians, that one of the major reasons for their difficulty in discussing critical illness and impending death with their patients is that they have not really come to terms with their own dying. Seravalli EP. The dying patient, the physician and the fear of death. N Engl J Med 1988; 319: 1728–1730 ("What a help it might be if physicians were to spend a few minutes in the room where a death has just occurred trying to find a place for it in their personal and professional lives") (page 1730). Thus, the more they understand about the dying process and the more they understand their own vulnerability to it, the better they will be able to discuss end-of-life treatment decisions with their patients. Nuland S. How we die: Reflections on life's final chapter. New York: Alfred A. Knopf, Inc., 1994, pages xvi–xvii. In connection with this awareness it is interesting to note that after the residency period of their training, many physicians seldom, if ever, are present when their patients die. (Even in residency programs, presence at the death of a patient generally occurs only when attempts at CPR have failed.) One cannot help but wonder if a change in this practice might alter discussions with patients.

6. Quint JC. Awareness of death and the nurse's composure. Nursing Research 1966; 15:49–55.

7. These issues, which are central to human life, were explored in chapter 4.

8. Engelhardt HT. The foundations of bioethics. 2d edition. New York: Oxford University Press, 1996, pages 296–300.

9. Engelhardt HT. Bioethics and secular humanism: The search for a common morality. London: SCM Press, 1991, pages 5–14.

10. Wolf SM et al. Sources of concern about the Patient Self-Determination Act. N Engl J Med 1991; 325:1666–1671.

11. In point of fact, compliance with the law has not been supervised by the government, but its regulation has been assumed by the Joint Commission for the Accreditation of Healthcare Organizations, which recently included Patient Self-Determination Act-related issues in its standards. Joint Commission on Accreditation of Healthcare Organizations. 1997 comprehensive accreditation manual for hospitals. Oakbrook Terrace, IL: Joint Commission on Accreditation of Healthcare Organizations, 1996, standards RI.1.2.4 and RI.1.4.

12. The Code of Medical Ethics articulated by the American Medical Association specifically states that physicians must deal honestly with their patients, act out of respect for the law, provide enough information for patients to make an intelligent choice, and help patients make choices from the available alternatives in ways that are consistent with good medical practice. Council on Ethical and Judicial Affairs, AMA. Code of Medical Ethics: Current opinions with annotations. Chicago: American Medical Association, 1996, page xiv. These obligations together would indicate that physicians have a significant professional role to play in implementing the Patient Self-Determination Act.

13. American College of Physicians. Ethics manual. 3d edition. Philadelphia: American College of Physicians, 1993, pages 3–4.

14. Zaner RM. Ethics and the clinical encounter. Englewood Cliffs, NJ: Prentice Hall, 1988, pages 55–56. See also Pellegrino ED. Humanism and the physician. Knoxville, TN: University of Tennessee Press, 1979, pages 123–124.

15. Annas GJ. The rights of patients: The basic ACLU guide to patients' rights. Carbondale IL: Southern Illinois University Press, 1989, page 83.

16. May WF. The physician's covenant: Images of the healer in medical ethics. Philadelphia: Westminster Press, 1983, pages 130–144.

17. Pellegrino ED, Thomasma DC. The Christian virtues in medical practice. Washington, D.C.: Georgetown University Press, 1996, page 85.

18. This phenomenon was discussed in chapter 3.

19. Lidz CW et al. Two models of implementing informed consent. Arch Intern Med 1988; 148:1385–1389. The role of processing information in the informed consent dynamics was discussed in detail in chapter 6.

20. Gamble ER et al. Knowledge, attitudes, and behavior of elderly persons regarding living wills. Arch Intern Med 1991; 151:277–280.

21. Tulsky JA et al. How do medical residents discuss resuscitation with patients? J Gen Intern Med 1995; 10:436–442.

22. Seckler AB. Substituted judgment: How accurate are proxy predictions? Ann Intern Med 1991; 115:92–98.

23. American Hospital Association. Values in conflict: Resolving ethical issues in hospital care. Chicago IL: American Hospital Association, 1985, pages 14–15.

24. Lo B. Improving care near the end of life: Why is it so hard? JAMA 1995; 274:1634–1636. See also Johnston SC et al. The discussion about advance directives: Patient and physician opinions regarding when and how it should be conducted. Arch Intern Med 1995; 155:1025–1030.

25. Lomas J et al. Opinion leaders vs audit and feedback to implement practice guidelines: Delivery after previous cesarean section. JAMA 1991;

265:2202–2207. See also Markon LJ et al. Implementing advance directives in the primary care setting. Arch Intern Med 1994; 154:2321–2327, which claims that "[t]eaching physicians about the law is not sufficient to change behavior; physicians also need practical experience discussing directives with patients." (page 2321).

26. Blumenthal D. Total quality management and physicians' clinical decisions. JAMA 1993; 269:2775–2778.

27. Council on Ethical and Judicial Affairs, AMA. Ethical issues in managed care. JAMA 1995; 273:330–335.

28. Rimler GW, Morrison RD. The ethical impacts of managed care. J Bus Ethics 1993; 12:493–501.

29. However, there is no reason why *physicians* cannot begin the conversations about advance directives and other end-of-life decisions. The only major obstacle may be the time such conversations take. But this obstacle can be overcome by efficient communication strategies. Carney MT, Morrison RS. Advance directives: When, why, and how to start talking. Geriatrics 1997; 52:65–73.

30. Pellegrino ED. Patient and physician autonomy: Conflicting rights and obligations in the physician-patient relationship. Journal of Contemporary Health Law and Policy 1994; 10:47–68.

31. Reilly BM et al. Can we talk? Inpatient discussions about advance directives in a community hospital: Attending physicians' attitudes, their inpatients' wishes, and reported experience. Arch Intern Med 1994; 154:2299–2308.

32. Edinger W, Smucker DR. Outpatients' attitudes regarding advance directives. J Fam Pract 1992; 35:650–653.

33. LaPuma J et al. Advance directives on admission: Clinical implications and analysis of the Patient Self-Determination Act, of 1990. JAMA 1991; 266:402–405. See also Carney MT, Morrison RS. Advance directives: When, why, and how to start talking. Geriatrics 1997; 52:65–73.

34. It can be argued that this model of the physician-patient relationship is becoming outdated by managed care and HMOs, where patients may not see the same physician on recurring visits to the clinic or office. Waymack MH, Health care as a business: The ethic of Hippocrates versus the ethic of managed care. Bus & Prof Ethics J 1990; 9:69–78. See also Sabin JE. Caring about patients and caring about money. Behavioral Science and the Law 1994; 12:317–330. Though this may be true, it does not mean that conversations in this climate between physicians and patients are of no value. Even in ICU, when patients or surrogates see treating physicians for the first time, effective communication is possible if physicians take the time and expend the effort to demonstrate to patients that they are trustworthy. Moss AH.

Informing the patient about cardiopulmonary resuscitation: When the risks outweigh the benefits. J Gen Intern Med 1989; 4:349–355.

35. This authority of physicians derives not just from their special social role but also from a cluster of features they bring to the clinical encounter. These include (1) the initial trust the patient brings to the clinical setting that the physician can address the source of the patient's vulnerability; (2) the physician's pledge to the healing profession, which includes *caring* for patients as well as attempting to cure them (see chapter 3, note 82); (3) the expert knowledge the physician possesses coupled with the experience with maladies, which combine in the ability to formulate clinical judgments; (4) the professional and personal virtues the physician has developed (see chapter 4); (5) the physician's direct contact with the patient (a feature that healthcare bureaucrats often ignore); and (6) the physician's *presence* to the patient as the patient becomes the focus of attention and as the physician accompanies the patient on the difficult road of vulnerability imposed by disease or injury.

36. This will also be an invaluable resource in situations where patients may be seen by a rotating group of physicians, as in managed care and HMOs.

37. Agich G. Professionalism and the ethics of health care. J Med Phil 1980; 5:187–199.

38. Greco PJ, Eisenberg JM. Changing physician's practices. N Engl J Med. 1993; 329:1271–1274.

39. Baker LC, Cantor JC. Physician satisfaction under managed care. Health Aff (Milwood) 1993; 12(suppl):258–270. See also Jellinek MS, Nurcombe B. Two wrongs don't make a right: Managed care, mental health, and the marketplace. JAMA 1993; 270:1737–1739.

40. This will often require a movement from bureucratic requirements imposed by third party payers to focusing more on discussing care plans with patients and the beliefs, values, and goals that underlie patients' decisions about them. See Woolhandler S, Himmelstein D. The deteriorating administrative efficiency of the U.S. health care system. N Engl J. Med 1991; 324:1253–1258.

41. Childress JF. Who should decide? Paternalism in health care. New York: Oxford University Press, 1982, page 40.

42. There are exceptions to this dimension of the physician-patient relationship. The President's Commission indicates that patient autonomy does not override the caregiver's judgment when the caregivers has some "deeply held" beliefs. President's Commission for the Study of Ethical Problems in Medicine and Biomedical and Behavioral Research. Making health care decisions: The ethical and legal implications of informed consent in the

patient-practitioner relationship. Washington, D.C.: U.S. Government Printing Office, 1982, page 3. Thus, the physician *may* refuse a patient's wish for assistance in suicide and, as some will say, *must* refuse such assistance as a matter of professional obligation. See Shapiro RS et al. Willingness to perform euthanasia: A survey of physician attitudes. Arch Intern Med 1994; 154:575–584.

43. Hood RW et al. The psychology of religion: An empirical approach. New York: Guilford Press, 1996, pages 174–179.

44. Saunders C. Spiritual pain. London: Fourth International Conference of St. Christopher's Hospice, 1987.

45. American College of Physicians. Ethics manual. 1st edition. Philadelphia: American College of Physicians, 1984, page 20.

46. Lo B. Assessing decision-making capacity. Law Med Ethics 1990; 18:193–203. See also Appelbaum PS, Roth LH. Clinical issues in assessment of competency. Am J Psych 1981; 138:1463–1467.

47. Lambert P. et al. The values history: An innovation in surrogate medical decision making. Law Med Health Care 1990; 18:202–212.

48. National Conference of Catholic Bishops. Ethical and religious directives for Catholic healthcare services. Washington, D.C.: United States Catholic Conference, 1995, Introduction to Part 2, "The pastoral and spiritual responsibility of Catholic healthcare."

49. The SUPPORT study does not indicate whether patients had the advantage of such extensive conversations with social services or even with the nurses involved in the study. They do conclude that the study "casts a pall over any claim that, if the health care system is given additional resources for collaborative decision making in the form of skilled professional time, improvements will occur" (page 1596). The study is inconclusive about what improvements might result from an improvement in the quality of the conversations between professionals and patients. See Connors AF et al. (SUPPORT principal investigators). A controlled trial to improve care for seriously ill hospitalized patients: The study to understand prognoses and preferences for outcomes and risks of treatments (SUPPORT). JAMA 1995; 274:1591–1598.

50. Hanson LC. The use of living wills at the end of life: A national study. Arch Intern Med 1996; 156:1018–1022.

51. Emanuel LL, Emanuel EJ. The medical directive: A new comprehensive advance care document. JAMA 1989; 261:3288–3293.

52. Hansen JC. Counseling. 3d edition. Boston: Allyn and Bacon, 1982, pages 343–371.

53. President's Commission for the Study of Ethical Problems in Medicine and Biomedical and Behavioral Research. Deciding to forego life-sustaining

treatment: Ethical, medical, and legal issues in treatment decisions. Washington, D.C.: U.S. Government Printing Office, 1983, pages 126–131.

54. Seckler AB et al. Substituted judgment: How accurate are proxy predictions? Ann Intern Med 1991; 115:92–98.

55. This is certainly one of the conclusions that can be drawn from the SUPPORT study. See Connors AF et al. (SUPPORT principal investigators). A controlled trial to improve care of seriously ill hospitalized patients: The study to understand prognoses and preferences for outcomes and risks of treatments (SUPPORT). JAMA 1995; 274:1591–1598.

56. Ethics Advisory Committee. Care to residents at life's end. South Bend IN: Holy Cross Care Services, 1989.

57. Garrett TM et al. Health care ethics. 2d edition. Englewood Cliffs, NJ: Prentice-Hall, Inc. 1993, page 23.

58. This problem is particularly aggravated by the fact that there are a number of nursing models that operate in the clinical setting. One can identify (1) the bureaucratic model, (2) the physician model, and (3) the patient advocate model. Thompson IE et al. Nursing ethics, 3d edition. New York: Churchill Livingstone, 1994, pages 45–53 and 113–115. Each model has its own peculiar intersection of loyalties, priorities, and duties. As healthcare changes, so do these interactions.

59. American Nurses' Association. Code for nurses with interpretive statements. Kansas City MO: American Nurses' Association, 1985.

60. Jameton A. Nursing practice: The ethical issues. Englewood Cliffs, NJ: Prentice-Hall Inc., 1984, pages 125–130.

61. Newton LH. In defense of the traditional nurse. Nursing Outlook 1981; 29:348–354.

62. Stein LI. The doctor-nurse game. Arch Gen Psy 1967; 16:699–703. In a later article the position was taken that the same dynamics are still occurring with little alteration. Stein LI et al. The doctor-nurse game revisited. N Engl J Med 1990; 322:546–549.

63. Kroeger-Mappes J. Ethical dilemmas for nurses: Physicians' orders versus patients' rights. In Mappes TA, DeGrazia D. (eds). Biomedical ethics. 4th edition. New York: McGraw-Hill, Inc. 1996, pages 139–146.

64. Haddad AH. The nurse/physician relationship and ethical decision making. AORN Journal 1991; 53:151–156.

65. Bates B. Doctor and Nurse: Changing roles and relations. N Engl J Med 1970; 283:129–134.

66. Cassileth BR et al. Informed consent: Why are its goals imperfectly realized? N Engl J Med 1980; 302:896–902.

67. Connors AF et al. (SUPPORT principal investigators). A controlled trial to improve care for seriously ill hospitalized patients: The study to

understand prognoses and preferences for outcomes and risks of treatments (SUPPORT). JAMA 1995; 274:1591–1598.

68. Ibid., page 1596.

69. Morrison RS et al. The inaccessibility of advance directives on transfer from ambulatory to acute care settings. JAMA 1995; 274:478–482. See also Teno JM et al. Do formal advance directives affect resuscitation decisions and the use of resources for seriously ill patients? J Clin Ethics 1994; 5:23–30. See also Teno JM et al. Advance directives for seriously-ill hospitalized patients: Effectiveness with the Patient Self-Determination Act and the SUPPORT intervention. J Am Geriatr Soc 1997; 45:500–507.

70. Connors AF et al. (SUPPORT principal investigators). A controlled trial to improve care for seriously ill hospitalized patients: The study to understand prognoses and preferences for outcomes and risks of treatments (SUPPORT). JAMA 1995; 274:1591–1598, page 1597.

71. The studies show only that previous attempts at conversations have not been successful. They do not suggest that *all* conversations are futile. The SUPPORT study suggests that while "the overall results are not encouraging," "[i]t is possible that the intervention would have been more effective if implemented in different settings, earlier in the course of illness, or with physician leaders rather than nurses as implementers . . . or if continued for more time." Ibid., page 1596.

72. Davis AJ, Aroskar MA. Ethical dilemmas and nursing practice. New York: Appleton-Century-Crofts, 1978, pages 60–61. See also Birnbaum B. Informed consent: Paradox, metacommunications, and the law. In Davis AJ, Krueger JC. Patients, nurses, ethics. New York: American Journal of Nursing Co., 1980, pages 103–108.

73. Levine S. Healing into life and death. Garden City, NY: Anchor Press/Doubleday, 1987, pages 283–290.

74. Hendin H. Selling death and dignity. Hast Cent Rept 1995; 25:19–23.

75. Quill TE, Brody RV. "You promised me I wouldn't die like this." Arch Intern Med 1995; 155:1250–1254.

9

The Role of the Responsible Patient

Setting the Stage

Much of what has been said in previous chapters has pointed in the direction of understanding the role of patients within the context of the Patient Self-Determination Act. It remains only to organize those issues around the central notion of the "responsible patient." Much of what will be said in this chapter has been explored earlier with different focal points. It is now a matter of articulating the importance of patients' exercising responsibility in healthcare decision making in light of all that has been said here about the Patient Self-Determination Act.

Even the Hippocratic corpus, which examines the authority and the multiple tasks of physicians, acknowledges the importance of patient responsibility. The first aphorism states: "It is not enough for the physician to do what is necessary, but the patient and the attendants must do their part as well, and circumstances must be favorable."[1] No doubt what the Hippocratic author had in mind was the patient's obligation to cooperate with the regimen determined by the physician.[2] And that has largely been the notion of patient responsibility until fairly recent times. Currently, the notion of patient responsibility has been enlarged and extends to, among other things, participation

293

in healthcare decision making, including such elements as good communication, expressing concerns to the physician, requesting further information, entering into agreements with the physician about the goals of therapy, discussion of end-of-life decisions with physicians, and the pursuit of a healthy lifestyle.[3]

For all that was said earlier about the authority of physicians[4] and the importance of understanding the vulnerability of patients,[5] it must always be kept in mind that "each patient is a free agent entitled to full explanation and full decision-making authority with regard to his/her medical care."[6] With this authority comes responsibility for its exercise when it is appropriate.[7] Hence, responsible self-determination plays an increasingly vital role in the clinical setting.[8] If, in psychotherapy, the assumption of responsibility is the necessary prerequisite for change,[9] then a similar assumption of responsibility on the part of patients for their healthcare decisions must occur if the goals of the Patient Self-Determination Act are to be met. The need for this enhanced role for patients does not place total responsibility on them and therefore total blame on them if the goals are not met. Rather, it only reinforces the notion that if patients and physicians make genuine efforts to work together in spite of their power inequities,[10] the goals of medicine, the goals of patients, and the goals of the Patient Self-Determination Act can be successfully achieved.

The Patient Self-Determination Act brings into focus some important rights that patients possess in healthcare.[11] As with all rights, the possessor of the rights is not obligated to exercise them. Obligations are imposed only upon those who have a duty to act or forbear in such a way that the values encased in the rights are protected.[12] Thus patients do not have to avail themselves of the protection the right offers them.

Patients may choose to avoid consenting to or refusing treatment by deferring to others to make decisions for them.[13] They may avoid any attempt to complete or even think about an advance directive. They may avoid any attempt to understand the policies of the healthcare facility. The only thing they will not be able to avoid is getting some information about these matters if the law is being implemented in the institution or organization to which they are seeking admission. But they can evade any incorporation of the information into their thinking. In other words, patients can escape from any impact of the Patient Self-Determination Act if they choose to do so.

The SUPPORT study indicates that, in spite of considerable communication effort, patients are not becoming more active in their decision making in the face of life-threatening illnesses.[14] It would be easy to conclude from this study either that intensive communicative efforts by allied health professionals are futile or that the health professionals themselves are deficient in their abilities to communicate, or that the power inequities in the clinical setting are such that patients are too intimidated to discuss the healthcare decisions they face. Perhaps there is an additional alternative—namely, that the problem lies with patients who are reluctant to receive discouraging news about their healthcare situation. As observed in chapter 4, patients have great difficulty in accepting their finitude.[15] In spite of the fact that we are continually being reminded of our limitations, we try to keep them at a distance.[16] In the previous chapter it was suggested that if efforts at increased patient involvement in healthcare decision making are going to succeed, physicians may have to make efforts to alter their culture.[17] Physicians and other caregivers can do only so much. Patients may have to change *their* culture if they wish to be better participants in the clinical decisions that affect them. Let us examine some of the characteristics of the cultural change in patients to which the Patient Self-Determination Act may contribute.

The Moral Responsibility for Making Decisions

We might characterize the change in patient culture as the culture of responsibility. It must be immediately noted that not all patients will want to engage in this cultural shift.[18] The experience of responsibility runs deep in the human condition.[19] On the one hand, individuals have a yearning for control over the events in their lives and their destinies. On the other hand, they often do not want to suffer the burden that this control brings them.[20] They want to be able to reflect on their actions, but at the same time they often want to shut down the reflective process when it becomes too difficult.[21]

The notion of responsibility can be characterized in a variety of ways. To be responsible is to intentionally initiate an action or series of actions that lead to specific consequences regardless of whether they are foreseen or unforeseen.[22] Thus, to be responsible is to be accountable to friends, society, and family for what one does.[23] Most of all it means to be accountable to oneself. To be responsible requires us to stand before the tribunal of our own minds and answer the most difficult of all questions: "Why?" It means that we cannot merely place the blame for undesirable consequences on another. We have to be able to say: "These are *my* consequences"; "These are the outcomes of *my* actions"; "*I* did it"; "*I* have produced the good results"; "The fault was *mine*." Considering the weight represented by these various expressions, it is no wonder that individuals often want to escape from this burden.

The ability to be responsible for one's actions is a feature of human existence, which we have examined in a preliminary way in chapter 4. The special character of human experience stems largely from this ability because responsibility keeps individuals from becoming totally dominated by forces outside themselves.[24] It allows them to react to situations in ways that are variable and that result from the individual's unique assessment of them. It allows individuals to differentiate themselves from others and, at the same time, "own" their decisions and actions independently of decisions made by others. Responsibility makes one's decisional process both attractive because of the power and sense of dignity it confers and, at the same time, fearful because of the accountability it entails.

Escaping responsibility in every phase of one's life is not an easy matter. But in times past healthcare presented a situation in which such an escape was relatively easy. When a patient became ill or injured, it seemed possible to blame a disease or an accident without carefully examining the causal influence the patient might have had on her condition. During an illness or recovery from injury there often seemed to be no end to solicitous family members who were willing to help and protect the patient from additional unpleasantness. Physicians and other caregivers seemed to be quite willing to exercise their parentalistic bent to keep the etiology of the disease or injury as distant from the patient as possible.[25] An obligation to make decisions about how diseases or injuries are to be treated brings the healthcare condition closer to the patient and often generates disturbing reflections about the patient's role in the process of disease or injury.

Never before has there been such a challenge to the patient to become involved in her disease process or injury as is presented by the Patient Self-Determination Act. This law, if properly implemented, masks none of the difficult decisions that patients or their authorized surrogates have to make. It brings end-of-life decisions into sharp focus and demonstrates the problems raised by simply acquiescing in our treatment decisions. The Patient Self-Determination Act affords patients the opportunity to transcend the role of passive consumers of healthcare, particularly at a time when the direction of therapy points to life-and-death decisions. Even to attempt to be passive often requires a decision.

The Patient Self-Determination Act assumes the possession of freedom that individuals are often believed to share to some degree.[26] It gives patients the opportunity to make choices that flow from the very foundations of our humanity. It gives direction to the way we can respond to the challenges of healthcare in a manner that embraces the basic finitude of human existence.

The responsibility that this law *invites* patients to exercise is not an easy calling. Like the role of healthcare professionals, the role of the responsible patient in the context of this law is an unfamiliar one. The Patient Self-Determination Act does not simply *expect* patients to take the initiative in exercising responsibility; it *challenges* them to do so.

The moral life itself sets the stage for this new texture in healthcare. To be moral is to accept the radical possibility of human freedom and the uncertainties it presents. Because we are moral agents, we do not have the luxury of merely following tendencies in our behavior without recriminations. Instead we have options in the decisional paths we wish to follow. This means that the choice of one path often forecloses the choice of another. It means that the choice often has unforeseen and even devastating consequences. Finally, it means that we accept the choices as our own.[27]

The reality of human freedom has been debated in myth, philosophy, and theology throughout the reflective life of humankind.[28] It is impossible to examine those arguments and their counterarguments in this analysis of the Patient Self-Determination Act. Whether or not there is adequate evidence for asserting the presence of freedom at the core of human existence, we cannot gainsay the terrible anguish we feel when we are confronted with our own sense of indetermination. Paths often look the same and there seems to be no safe or sure way to make the choice to go in one direction or the other. Often they look either equally risky and undesirable or similarly beneficial.

Surely this is the feeling many patients have when confronted with critical conditions in healthcare and when the invitation is extended to them to consider refusing treatments either directly or through an advance directive.[29] At this time they are called upon to confront their finitude in its most essential dimension and possibly to surrender the life that has been their most precious possession. The courage required to *respond* to this situation—to be *responsible*—can cause even the most insensitive to shudder. And yet this is what the Patient Self-Determination Act calls upon patients to consider. It beckons them to reach into their innermost selves and summon the courage to make the most difficult decisions they will ever have to face.

Developing a Life of Virtue

To engage successfully in the test presented by the Patient Self-Determination Act, patients have one very powerful resource at their disposal. This is their life of virtue.[30] Earlier we saw that virtues can be described as character traits or habits that individuals choose to accomplish the goals they have set for themselves.[31] Any new experience occurs within the context of the personal history of experiences and virtues that an individual brings to a situation. It is that personal historical narrative that allows an individual to make sense out of a new situation or plot a course of action that will allow that situation to be turned to the individual's advantage.[32]

Individuals possess an important resource to guide them in making an important decision. The resource could be characterized as the beliefs and values to which the individual subscribes, the features of our experience that enrich our lives. Some patients may wish to surrender humbly to a divine being who is believed to have decreed death at a particular time. Certain actions, such as the ability to listen to or produce music, may hold a particular value for us. We may particularly value characteristics such as physical beauty or mental prowess. Certain possessions, such as an art collection, may have a particular value that gives meaning to our lives. Certain qualities of our lives, such as protecting our loved ones, may have a particular value. All these objects of value orient our lives and influence the direction of the choices we make. Their relative importance will be weighed in a given situation, and courses of action will be designed to safeguard the values we hold or the valued objects we wish to protect.

Just as the values one cherishes act as a gyroscope for the conduct of one's life, virtues have a similar function. The virtues one has chosen to practice give guidance to the decisions with which one is confronted in everyday life. For example, the individual who has chosen the goal of financial security develops the virtues required to hold a job, including industriousness and punctuality. When faced with a choice to show up for work at the assigned time or go off for a day's fishing trip, the person relies on these virtues to guide him in the direction of accomplishing the goal of economic security. And, appealing as the fishing trip might be, he goes to his job.

Admittedly, some patients will present themselves in the clinical setting with a limited—sometimes very limited—set of virtues. Their ability to participate in decisions about their healthcare may be equally limited. Such patients cannot be abandoned, for they have a very special vulnerability and may even have a particular claim to limited parentalistic interventions.[33]

The responsible person takes the initiative to set goals for her life, selects the values that will allow her to discriminate among her goals and the paths for achieving them, and chooses the virtues to exercise when making decisions about the accomplishment of the goals that have been chosen. This exercise of responsibility requires a reflective life on the part of individuals, a life that is not lived by merely automatic responses to situations that arise.

Until recently healthcare has not nurtured this notion of responsibility in patients.[34] Decision making has generally been in the hands of physicians rather than patients. Particularly unpleasant decisions might have incorporated family members, but they often excluded the patients themselves. And even when family members were included, the authority of the physician was the dominant factor in making decisions. The tendency to displace responsibility away from patients has taken the form of default therapy as advanced technology developed more and more of a grip on healthcare interventions.[35]

One of the major promises of the Patient Self-Determination Act has been to give patients central authority in making healthcare decisions and thereby encourage them to take more responsibility in those decisions. In this context responsible patients can affirm the continuity between the attention they give to their beliefs, goals, values, and virtues and the issues they face in the healthcare setting. Responsible patients can reflect on the goals they wish to accomplish in their lives as they are conditioned by their healthcare situations. They can also establish a priority of values that will help them discriminate among outcomes that can result from the healthcare interventions that may be considered. Finally, they can utilize and nurture the virtues that will help them make healthcare decisions that are appropriate for their values and goals.

It is inappropriate for patients to simply surrender their life of virtue as they enter a clinical setting or a healthcare institution. Rather, they must both reflect upon the virtues they have chosen to practice and reconsider the adequacy of their virtues for making the decisions with which they are confronted. They may even understand the need for developing new virtues to address the situations they face.[36] They can determine the appropriate level of curiosity, communicativeness, and assertiveness. They can decide upon the parameters for practicing perseverance, acceptance, or detachment. They can establish the limits of hope, risk taking, and self-restraint. If they need assistance in practicing the virtues, they can solicit that help from the appropriate healthcare professionals.

Since the Patient Self-Determination Act encourages patients to exercise responsibility in healthcare decisions, it sets the stage for them to be true partners in the fiduciary relationship. One cannot be a genuine collaborator with another unless both have tools with which to work. We have seen that it is the life of virtue that places the physician and patient on relatively equal grounds for negotiating approaches to the patient's healthcare.[37] Though both have a life of virtue, they do not always choose to practice the same virtues with the same intensity. Thus, responsible patients are in a better position to work out differences with their physicians and others if they have already developed a background of virtue to use as a standard or a context. Without the conscious effort to identify, develop, and employ a set of virtues, patients will be dominated by the virtues of others who have developed a set of virtues that may not be to the patient's liking.

Taking responsibility for developing a life of virtue and employing it in healthcare decisions, then, is a sure way of affirming one's dignity and promoting it in a manner that is certain to enhance it. Responsibility, as a major hallmark of the moral life, touches us at the fundamental core of our humanity. It both incorporates us into the family of human beings, thereby enhancing the quality of our interpersonal relationships, and establishes our particular individuality, which is the touchstone for our personal dignity.

Essential Virtues of the Responsible Patient

Now let us briefly examine some of the particularly important manifestations of patient responsibility that can arise in the healthcare setting. This examination may help patients understand their roles better, and improve healthcare professionals who assist patients in the implementation of the Patient Self-Determination Act with a perspective in promoting the decision-making responsibility of patients. The identification of the following virtues is by no means an attempt to claim that all patients need to practice them either singly or collectively. The following is only an attempt to develop a possible profile of a patient who will be an active (i.e., responsible) participant in clinical decision making within the context of the Patient Self-Determination Act.

Exercising Autonomy

The exercise of autonomy, which is the foundation of the Patient Self-Determination Act, entails the ability of an individual to consider options for actions, make decisions that will determine the preferred option within a particular value context, and effectively carry out the decision that is made.[38] The autonomy of an individual must be set within the perspective of personal dignity. As a part of this dignity we saw earlier that there is an historical dimension that cannot be ignored.[39] Thus, autonomy is exercised within the historical context of the individual's selection of values and choice of virtues. To ignore the latter is to ignore an essential element of patient autonomy. The historical context plays a central role in the drafting of an advance directive that truly reflects the dignity of the patient who has elected to formulate it.

The notion of patient autonomy has become a central issue in the practice of medicine in the past two generations. This new emphasis on the authority and power of the patient in the decisional process has often led patients to believe that their authority is absolute. But patient autonomy is not without its limits.[40]

To practice autonomy as a virtue requires moderation.[41] The approach of moderation dictates that the exercise of autonomy does not require the same practice in every case. To practice the virtue of exercising autonomy requires that one must determine its suitableness in various situations. The virtue of exercising one's autonomy requires a responsible judgment both about whether and when it is suitable and about the intensity with which one should cling to its practice. In other words, moderation in the practice of autonomy might call for one to consent to treatments that are beneficial and to refuse treatment in cases, such as a terminal illness, where it is appropriate to do so. It would also call for one to refrain from demanding treatment in cases of clinical futility. Furthermore, the practice of autonomy does not call for patients to exercise their decisional authority in every healthcare decision.[42] The prudence of negotiation may require one to modify his tendencies to practice autonomy unswervingly in order to further his collaborative efforts with the healthcare professionals who are legitimate participants in the healthcare decisions that must be made.

The practice of autonomy entails not just the self-determination of the patient. It also requires that patients accept the responsibility for their decisions and bear the consequences of those decisions as their own. When good outcomes occur, they are the result of the patient's decisions; the same applies to negative outcomes. The responsible patient who exercises his autonomy holds others accountable only for negligence. He holds *himself* accountable for outcomes that flow from his own decisions.

Finally, as was mentioned earlier,[43] individuals often wish to evade responsibility, and that particularly happens when healthcare decisions need to be made. This tendency may result from the complexities involved in healthcare decision making and/or the enormity of the consequences that often flow from those decisions. The responsible patient who wishes to practice the virtue of exercising autonomy does not evade her role in the decisional process but rather accepts its centrality in the decisions to be made. This patient will not project responsibility onto others, thereby diminishing her own part in the decisional process. If the patient decides to forgo the practice of autonomy, such a decision is still a matter of the responsibility of the patient. Some individuals are willing to surrender to the decisions and actions of others, as in the appointment of an attorney-in-fact. They lose their right to complain if adverse consequences follow from the decisions of others, since they have authorized others to make decisions in their stead.[44] Patients need to understand that even when they yield their decisional authority to others, their responsibility is a central factor. They have the right to complain if they are deceived in the exercise of their responsibility but not when they consciously place their own obligations on others.

The Patient Self-Determination Act dramatically presents patients with the opportunity to behave responsibly and to practice the virtue of exercising autonomy with reflective care regardless of the burden it places on them. The spirit of healthcare practice today is directed more and more to this end.[45] The shortcomings of default therapy are becoming increasingly apparent, as are the limitations of allowing physicians to make decisions for patients.[46] Finally, any movement toward healthcare reform will probably demand that patients become more responsible in the decisions about the healthcare they will receive.

Being Informed

The expectation of informed consent in healthcare is often seen initially as the responsibility of the physician.[47] The physician is expected to make a judgment about the range of information the patient needs to make a sound decision about the direction of her healthcare[48] and to provide that information, including recommended alternatives to treatments. Finally, the physician is expected to provide the patient with the necessary information in language that is understandable and will facilitate the patient's participation in the decisional activity. If the process model discussed in chapter 6 is followed,[49] the physician is also supposed to help the patient situate the informational elements in her value context so that the final decision will reflect the value agenda of the patient rather than that of someone else.

In the more traditional model of informed consent the responsibility of the patient would seem to extend only to the giving or refusing of consent.[50] The patient waits for the information to be channeled to her and responds primarily by giving consent. Of course, this can be an issue of considerable significance because the patient could always bypass the responsibility of giving or refusing consent by redirecting that dimension of informed consent to someone else, such as the physician or a family member or another surrogate.

In the context of the Patient Self-Determination Act, the role of the responsible patient underscores not only the matter of consent, or its refusal, but also the acquisition of information.[51] The virtue of curiosity looms large in this dimension of patient responsibility. In discharging this role, the patient is not a mere passive recipient of information who waits for the physician to decide what information to communicate and how to deliver it in the appropriate form. The patient is invited to take the responsibility of communicating to the physician her interest in acquiring information and to adopt a positive attitude toward receiving the information given. This active interest in gaining information extends to requesting clarity when the information is obscure for some reason.

Furthermore, when considering the information dimension, the responsibility of the patient requires that the patient take the initiative in achieving or seeking clarification of her values and beliefs,[52] so the information provided by the healthcare professionals can be placed in the patient's value context in some meaningful way. This activity further embraces the patient's taking the initiative in incorporating the information acquired in the experience she has with the disease or therapeutic modalities in order to monitor whether the additional experience reinforces the realization of her values or whether a new approach should be attempted in managing her disease or injury.

On the consent side, the role of the responsible patient does not merely apply to the right to consent to or refuse treatment. It may also extend to the formation and articulation of the patient's individual reasons for her response, particularly if the response takes the form of refusal of treatment. Although giving reasons is not required for a competent patient to refuse treatment,[53] the responsible patient will develop a framework for such refusals when this is possible. If help is required to reach a conclusion in the matter of consent, the virtue of curiosity prompts the patient to seek help from qualified professionals in forming this framework. This may include asking the physician for a recommendation regarding therapy.[54]

In the matter of advance directives, the responsible patient will carefully reflect on the role of an advance directive in her life and on her plans for managing the dying process.[55] She will take the initiative in entering into a meaningful conversation with her physician and others in order to acquire all the pertinent information necessary to draft or sign an advance directive in order to help her accomplish her goals in this area. The responsible patient will not indefinitely delay the attainment of this information so that others will then be burdened with making decisions the patient herself could have made with a deliberate exercise of curiosity and responsibility.

Finally, the responsible patient will seek clarifications of hospital policies pertaining to the Patient Self-Determination Act so that she can make healthcare decisions in an atmosphere conducive to the attainment of her goals. Gaining this information will not only help the patient be sure that she is being admitted to a facility or program that will allow her to achieve her purposes but will also reduce the number of obstacles that could arise in her path if and when she wishes to exercise her rights as identified in the context in the Patient Self-Determination Act.

It can be seen from this brief exploration of responsibility in the dynamics of informed consent that this process is a complex one. Responsibility is many-sided, and the patient bears a major portion of it. If patients seem to avoid their role in this process, the Patient Self-Determination Act, if properly implemented as outlined earlier in this book, can remind them that being a passive recipient of healthcare reduces their ability to be a full partner in achieving their healthcare goals. In the final analysis, a reluctance on the part of the patient to engage in the process of informed consent compromises not only her role as a patient but her moral agency as a human being.

Being Assertive

One of the most difficult virtues to practice in healthcare is assertiveness. The difficulty stems largely from the basic vulnerabilty that disease and injury impose on the patient. In chapter 3 we examined this vulnerability in the clinical encounter and noted its inevitability.[56] Patients feel at a loss because of the lack of familiarity with the nature and causes of their conditions and the remedies that might be pursued in attempting to correct them. They also lack the requisite expertise for effectively addressing the issues raised by their healthcare conditions and the authority to introduce the resources of medicine into the situation.

This vulnerability, together with the intimidation that patients frequently feel, often leads them to adopt a passive posture in their clinical encounter with their physicians or other healthcare professionals.[57] The tendency is to believe that since the professional has so much information at his disposal, he knows best what will benefit the patient regardless of any misgivings the patient may have.

Patients often fail to reflect on the fact that they are in the best position to identify or design the goals they wish to accomplish in their lives as they are coping with a particular healthcare condition and that they have the most direct stake in the outcomes of the disease, injury, and therapeutic remedies being considered. One's life goals and a pivotal stake in treatment outcomes are reasons enough for a patient to diligently pursue the practice of assertiveness.

Assertiveness directs patients in the exercise of their autonomy and keeps them on target in its pursuit. It assures them of retaining a vital measure of control over the healthcare decisions being made. The responsible patient will practice assertiveness as an ongoing dimension of her participation in the decision making that directs her care. She will not simply yield to the agenda of healthcare professionals or family members because they do not know, as a matter of direct experience, the patient's feelings about the direction of her healthcare.[58] The responsible patient will continually affirm her goals, take the initiative in reexamining them, articulate them to those involved in her care, and reiterate her stake in what will happen to her in her particular healthcare situation.

Healthcare professionals, family members, and surrogates must practice self-restraint in the presence of the patient's assertiveness. Their self-restraint in imposing their beliefs about what they think should occur in the patient's healthcare situation will allow patients who wish to practice assertiveness to do so without conflict.[59] It will also encourage those who might be hesitant in practicing the virtue to promote their autonomy and fulfill their role of responsibility by being assertive.

Being assertive is particularly important to patients who wish to draft or sign advance directives. It was noted in chapter 7 that one of the most important functions of an advance directive is to act as an instrument of communication. The communication is directed to both physicians and family members or surrogates. It is possible that these individuals may be reluctant to enter into the necessary discussions with patients if the patient is not sufficiently assertive. Lack of communication may reduce the effectiveness of the advance directive if it should ever have to be employed.

Physicians may have difficulties either because they do not believe that advance directives are effective tools for healthcare decisions for those lacking decisional capacity or because they have difficulty dealing with discussions about death and dying with their patients.[60] Family members or surrogates have difficulties because the prospect of the loss of a loved one can distress them to the point of shutting down communication. In the face of these obstacles to communication, the need for patients to practice the virtue of assertiveness in order to effectively discharge their role as responsible patients becomes apparent.

If individuals wish to fulfill their roles as responsible patients, they must nurture their assertiveness even at a time when their vulnerability might make it most difficult to do so.[61] Utilizing the skills of those trained in communication and the affirmation of assertiveness could help break down the barriers to the patients' practice of this virtue in their interaction with physicians and others.[62] For this reason, the role of healthcare professionals in implementing the Patient Self-Determination Act takes on added significance. Patients who have difficulty with being assertive may utilize the skills and training provided by ancillary healthcare professionals employed by healthcare facilities, if the facilities have demonstrated their willingness to fulfill the spirit of the Patient Self-Determination Act in this way. The responsible patient will pursue the use of such caregivers.

Finally, the understanding of hospital policies governing the withholding and withdrawing of life-sustaining treatments will be a matter of concern to the patient who wishes to practice the virtue of assertiveness in the role of a responsible patient. Many hospital policies are couched in language that is unfamiliar to patients. Even attempts to summarize them for patients in compliance with the Patient Self-Determination Act may not dispel all technical language or achieve maximum clarity. Patients must be cautious about simply accepting summaries of policies they do not understand. The virtue of assertiveness will serve them well in pursuing the understanding of unclear policies and in learning precisely how the policies might affect them in their role as patients in the healthcare facility.

The virtue of assertiveness is particularly important to cultivate when individuals in a relationship occupy radically different social roles. Along with different social roles come unequal positions of power. The illusion of the "powerlessness" of the patient must be dispelled in contemporary healthcare, and the Patient Self-Determination Act has gone a long way in doing so. But in accepting the power of patients acknowledged by the Patient Self-Determination Act, patients must also accept the responsibility entailed by their roles in contemporary healthcare. Developing the virtue of assertiveness is a major step in discharging this responsibility.

Being Communicative

Just as the virtue of assertiveness is difficult to practice in the clinical setting, so also is the virtue of communicativeness. Being communicative is difficult for patients because of uncertainty about what to discuss and fear of what they might learn. When we reflect upon the process of communication, we discover that there is a significant ethical dimension to it that underscores the importance of practicing this virtue.

Communicativeness is essential for caregivers if they are to maximize respect for their patients. This ethical underpinning of communication was the foundation for the considerations explored in chapter 8, which focused on the assistance given to patients in the implementation of the Patient Self-Determination Act.[63] This virtue, as practiced by caregivers, is expressed not only in talking but in listening to patients and in conveying the attitude that they are open to their patients' expressing their concerns.

Being communicative is a major way for patients to express their dignity. The Patient Self-Determination Act, with its ethical emphasis on patient dignity through self-determination, encourages the development and practice of this virtue. But the responsible patient does not passively communicate with a mere nod of the head or a signature on a piece of paper. Being responsible requires patients to be willing to express their concerns about whatever troubles them in relation to their clinical condition. To remain silent because they may think they would be "too much trouble" if they spoke out is a betrayal of their responsibility. Patients cannot expect caregivers to be able to guess about their needs and concerns.[64] If they wish to have their dignity respected, they must assume the responsibility to express it in clear and unambiguous ways.

A great deal of emphasis has been placed in this book on the importance of conversations in the implementation of the Patient Self-Determination Act. It has been suggested that having these conversations as essential supplements to the technical requirements of the Patient Self-Determination Act is vastly superior to implementing merely the letter of the law, particularly when this is done with a shuffling of papers. However, these conversations will fail if, in spite of the best efforts of the healthcare professionals, patients do not take an active and responsible part in engaging in these conversations.[65] The responsible patient communicates with the healthcare professionals about those matters related to the Patient Self-Determination Act that touch the patient and will have an impact on the quality of the care he will receive. Furthermore, the responsible patient will converse about matters that may not be of direct significance at the particular time of admission but that may need to be considered for future involvements with healthcare institutions.

For the reasons just outlined, the responsible patient will not casually ignore conversations about advance directives. Even if the patient does not consider an advance directive entirely appropriate at a particular point in his life, the practice of the virtue of communicativeness will keep the avenues of inquiry and information open so that the significance of an advance directive can be explored at a later date.[66]

For those patients who do choose to draft or sign an advance directive, the virtue of communicativeness is essential. The responsible patient does not simply draft or sign an advance directive and then file it away; rather, he creates and pursues avenues of communication that will ensure that all those affected by the advance directive clearly understand the significance the patient places upon it. The responsible patient realizes that the more specific he can be about the wishes that underlie or are imbedded in the advance directive, the more help the advance directive will be to those who must rely upon it for future healthcare decisions. Finally, he appreciates the role of the advance directive as a serious expression of his personal dignity rather than as a mere convenience for others in healthcare decision making. Accordingly, he takes the time to reflect carefully on the decisions and contingencies the advance directive expresses.

In chapter 6 it was noted that when patients demand futile treatments, the appropriate response is not to initiate the treatment automatically but rather to enlist the aid of skilled communicators to explore the patient's feelings.[67] If it is important for healthcare professionals to take this approach in dealing with patients, it is equally important for patients in dealing with healthcare professionals. For caregivers often desire to initiate or continue treatments that patients wish to refuse either directly or through an advance directive.[68] When this happens, patients do not always have the necessary communication skills or decisional capacity to make their wishes known to the caregivers or to persuade caregivers that they should follow the patients' wishes. The responsible patient or surrogate will realize when this occurs and will request help from those professionals who are especially skilled in communication processes, utilizing them to affirm the patient's wishes and guarantee that they will be respected.

Of all human interactions, communication is one of the most difficult. To many it comes neither automatically nor easily. This is particularly true when the situation in which the communication must occur is serious or highly charged, or when the patient's condition is severely compromised by critical illness. The practice of its related virtues requires determination and skill. The responsible patient will not simply "wait" for communication in the clinical setting to develop. He will work to develop the virtue in all of his life situations so that he can draw upon the skill he has developed when the time comes to communicate in the clinical setting. Skillful practice of the virtue of communicativeness is an important ingredient for the achievement of successful outcomes in a clinical situation, and often is a matter of life or death.

Taking Risks

If there is one virtue besides the practice of autonomy that lies at the heart of the Patient Self-Determination Act, it is the virtue of risk taking. We saw in chapter 4 that one of the fundamental features of our finitude is uncertainty. Since human life is so replete with uncertainty, one must develop the appropriate virtues to cope with it. Risk taking is one of the basic ways of dealing with uncertainty in the moral life and its accompanying decisional opportunities.

It is not just that our personal lives possess uncertainty. This burden alone may not be so difficult to bear. But what may be more difficult to endure and more directly at issue in the Patient Self-Determination Act is the fact that the outcomes of the decisions we make are often unpredictable. Although we often delude ourselves into thinking that the outcomes we expect will flow directly from our decisions, we can never be quite sure that this will happen. There is also an additional dimension of our decisional activity—that we are often faced with probabilities that may or may not be accurate. Furthermore, we may be faced with a moment of decision where the different outcomes have a relatively equal chance of occurring. Finally, we may be faced with a decision whose outcome is not likely but that we might wish to try to achieve.

All these considerations are dramatically illustrated in medical practice partly because of the nature of the human condition and partly because medicine is an art rather than a science.[69] Nothing reminds us quite so directly or so frequently of the finitude of our human condition as do disease and injury.[70] The technological possibilities open to healthcare practice offer only limited escape from the human condition and the contingencies of our decision making that play a central role in it. Thus, every time we make a healthcare decision, we are taking a risk. Fortunately, the risks are often not serious and are frequently reversible. Unfortunately, however, this often creates the illusion that our decisions entail little or no risk at all.

However, the Patient Self-Determination Act relates to decisions that are often critical and that are not always reversible. When a patient consents to treatment, the result may be more intolerable than the patient anticipated.[71] When a patient decides to refuse treatment, the result may be that it simply takes her longer to recover. On the other hand, however, it may shorten or cost the patient her life. This possibility applies to refusals of treatment both by patients with decisional capacity and through an advance directive.

The responsible patient reflects carefully not only upon the uncertainties of the human condition but also on the consequences of treatment consents and refusals and the effects of an advance directive. She will not be seduced into surrendering her responsibility in the pursuit of default therapy. In this role the patient accepts the outcomes as a result of her own decisions rather than assigning them to the decisions of others. The patient holds *herself* accountable rather than others. And the responsible patient willingly accepts this as an inevitable feature of human decision making in the healthcare setting.

The responsible patient assumes the risks that accompany healthcare decisions within a context of practicing the virtues of acceptance and detachment.[72] The patient identifies the limits she faces and the range of choices open to her within those limits. She realizes that her responsibility can extend only to those limits and that self-restraint in attempting to move those limits is also a responsible decision on her part.

Summary

In taking and assuming responsibility in healthcare decision making, patients discover a fundamental feature of being human. They turn this element to their advantage by practicing virtues that allow them to enter more fully into the human project and create a dimension of themselves through their moral lives that contributes substantially to their personal dignity. Without responsibility they would be severely impoverished because they would fail to develop a core feature of their humanity. The development of personal responsibility and one of its central virtues, risk taking, allows patients to be truly individuals because it allows them to be responsible for themselves in the most difficult of all decisions to make, those that may result in their deaths.

NOTES

1. Lloyd GER (ed.) Hippocratic writings. New York: Penguin Books, 1983, page 206.

2. This notion continues to be reflected in some of the ethics codes in contemporary medicine, illustrated by the statement: "The patient should be informed and educated about his condition and should understand and

approve of his treatment. In turn, he should participate *responsibly* in his own care." [emphasis added]. American College of Physicians. Ethics manual. 3d edition. Philadelphia: American College of Physicians, 1993, page 4.

3. Council on Ethical and Judical Affairs, AMA. Code of Medical Ethics: Current opinions with annotations. Chicago IL: American Medical Association, 1996, pages xliv–xlv.

4. Chapter 8, note 35.

5. Pellegrino ED. Humanism and the physician. Knoxville TN: University of Tennessee Press, 1979, pages 123–126.

6. American College of Physicians. Ethics manual. 1st edition. Philadelphia: American College of Physicians, 1984, page 25.

7. It is clear that competent patients can directly exercise their decisional responsibility. But many times patients cannot do so because they are compromised by critical illness, pain, altered states of consciousness, limited access to surrogates, etc. It is for just such times that advance directives and healthcare proxies have been developed. Competent patients can provide for these situations by entering into conversations with their caregivers and family members about making provisions for their compromised clinical circumstances through the development of advance directives or the appointment of a healthcare proxy. The Patient Self-Determination Act opens the door to these conversations and provides another pathway to patients who wish to exercise their responsibility, which is supported by the principle of autonomy.

8. President's Commission for the Study of Ethical Problems in Medicine and Biomedical and Behavioral Research. Making health care decisions: The ethical and legal implications of informed consent in the patient-practitioner relationship. Washington, D.C.: U.S. Government Printing Office, 1982, pages 45–47.

9. Yalom ID. Existential psychotherapy. New York: Basic Books, Inc., page 226.

10. American College of Physicians. Ethics manual. 3d edition. Philadelphia: American College of Physicians, 1993, pages 3–4.

11. As far back as 1973 the American Hospital Association identified certain rights of patients, which are now connected with the Patient Self-Determination Act: (1) the right to considerate and respectful care, (2) the right to information and informed consent, (3) the right to refuse treatment, and (4) the right to know what hospital rules and regulations (update this to policies on withholding and withdrawing life-sustaining treatments) apply to the conduct of patients. American Hospital Association. A patient's bill of rights. In Values in conflict: Resolving ethical issues in hospital care. Chicago IL: American Hospital Association, 1985, pages 77–79.

12. Facione PA et al. Ethics and society. 2d edition. Englewood Cliffs, NJ: Prentice Hall, 1991, pages 108–110.

13. President's Commission for the Study of Ethical Problems in Medicine and Biomedical and Behavioral Research. Making health care decisions: The ethical and legal implications of informed consent in the patient-practitioner relationship. Washington, D.C.: U.S. Government Printing Office, 1982, page 51.

14. Connors AF et al. (SUPPORT principal investigators). A controlled trial to improve care for seriously ill hospitalized patients: The study to understand prognoses and preferences for outcomes and risks of treatments (SUPPORT). JAMA 1995; 274:1591–1598.

15. McCue JD. The naturalness of dying. JAMA 1995; 273:1039–1043.

16. Callahan D. The troubled dream of life: Living with mortality. New York: Simon & Schuster, 1993, pages 71–73.

17. Lomas J et al. Opinion leaders vs audit and feedback to implement practice guidelines: Delivery after previous cesarean section. JAMA 1991; 265:2202–2207.

18. Strull WM et al. Do patients want to participate in medical decision-making? JAMA 1984; 252:2990–2994.

19. Dewart L. Evolution and consciousness: The role of speech in the origin and development of human nature. Toronto: University of Toronto Press, 1989, pages 346–347.

20. This is not to say that there should not be cultures that do not value responsibility in the same way that Western industrial democracies value it. There can be and are many flourishing cultures that do not have the sense of autonomy or responsibility we find in the West. Carmody, DL, Carmody JT. Ways to the center: An introduction to world religions. Belmont, CA: Wadsworth Publishing Co., 1981, pages 337–339. To respect the dignity of individuals belonging to such cultural communities requires a respect for a value system that admits of no concept of autonomy or responsibility. This is a challenge for Western medical practice. See Pellegrino ED. Intersections of Western biomedical ethics and world culture: Problematic and possibility. Cambridge Quarterly of Healthcare Ethics 1992; 3:191–196. A secular society would allow for a tolerance for such a variety of cultural communities. See Engelhardt HT. The foundations of bioethics. 2d edition. New York: Oxford University Press, 1996, pages 418–422. Nothing in this chapter should be interpreted as a criticism of patients who consciously operate in an alternative culture to that of Western medical practice. They have a rich source of dignity that may serve them well. See Ulrich LP. The Patient Self-Determination Act and cultural diversity. Cambridge Quarterly of Healthcare Ethics 1992; 3:410–413. This chapter merely attempts to develop

a view of patient attitudes and behaviors that invites but does not compel patient participation in healthcare decision making. If patients in Western medical practice fail to participate in decisions about their healthcare, they frequently surrender their well-being to the choices of others. If they consciously forgo responsible participation when to do so would bring about a result that they might otherwise consider undesirable, then they also forgo their right to complain about the adverse consequences.

21. Plato. The apology. Grube GMA (trans). Indianapolis, IN: Hackett Publishing Co. Inc., 1985, page 27.

22. Aristotle. Nicomachean ethics. Irwin T (trans). Indianapolis, IN: Hackett Publishing Co., Inc., 1985, pages 54–55.

23. Facione PA et al. Ethics and society. 2d edition. Englewood Cliffs, NJ: Prentice Hall, 1991, pages 161–163.

24. Those who have a strong commitment to the belief that human freedom is a myth do not accept this claim. See Skinner BF. Beyond freedom and dignity New York: Bantam Books, 1972, pages 24–40. See also Wilson, EO. On human nature. Cambridge, MA: Harvard University Press, 1978, page 71. On the other hand, humanistic psychologists hold that freedom is a viable concept that adds texture and important dimensions of meaning to our lives. See Maslow AH. Toward a psychology of being. Princeton, NJ: D. Van Nostrand Co., Inc., 1962, pages 10–11. See also Rogers CR. On becoming a person. Boston, MA: Houghton Mifflin Co., 1961, pages 107–124. It is not our purpose to try to settle this long-standing controversy. The fact remains that we do behave as though the notion of responsibility has some meaning in our lives; witness the language of praise and blame that presumes a concept of responsibility. Facione PA et al. Ethics and society. 2d edition. Englewood Cliffs, NJ: Prentice Hall, 1991, page 162. This belief in responsibility stemming from "freedom" is sufficient to guide our actions in many situations.

25. As we became more sophisticated in plotting the etiology of diseases, it became more and more difficult to distance ourselves from our responsible role in their etiologies—for example, smoking and lung cancer, chronic obstructive pulmonary disease (COPD; i.e., emphysema), and heart disease; ingesting fatty foods and coronary artery disease, etc. See Engelhardt HT. Human well-being and medicine: Some basic value-judgments in the biomedical sciences. In Engelhardt HT, Callahan D (eds). Science, ethics, and medicine. New York: Institute of Society, Ethics and the Life Sciences, 1976, pages 120–139.

26. But see note 24.

27. Sartre JP. Existentialism is a humanism. In Kaufman W (ed). Existentialism from Dostoevsky to Sartre. New York: World Publishing Co., 1965, page 293.

28. Abel DC. Theories of human nature. New York: McGraw-Hill, Inc., 1992, pages 1–2.

29. Gamble ER et al. Knowledge, attitudes, and behavior of elderly persons regarding living wills. Arch Intern Med 1991; 151:277–280.

30. The issue of the virtue life of patients was examined in chapter 4.

31. Aristotle. Nicomachean ethics. Irwin T (trans). Indianapolis, IN: Hackett Publishing Co., Inc., 1985, page 33.

32. Hauerwas S. A community of character: Toward a constructive Christian social ethic. Notre Dame, IN: University of Notre Dame Press, 1981, pages 131–145.

33. Zembaty JS. A limited defense of paternalism in medicine. Geneseo, NY: In Mappes TA, Zembaty JS. Biomedical ethics. 2d edition. New York: McGraw-Hill Book Co., 1986, pages 60–66.

34. Katz J. The silent world of doctor and patient. New York: Free Press, 1984, 100–103.

35. The issue of "default therapy" was examined in chapter 3.

36. Patients often recount their discovery of new virtues that are needed in terminal situations and that they develop as part of the process of dying. See Levine S. Meetings at the edge: Dialogues with the grieving and the dying, the healing and the healed. New York: Anchor Books/Doubleday, 1984.

37. See chapter 4.

38. Miller B. Autonomy and the refusal of life-saving treatment. Hast Cent Rep 1981; 11:22–28.

39. See chapter 4.

40. These limits were outlined in chapter 6. See President's Commission for the Study of Ethical Problems in Medicine and Biomedical and Behavioral Research. Making health care decisions: The ethical and legal implications of informed consent in the patient-practitioner relationship. Washington, D.C.: U.S. Government Printing Office, 1982, page 3.

41. Hitting the mean is important in the practice of any virtue, but it is particularly important when exercising autonomy in clinical decision making because it is easy to go to either extreme—either to surrender to the agenda of others (either surrogates or caregivers) or to demand total control of every element related to the situation about which the decision must be made. See Aristotle. Nicomachean ethics. Irwin T (trans). Indianapolis, IN: Hackett Publishing Co., Inc., 1985, pages 49–53.

42. President's Commission for the Study of Ethical Problems in Medicine and Biomedical and Behavioral Research. Making health care decisions: The ethical and legal implications of informed consent in the patient-practitioner relationship. Washington, D.C.: U.S. Government Printing Office, 1982, page 51.

43. See the section on moral responsibility, above.

44. It is for this reason that patients must be careful in choosing their healthcare surrogates. They must be able to *trust* them to make the best possible decision for the patient, knowing full well that all decisions are fallible to some degree.

45. Blackhall LJ et al. Discussions regarding aggressive care with critically ill patients. J Gen Intern Med 1989; 4:399–402.

46. Hofmann JC et al. Patients' preferences for discussing cardiopulmonary resuscitation with their physicians. J Gen Intern Med 1995; 10(suppl):69.

47. Informed consent was discussed in some detail in chapter 6.

48. Brunetti LL, Stell LK. A physician's guide to the legal and ethical aspects of patient care. Charlotte, NC: Department of Internal Medicine, Carolinas Medical Center, 1994, pages 44–50.

49. Lidz CW et al. Two models of implementing informed consent. Arch Intern Med 1988; 148:1385–1389.

50. This model is called the "event" model. Ibid.

51. "Patients have the responsibility to request information or clarification about their health status or treatment when they do not fully understand what has been described." Council on Ethical and Judicial Affairs, AMA. Code of Medical Ethics: Current opinions with annotations. Chicago: American Medical Association, 1996, page xliv, number 3.

52. Clarification of beliefs is particularly important for patients who are members of religious congregations that may have particular beliefs about treatments at the end of life. This clarification process may apply to Roman Catholics, who will need clarification about the difference between ordinary/proportionate and extraordinary/disproportionate means of extending life as one approaches death. See National Conference of Catholic Bishops. Ethical and religious directives for Catholic health care services. Washington, D.C.: United States Catholic Conference, 1995, directives 56 and 57. It may also apply to Eastern Orthodox who have to make the determination of accepting end-of-life treatments that can help them maintain their spiritual orientation toward death, or Orthodox Jews, who are expected to consult with their rabbi about appropriate end-of-life care.

53. President's Commission for the Study of Ethical Problems in Medicine and Biomedical and Behavioral Research. Deciding to forego life-sustaining treatment: Ethical, medical and legal issues in treatment decisions. Washington, D.C.: U.S. Government Printing Office, 1983, pages 30–32. See also Council on Ethical and Judicial Affairs, AMA. Code of Medical Ethics: Current opinions with annotations. Chicago, IL: American Medical Association, 1996, page xxxix, number 2, and most recently Vacco v. Quill. 117 S. Ct. 2293 ad 5 (1997).

54. Council on Ethical and Judicial Affairs, AMA. Code of Medical Ethics: Current opinions with annotations. Chicago: American Medical Association, 1996, xxxix, number 2. Physicians are encouraged to make recommendations as part of the informed consent process, but the recommendation should not be presented in a coercive fashion. See also American College of Physicians. Ethics manual. 3d edition. Philadelphia: American College of Physicians, 1993, page 7.

55. Stelter KL et al. Living will completion in older adults. Arch Intern Med 1992; 152:954–959.

56. Pellegrino ED, Thomasma DC. The Christian virtues in medical practice. Washington, D.C.: Georgetown University Press, 1996, page 108.

57. Sachs GA et al. Empowerment of the older patients: A randomized controlled trial to increase discussion and use of advance directives. J Am Geriatr Soc 1992; 40:269–273.

58. Seckler AB et al. Substituted judgment: How accurate are proxy predictions? Ann Intern Med 1991; 115:92–98.

59. The practice of self-restraint in this context does not mean that others should not express their views to the patient. Physicians are expected to make therapeutic recommendations. See Council on Ethical and Judicial Affairs, AMA. Code of Medical Ethics: Current opinions with annotations. Chicago: American Medical Association, 1996, page xxxix, number 2. Family members and surrogates also have a stake in what happens to patients, and so they have an interest in expressing their opinions as well. See Hardt DV. Death: The final frontier. Englewood Cliffs, NJ: Prentice-Hall, Inc., 1979, pages 126–127. But since the interest of others is only indirectly related to treatment interventions and the patient has the most direct interest, the patient occupies the position of decisional authority. In this kind of situation an *expression* of an opinion should not lead to an *imposition* of the opinion. This approach to patient authority is, of course, the reasoning behind the substituted-judgment criterion for surrogate decision making.

60. Brunetti LL et al. Physicians' attitudes towards living wills and cardiopulmonary resuscitation. J Gen Intern Med 1991; 6:323–329.

61. See note 7 above.

62. Ruark JE et al. Initiating and withdrawing life support: Principles and practice in adult medicine. N Engl J Med. 1988; 318:25–30.

63. See Tomlinson T, Brody H. Ethics and communication in DNR orders. N Engl J Med 1988; 318:43–46. See also Quill TE. Recognizing and adjusting to barriers in doctor-patient communication. Ann Intern Med 1989; 111:51–57.

64. This is particularly true since caregivers are so poor at guessing what

their patients would want. See Seckler AB et al. Substituted judgments: How accurate are proxy predictions? Ann Intern Med 1991; 115:92–98.

65. The importance of the responsibility of the patient to be actively communicative with her caregivers about the direction of treatments, particularly life-sustaining treatments and the use of advance directives, may be one of the most significant clues that can be derived from the SUPPORT study. See Connors AF et al. (SUPPORT principal investigators). A controlled trial to improve care for seriously ill hospitalized patients: The study to understand prognoses and preferences for outcomes and risks of treatments (SUPPORT). JAMA 1995; 274:1591–1598.

66. A developing interest in a personal advance directive may occur as patients become more reflective about the quality of life they hope to enjoy in the future and the way they may wish to address obstacles to their desired quality of life. See Callahan D. What kind of life: The limits of medical progress. New York: Simon and Schuster, 1990, pages 25–26.

67. Ruark JE et al. Initiating and withdrawing life support: Principles and practice in adult medicine. N Engl J Med 1988; 318:25–30.

68. Quill TE. Utilization of nasogastric feeding tubes in a group of chronically ill, elderly patients in a community hospital. Arch Intern Med 1989; 149:1937–1941.

69. Pellegrino ED, Thomasma DC. A philosophical basis of medical practice: Toward a philosophy and ethic of the healing professions. New York: Oxford University Press, 1981, page 61.

70. Engelhardt HT. The counsels of finitude. Hast Cent Rep 1975; 5:29–36.

71. A good example is doing CPR on elderly patients who are at high risk not only for not surviving CPR but for surviving CPR in a severely compromised state. See Murphy DJ et al. Outcomes of cardiopulmonary resuscitation in the elderly. Ann Intern Med 1989; 111:199–205. In this study 8 percent of the patients survived to be discharged from the hospital, but more than 50 percent of the survivors went to extended care facilities with extensive deficits.

72. Acceptance and detachment were discussed in chapter 4.

Conclusion

This exploration of the Patient Self-Determination Act began with the observation that its implementation could be construed as a relatively simple matter. The basic notification required by the law can occur at the time of admission to healthcare institutions and programs with little fanfare. It does not take much effort to "read patients their rights" and give them a written statement about them.

However, this closer scrutiny of the spirit and possibilities of the law, and the ethical issues that underlie it, reveals a richness in the law that is not always understood. It can produce an opportunity for patients to become much more reflective in their role as patients and in determining their destiny. The law can involve a highly complex interaction between caregivers and patients in, and out of, the institutional setting. It creates the setting for the intersection of a whole host of issues that have preoccupied bioethical studies and discussions for the last two generations. In a very real way the Patient Self-Determination Act is the culmination and integration of those ethical concerns, which have attempted to move the practice of healthcare beyond a technological and mechanistic response to disease and injury to a genuine concern about personal dignity together with the strategies to preserve that dignity.

The real challenge of the Patient Self-Determination Act is for institutions and healthcare professionals to decide how far beyond the basic requirements of the law they are willing to go. Patients' becom-

ing more reflective consumers of healthcare and more active participants in the decision-making process is an increasingly important goal
in our society. Special assistance for patients in these activities may be
required. The technological and social forces that come into play in
healthcare decision making can easily overwhelm patients who already enter the healthcare setting with a basic vulnerability, often
leaving them limited in their decision-making role.

In the current social situation there is often confusion and inconsistency about whose agenda should govern decisions, particularly when
it comes to end-of-life decisions, which often involve a convergence of
the wishes and goals of the patient and the perceived futility of further
medical interventions. Patients, families, and caregivers often have
different agendas. Even when those directly involved in the outcome
of the healthcare decision-making process are closely aligned, special
interest groups sometimes interpose themselves in the implementation
of decisions made in the clinical setting. To help resolve actual or
possible disputes that have arisen, the courts and legislatures have
become involved, often setting their own agendas. We have seen how
many of these conflicts occur within a broader context of the technological imperative that is advanced to alter the processes of nature or,
for those theologically inclined, to interfere with a divine plan.

There is little wonder that patients need considerable protection in
order to find their way through the intricacies, uncertainties, and
probabilities of healthcare practices. They need similar protection
when confronted with the labyrinth of conflicting interests in trying
to decide what is best for them. The Patient Self-Determination Act is
a major step in providing this much needed protection. The development of informed consent was certainly the first major line of protection for patients. It held out the promise of helping patients make
better healthcare decisions because they were grounded in appropriate
information.

The Patient Self-Determination Act follows in that tradition by
recognizing the importance of refusing as well as consenting to treatments from a sound information base. In this way it gives a perspective on the use of technological interventions in healthcare, which is
becoming critical in an age when technology can extend the length of
an individual's life without significantly improving its quality—and
this at great expense. Furthermore, the Patient Self-Determination Act

acknowledges that the interests of patients in determining what will happen to them in the process of their healthcare do not cease to be a significant factor when decisional capacity is lost. The emphasis on advance directives gives patients the opportunity to exercise fully and actively their responsibility in the entire range of healthcare decisions that must be made in their living and dying.

Current research has raised challenges to the implementation of the Patient Self-Determination Act in two special areas. The effectiveness and adequacy of communication strategies about end-of-life decisions have been seriously challenged by the SUPPORT study. The possibility of a significant residual effect of resource savings resulting from patients' refusing treatment and utilizing advance directives has not been decisively demonstrated. Conflicting studies, anecdotal accounts, and intuitions still leave open the possibility that the Patient Self-Determination Act may truly provide the foundation for better-quality communication in the clinical setting and some significant impact on the resource issue. Further experience and research in these two areas will have to occur before totally convincing conclusions can be drawn. It is clear, however, that caregivers are taking advance directives seriously and honoring them in ways that truly promote patient autonomy. It is also clear that the right to refuse treatment is becoming much better understood and the duty to honor it is being taken very seriously in the clinical setting.

All things considered, the Patient Self-Determination Act has the potential of initiating a radical change in the way healthcare is practiced. If the spirit of the law is taken seriously, patients and caregivers (who will eventually become patients) will converse on a much more comprehensive plane and with deeper understanding, not only of each other but of themselves as well. They will realize that signatures on pieces of paper are only the first step, and not the final goal, of sound healthcare decision making. They will be better able to face the limitations of their human existence and make more discerning judgments about the technological interventions that alter the natural course of their lives. They will enrich their dignity as persons by reflecting on their values and by conscientiously practicing the virtues that guide them in the achievement of their goals. And, finally, they will be able to move beyond the exercise of their rights to an appreciation of their responsibilities as patients and as human beings.

Index

www.ingramcontent.com/pod-product-compliance
Lightning Source LLC
Chambersburg PA
CBHW022101210326
41518CB00039B/353